Advances in Cancer Drug Targets

Volume 2

Editor

Atta-ur-Rahman, *FRS*
Honorary Life Fellow
Kings College
University of Cambridge
UK

Bentham Science Publishers Ltd.
Executive Suite Y - 2
PO Box 7917, Saif Zone
Sharjah, U.A.E.
subscriptions@benthamscienc.org

CONTENTS

contd…..

PREFACE

As the discovery and classification of novel human drug targets for anti-cancer drugs continue to grow, the eBook Series "**Advances in Cancer Drug Targets**" has become essential for all pharmaceutical scientists. This eBook series is a compilation of recent expert reviews published in ***Current Cancer Drug Targets*** on the subject with a focus on novel strategies. The current volume covers reviews on contemporary molecular drug targets involved in cancer, including medicinal chemistry, pharmacology, molecular biology, genomics and biochemistry.

The 'cancer chaperone' heat-shock protein 90 (Hsp90) plays a crucial role in maintaining the stability and activity of numerous signaling proteins. In chapter 01, Bruserud *et al.* explain the role of Heat Shock Protein 90 (HSP90) as a potential target in the treatment of Acute Myelogenous Leukaemia (AML). The HSP90 inhibition targets several intracellular signalling pathways, leading to the degradation of client proteins and hence exhibits multiple antileukaemic effects. This has been comprehensively reviewed.

The mitotic spindle assembly checkpoint (SAC) is a vital regulatory system of the eukaryotic cell cycle. Mutations in Spindle Assembly Checkpoint (SAC) lead to a condition that is associated with various types of cancers. Kapanidou & Bolanos-Garcia in chapter 02 explain the organization, structure and function of SAC components as this molecular understanding is essential to identify and evaluate new targets and novel strategies for the treatment of cancer.

Excessive ErbB signaling is associated with the development of a diverse range of solid tumours. The involvement of the ErbB receptor tyrosine kinases in human cancer has motivated the interest in this receptor family. In chapter 03, Angelucci explains the role of ErbB receptors as a potential therapeutic target in metastasis. This review summarises the recent molecular evidence and the outcome of clinical examinations to demonstrate the potential of ErbB family members.

At least 25% of patients with breast cancer develop skeletal metastases, with bone cancer resulting in the greatest morbidity. Bisphosphonates are the treatment of choice in tumour-induced hypercalcaemia, and they can lessen bone tenderness and skeletal complications. Chapter 04 by Brown & Holen summarizes anti-tumour effects of bisphosphonates reported from *in vivo* models, alone and in combination with other anti-cancer agents.

Caveolin-1 (cav-1) is a major structural component of caveolae and it affects diverse signaling pathways regulating cell proliferation, apoptosis, differentiation, migration and growth. Kasper & Barth in chapter 05 elaborate on the role of Bleomycin in inducing apoptosis and senescence in Alveolar Epithelial Lung Cells. This review highlights the issue that bleomycin-induced injury of lung cells is accompanied by altered expression levels of caveolin-1.

Chapter 06 by Cazzaniga *et al.* summarizes the vast array of molecules involved in carcinogenesis and the role of candidate biomarkers in risk assessment and prevention of breast cancer.

Costelli *et al.* in chapter 07 discuss the efficacy of two histone deacetaylase inhibitors, valproic acid and trichostatin A in preventing muscle atrophy associated with certain cancers.

Indoleamine-2, 3-dioxygenase (IDO) is an immunosuppressive enzyme and its expression is evident in tumours. Chapter 08 by Liu *et al.* explains the role of IDO as a mediator of peripheral immune tolerance, and the potential of inhibition of IDO serves as a novel anti-cancer therapy.

Association of p53 with Bid induces cell death in response to etoposide treatment. Chen *et al.* in chapter 09 discuss a novel mechanism of facilitation of Bid nuclear export by p53 and their interaction in the nucleus and the mitochondria to induce apoptosis in response to etoposide-induced DNA damage.

Daunorubicin belongs to the group of chemotherapy drugs known as *anthracycline antibiotics* and is a toxic analogue of anthracycline which is reduced to daunorubicinol (less toxic) by the action of AKR1B10. It was discovered that the enzyme AKR1B10 is overexpressed in some types of cancer. Balendiran in chapter 10 presents the chemical mechanism of action of daunorubicin and proposes a method to advance the effectiveness of daunorubicin by modulating the catalytic activity of AKR1B10.

I hope the current volume will provide insights into the development of new approaches to anti-cancer therapy for interested researchers and pharmaceutical scientists. I greatly appreciate the assistance from the editorial staff, particularly Mr. Mahmood Alam (Director Publication) and Mr. Shehzad Naqvi (Senior Manager) for their hard work and determined efforts.

Atta-ur-Rahman, *FRS*
Honorary Life Fellow
Kings College
University of Cambridge
UK

LIST OF CONTRIBUTORS

A. Brenner
Department of Clinical Science, University of Bergen, Bergen, Norway

Adriano Angelucci
Department of Biotechnological and Applied Clinical Sciences, University of L'Aquila, L'Aquila, Italy

Alberto Luini
Division of Breast Surgery, European Institute of Oncology, Milan, Italy

Andrea Bonetto
Department of Surgery, Indiana University School of Medicine, IUPUI, Indianapolis, IN, USA

Andrea Decensi
Medical Oncology, E.O. Ospedali Galliera, Genoa, Italy

Baoguang Hu
Department of Surgery, Faculty of Medicine, The Chinese University of Hong, Kong, Hong Kong, China; Department of Gastrointestinal Surgery, the Affiliated Hospital of Binzhou Medical University, Binzhou, Shandong, China

Bernardo Bonanni
Division of Cancer Prevention and Genetics, European Institute of Oncology, Milan, Italy

E. Ersvær
Department of Clinical Science, University of Bergen, Bergen, Norway

Fabio Penna
Department of Clinical and Biological Sciences, University of Turin, Italy; Interuniversitary Institute of Myology, Italy

Francesco M. Baccino
Department of Clinical and Biological Sciences, University of Turin, Italy

Gabriella Bonelli
Department of Clinical and Biological Sciences, University of Turin, Italy

Ganesaratnam K. Balendiran
Department of Chemistry, Youngstown State University, One University Plaza, Youngstown, OH 44555, USA

Gang Song
Department of Surgery, Faculty of Medicine, The Chinese University of Hong, Kong, Hong Kong, China; Cancer Research Center, Medical College of Xiamen University, Xiamen, People's Republic of China

George G. Chen
Department of Surgery, Faculty of Medicine, The Chinese University of Hong, Kong, Hong Kong, China

H. Reikvam
Department of Clinical Science, University of Bergen, Bergen, Norway; Department of Medicine, Haukeland University Hospital, Bergen, Norway

Hannah K. Brown
Academic Unit of Clinical Oncology, University of Sheffield, Sheffield, UK

Ingunn Holen
Academic Unit of Clinical Oncology, University of Sheffield, Sheffield, UK

K.J. Hatfield
Department of Clinical Science, University of Bergen, Bergen, Norway

Kathrin Barth
Institute of Anatomy, Medical Faculty "Carl Gustav Carus", Technische Universität Dresden, 01307 Dresden, Germany

Liping Liu
Department of Surgery, Faculty of Medicine, The Chinese University of Hong, Kong, Hong Kong, China; Department of Hepatobiliary and Pancreas Department of Hepatobiliary Surgery, the Second Clinical Medical College of Jinan University (Shenzhen People's Hospital), Shenzhen, Guangdong Province, China

Maria Kapanidou
Faculty of Health and Life Sciences, Department of Biological and Medical Sciences; Oxford Brookes University, Oxford, England, OX3 0BP, UK

Massimiliano Cazzaniga
Division of Cancer Prevention and Genetics, European Institute of Oncology, Milan, Italy

Michael Kasper
Institute of Anatomy, Medical Faculty "Carl Gustav Carus", Technische Universität Dresden, 01307 Dresden, Germany

Ø. Bruserud
Department of Clinical Science, University of Bergen, Bergen, Norway; Department of Medicine, Haukeland University Hospital, Bergen, Norway

Oreste Gentilini
Division of Breast Surgery, European Institute of Oncology, Milan, Italy

Paola Costelli
Department of Clinical and Biological Sciences, University of Turin, Italy; Interuniversitary Institute of Myology, Italy

Paul B.S. Lai
Department of Surgery, Faculty of Medicine, The Chinese University of Hong, Kong, Hong Kong, China

Peggy A. Scherle
Incyte Corporation, Wilmington, DE 19880, USA

R.B. Forthun
Department of Clinical Science, University of Bergen, Bergen, Norway

Robert C. Newton
Incyte Corporation, Wilmington, DE 19880, USA

Steven M. Friedman
Incyte Corporation, Wilmington, DE 19880, USA

Victor M. Bolanos-Garcia
Faculty of Health and Life Sciences, Department of Biological and Medical Sciences; Oxford Brookes University, Oxford, England, OX3 0BP, UK

Xiangdong Liu
Incyte Corporation, Wilmington, DE 19880, USA

CHAPTER 1

Heat Shock Protein 90 – A Potential Target in the Treatment of Human Acute Myelogenous Leukemia

H. Reikvam[1,2], R.B. Forthun[1], A. Brenner[1], E. Ersvær[1], K.J. Hatfield[1] and Ø. Bruserud[*,1,2]

[1]Department of Clinical Science, University of Bergen, Bergen, Norway; [2]Department of Medicine, Haukeland University Hospital, Bergen, Norway

Abstract: Heat shock proteins (HSPs) are molecular chaperones that stabilize folding and conformation of normal as well as oncogenic proteins. These chaperones thereby prevent the formation of protein aggregates. HSPs are often overexpressed in human malignancies, including AML. HSP90 is the main chaperon required for the stabilization of multiple oncogenic kinases involved in the development of acute myelogenous leukemia (AML). HSP90 client proteins are involved in the regulation of apoptosis, proliferation, autophagy and cell cycle progression; several of these proteins are in addition considered as possible therapeutic targets for the treatment of AML. HSP90 inhibition thereby offers the possibility to modulate several of the intracellular regulatory pathways through targeting of a single molecule. Several inhibitors of HSP90 have been developed, and they are classified into four groups: geldanamycin derivatives, radicicol derivates, synthetic inhibitors and a final group of others. The HSP90 activity is in addition regulated by posttranscriptional modulation; HSP90 inhibition can thereby be indirectly achieved through increased acetylation caused by histone deacetylase inhibitors. Many of these agents have entered clinical trials, and the results from these initial studies have documented that HSP90 inhibition can mediate antileukemic effects *in vivo*. However, one would expect immunosuppressive side effects because HSP90 inhibitors have both direct and indirect inhibitory effects on T cell activation. Thus, future clinical studies are needed to clarify the efficiency and toxicity of HSP90 inhibitors in the treatment of human AML, including studies where HSP90 inhibitors are combined with conventional chemotherapy.

Keywords: Acute myelogenous leukemia, apoptosis, chaperone, client proteins, heat shock protein, heat shock protein 90 inhibitors.

***Corresponding Author Ø. Bruserud:** Medical Department, Haukeland University Hospital, N-5021 Bergen, Norway; Tel: 55 97 50 00; Fax: 55 97 29 50; E-mail: oystein.bruserud@haukeland.no

INTRODUCTION

Acute myeloid leukemia (AML) is a heterogeneous group of hematopoietic disorders characterized by bone marrow accumulation of immature leukemic cells [1]. Although progress has been made in the management of AML, especially for the acute promyelocytic leukemia (APL) variant [2], the overall outcome is still poor. This is especially true for the majority of elderly patients who cannot receive the most intensive therapy and have increased frequencies of high-risk genetic abnormalities [3]. The average survival for those patients who can receive only supportive or disease-stabilizing therapy is 3-4 months and very few survive longer than 12 months [1, 4]. Thus, new molecular diagnostics have improved the characterization and classification of patients [5, 6], but this has not yet been accompanied by the design of new effective therapeutic strategies.

Molecular chaperones are a class of proteins that interact with diverse protein substrates to assist in their folding [7]. They have a critical role during cellular stress to prevent the appearance of misfolded or otherwise damaged molecules. Heat shock proteins (HSPs) act as molecular chaperones and the HSPs assist in the recovery from stress either by repairing damaged proteins (protein refolding) or by degrading them and thereby restoring protein homeostasis [7]. The HSPs have been implicated in carcinogenesis by promoting tumor cell proliferation as well as inhibiting cellular death pathways [8].

Chemoresistant leukemia relapse is an important cause of death in AML [1]. Exposure to anticancer therapies can induce expression of HSPs and thereby enhance cellular recovery from stress conditions. With the known roles of such stress proteins in the regulation and remodeling of a wide range of client proteins (*e.g.* hormone receptors, protein kinases, several caspases), it is not surprising that molecular chaperones have been implicated in resistance to anticancer treatments. Several HSP client proteins have been validated as possible therapeutic targets in cancer treatment, and HSP90 inhibitors have emerged as potentially beneficial anticancer agents [9]. This represents a new therapeutic strategy by altering several signalling pathways through a single target. Some of the HSP90 inhibitors have entered clinical trials also in AML [10, 11]. This article focuses on the potential role of HSPs in leukemogenesis and HSP inhibitors in the treatment of AML.

EXPRESSION AND FUNCTION OF HEAT SHOCK PROTEINS

Classification and Function of HSPs

HSPs are also called stress proteins and represent a group of ubiquitous proteins that are expressed at low levels under normal physiological conditions, but production of high levels is triggered by exposure to environmental stress [12]. This is often referred to as the heat shock response [12]. This response can be triggered by malignant transformation, infections, inflammation, exposure to toxins, starvation, oxygen deprivation, nitrogen deficiency or water deprivation [13]. Consequently, the HSPs are also referred to as stress proteins.

HSPs are usually cytoplasmic proteins, but their functions involve various intracellular compartments and processes [14]. They act as molecular chaperons together with a group of cochaperones, they play important roles in protein-protein interactions and assist in establishing proper protein conformation with prevention of unwanted protein aggregation. The last process also depends on ubiquitin that serves as a tag for proteasomal protein destruction. One major function of the ubiquitin-proteasome system is to prevent accumulation of non-functional and potentially toxic proteins [15]. To summarize, HSPs prevent formation of protein aggregates whereas ubiquitination facilitates removal of aggregates.

The HSPs are named according to their molecular weights, *e.g.* HSP60, HSP70 and HSP90 (the most widely studied HSPs) (Table **1**). In contrast to HSP70 that controls folding of all newly synthesized proteins, HSP90 has a more restricted repertoire of client proteins mainly including various protein kinases [14, 16]. HSP90 seems to be important for cellular proliferation, survival and adaptation to unfavorable microenvironments, and HSP90 inactivation results in inappropriate functioning and rapid degradation of its client proteins. Its normal chaperoning activity is strongly dependent on its cochaperones, *i.e.* accessory proteins that interact with HSP90 and induce conformational changes (Table **2**). Many cochaperones have been detected, but the molecular details in their interactions with HSP90 are not known.

Table 1: The Major HSPs and their Main Functions

Heat Shock Protein	Main Function
HSP27	Protection against protein aggregation, regulation of signaling in the apoptotic pathway, regulation of cell movement, involved in embryogenesis.
HSP60	Promotes efficient mitochondrial protein folding, the main function in cytosol is to induce folding of actin and tubulin.
HSP70	Stabilizes proteins prior to complete folding, regulate transport across membranes and proteolysis.
HSP90	Stabilizes kinases prior to complete folding or activation; forms stable complexes with several transcription factors.
HSP110	Dissociates protein aggregates, facilitates proteolysis, essential for thermotolerance.

Table 2: The Most Important Cochaperones of HSP90 and their Main Function

Cochaperone	Main Function
Activator of HSP90 ATPase 1 (Aha 1)	Stimulate ATPase activity.
Cell division cycle 37 homologue (Cdc37)	Recruit kinases to the HSP90 machinery.
Cyclophilin-40 (CyP40)	Essential for modulation of steroid receptors.
FK506 binding protein 52 (FKBP52)	Potentiate receptor function.
HSP organizing protein (HOP)	Mediate interactions between HSP70 and HSP90, modulate ATPase activity and facilitate client protein transfer between the HSP70 and HSP90.
p23	Stimulate ATPase activity and enhances the maturation of client proteins.
Protein phosphatase 5 (PP5)	Stabilize the interaction between HSP90 and its clients.

HSP90 has three structural domains; (i) an N-terminal nucleotide binding domain, (ii) a middle segment that interacts with client proteins, and (iii) a C-terminal domain that is implicated in homodimerization (Fig. **1**). HSP synthesis is strictly regulated both through (i) activation and nuclear translocation of the transregulatory heat shock transcription factors (HSFs), and (ii) at the level of translation of mRNA into protein [17]. In vertebrates four members of the HSF family (HSF1-4) have been identified, but only HSF1 and HSF2 are ubiquitously expressed and conserved. HSF1 is rapidly activated though protein-damaging stress, whereas HSF2 is a less active regulator that is inhibited by heat shock [18].

Transcription is initiated through HSF binding to the heat shock promoter elements (HSEs) that are present upstream to all HSP genes [19].

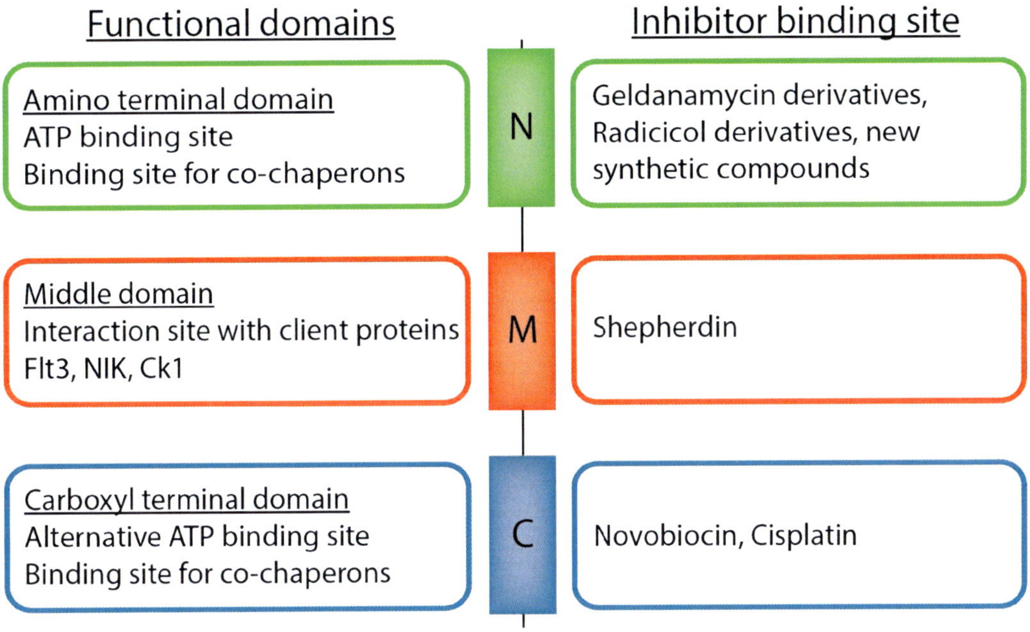

Fig. (1): The three structural domains of HSP90. N refers to the amino terminal binding domain that also is the binding site for ATP, some of the cochaperones and most HSP90 inhibitors. M refers to the middle segment, whose main function is interactions with client proteins. C refers to the carboxy binding terminal domain that is an alternative binding site for ATP, binds some cochaperones and some HSP90 inhibitors.

Cells constitutively express HSF proteins, but these proteins do not induce HSP expression genes in the absence of stress reactions. In mammalian cells, HSF1 is maintained in the cytoplasmatic HSP90 complex as a monomer that lacks DNA binding activity [20]. This complex dissociates in response to stress and releases the HSF1 monomer (Fig. **2**). The monomer then forms a trimer capable of DNA binding [20]. Sequestering of HSP90 itself also seems to be a signal for HSF1 activation. Further, HSF1 is activated by multiple phosphorylations [21] and thereby concentrated in two large foci in the nucleus of normal cells. In contrast HSF1 display several foci in cancer cells, probably correlating to the ploidy of the cells [22].

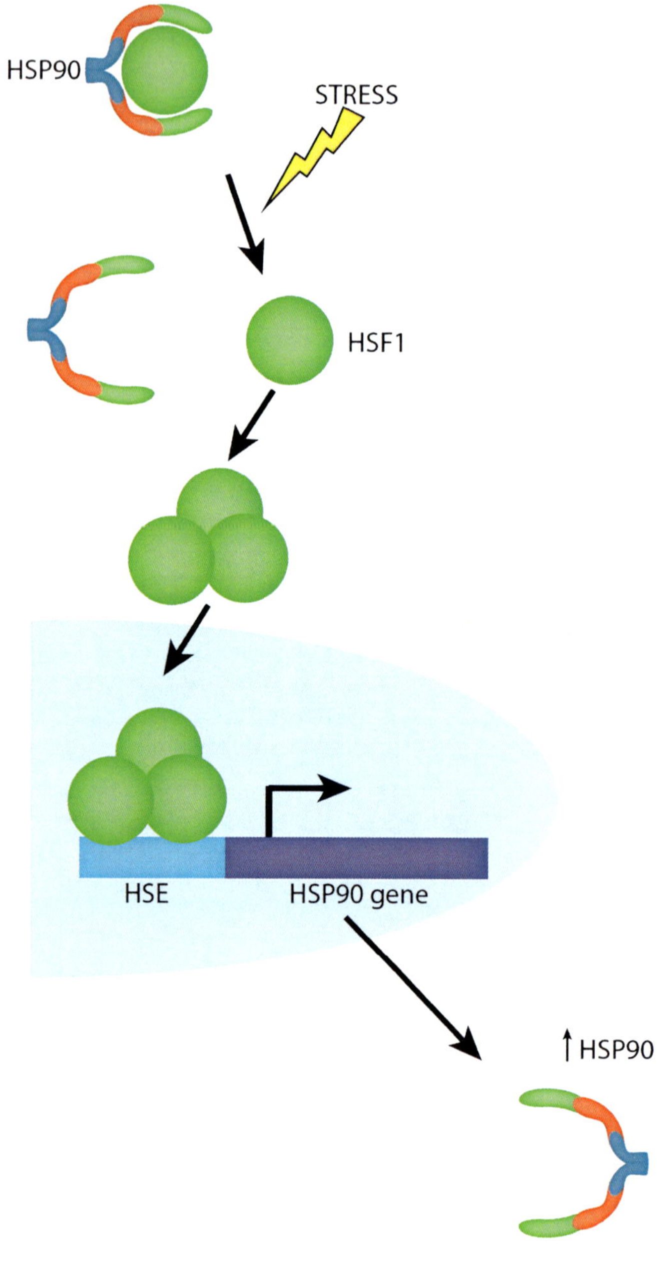

Fig. (2): Activation of HSP90 transcription. HSF1 is maintained in the cytoplasmatic HSP90 complex as a monomer that lacks DNA binding activity. This complex dissociates in response to accumulation of denaturated proteins, and releases the HSF1 monomer. The monomer then forms a trimer that translocates to the nucleus and binds to HSE. Transcription is initiated resulting in increased HSP90 translation in cancer cells. (Abbreviations: HSE -Heat shock element; HSF1 - Heat shock transcription factor 1).

It is largely unknown how the various regulatory mechanisms contribute to the HSPs overexpression in malignant cells. One initial signal for HSP induction in malignant cells is probably the accumulation of denatured proteins, including HSP90 itself [23]. It is also postulated that the pathophysiological features of the tumor microenvironment facilitate HSP induction. This last possibility is supported by a study of prostate carcinoma cells demonstrating that HSP90 expression declined markedly when the cells were transferred from tissue culture to growth as xenografts *in vivo* [24]. However, observations in other tumor models suggest that these increased levels are a fundamental characteristic that is regulated at the post-mRNA level [24]. Results from *in vitro* studies suggest that interactions between leukemic and stromal cells also support leukemogenesis [25], but it is not known whether this crosstalk affects the expression of HSPs. Interestingly, combination of a HSP90 inhibitor with either a serine/threonine kinase (Akt) inhibitor [26] or rapamycin [27], inhibited angiogenesis in myeloma bone marrow, and similar effects may also be important in AML [28].

Potential Role of HSP90 in Apoptosis, Autophagy and Cell Cycle Regulation

Treatment failures in AML can be either primary resistance or later relapse [29]. Failure is often associated with defects in apoptotic pathways [30, 31], and a variety of genes are now recognized as pro- or antiapoptotic. Apoptosis is a very frequent type of cell death observed in hematological malignancies after treatment with cytotoxic drugs [32], probably through simultaneous activation of several pathways. Two distinct pathways can initiate apoptosis through common downstream steps mediated by cysteine proteases known as caspases: the intrinsic or mitochondrial pathway and the extrinsic or death receptors pathway [30, 31]. HSPs block apoptosis by interfering with caspase activation. Overexpression of HSP27, HSP60, HSP70 or HSP90 inhibits stress-induced apoptosis through prevention of caspase activation [33].

Expression of HSPs correlates with increased resistance to apoptosis induced by a range of diverse cytotoxic agents and has therefore been implicated in chemoresistance [34]. However, high HSP90 levels were associated with increased apoptosis when an AML cell line was treated with a combination of tumor necrosis factor-α (TNF-α) and cycloheximide [35]. In contrast, high apoptosis/low viability was associated with low levels of HSP70 and HSP90 in a model of spontaneous *in vitro* apoptosis of primary human AML cells [25]. Thus, the final effect of HSP90 on regulation of apoptosis depends on the intra- and extracellular context and not only on the HSP level alone.

Autophagy has a potential role in cancer therapy [36]. This is a dynamic system of protein degradation, in which cellular proteins and organelles are sequestered, delivered to lysosomes and finally digested by lysosomal enzymes. An isoform of the constitutively expressed HSP70 is associated with the cytoplasmic side of the lysosomal membrane where it binds to substrates of this proteolytic pathway. Results from coimmunoprecipitation and colocalization studies indicate that this molecular chaperone forms complexes with other chaperones and cochaperones, including HSP90 [37]. Furthermore, the I-κB kinase (IKK) that is an essential activator of the transcription factor Nuclear factor-κB (NF-κB), is selectively degraded by autophagy in the presence of HSP90 inhibition [37]. These observations provide evidence for a molecular link between HSP90, NF-κB and autophagy [38]. For multiple myeloma the combination of rapamycin, an agent known to interfere with autophagy, and a HSP90 inhibitor synergistically inhibits proliferation, induces apoptosis and cell cycle arrest and inhibits angiogenesis and osteoclast formation in the bone marrow [27]. However, it is not known whether such synergism between rapamycin and HSP90 inhibition is a general effect or a specific phenomenon for myeloma cells.

HSP90 INHIBITION

The Molecular Basis for HSP90 Inhibition

HSP90 possesses two binding sites for client proteins located in the N- and C-terminal fragments, respectively. The C-terminal fragment binds partially folded proteins in an ATP-independent way potentially regulated by cochaperones. The N-terminal domain contains a peptide-binding site that seems to bind preferentially peptides longer than 10 amino acids, and peptide dissociation is induced by ATP binding [39, 40]. HSP90 operates as a dimer in a conformational cycle driven by ATP binding and hydrolysis at the N-terminal end; the cycle is in addition regulated by cochaperones and accessory proteins (Fig. **3**). Through its binding of a wide range of client proteins HSP90 displays a multifaceted influence on several signalling pathways in addition to epigenetic regulation and differentiation. The inhibitors of HSP90 can be divided into four classes; benzoquinone ansamycin and their derivates, radicicol and its derivates, small synthetic inhibitors and others (Table **3**) [41].

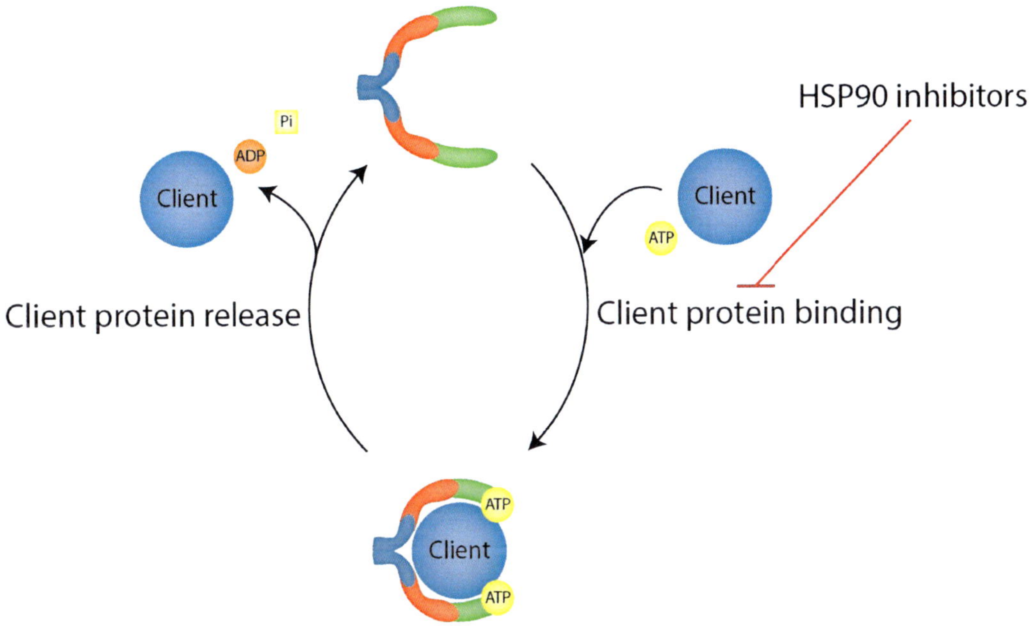

Fig. (3): Conformational status of HSP90. HSP90 operates as a dimer in a conformational cycle driven by ATP binding and hydrolysis at the N-terminal end; the cycle is in addition regulated by cochaperones and accessory proteins. Client proteins (CP) bind to HSP90 in the "open" state and undergo stabilization and folding. At the same time ATP is bound and this trigger an alternation in the conformational state to a "closed" form. ATP is later hydrolysed, the client proteins are released after folding and stabilization and HSP90 is returned to the open state. Most HSP90 inhibitors interact with the ATP or client protein binding to HSP90.

- **Inhibitors of N-terminal ATPase.** The benzoquinone amsancines such as herbimycin and geldanamycin were the first HSP90 inhibitors to be developed [42, 43]. Geldanamycin has several pharmacological limitations, including poor solubility, limited *in vivo* stability and hepatic toxicity, and it is not for clinical use [44]. The semisynthetic analogue 17-allylamino-17-demethoxygeldanamycin (17-AAG, tanespimycin) [45-50] and its more

Table 3: Classification and Characterization of HSP90 Inhibitors. The Table Shows the Four Different Families HSP90 Inhibitors, the Most Important Compounds in each Family and Some Important Pharmacological Characteristics of Each Compound

Functional Classification / Molecular Subclassification	Name of Inhibitor	Main Administration	Key References
Inhibition of N-terminal ATPase			
Benzoquinones ansamycines	Geldanamycin	Not for further clinical development	[42]
	Tanespimycin, 17-AAG, KOS-953, CNF110	Intravenous	[45-50]
	Alvespimycin, 17-DMAG, KOS-1022	Intravenous	[51, 52]
	Retaspimycin, IPI-504	Intravenous	[53, 54]
	IPI-493, 17-AG	Oral	[189]
Radicicol and its derivatives	Radicicol	Not for further clinical development	[55]
	AT13387	Oral	[57]
	NVP-AUY922	Intravenous	[56, 97]
Synthetic	MPC-3100	Oral	[61]
	BIIB021, CNF2024	Oral	[62, 63]
	Debio 0932, CUDC-305	Oral	[64]
	PU-H71	Oral	[65]
	SNX-2112, PF-04929113	Oral (by prodrug SNX-5422)	[66, 67]
	STA-9090	Intravenous	[68-70]
	XL888	Oral	[71]
	NVP-BEP800	Oral	[72]
	KW-2478	Intravenous	[73]
Inhibition of C-terminal ATPase			
Aminocoumarin antibiotic	Novobiocin	High rates of hypersensitivity reactions. Withdrawn from the market	[75]
Platinum-based chemotherapy	Cisplatin	Intravenous	[76]
Inhibition of client protein interaction			
Synthetic drugs	Shepherdin		[78]
Molecular modulation			
HDAC-inhibitors		Oral	[80, 81, 92]

soluble derivatives such as 17-dimethylalaminoethylamino-17-demethoxy-geldanamycin (17-DMAG, alvespimycin) [51, 52] and retaspimycin (IPI-504) [53, 54] have in contrast been tried in clinical studies. The latest development of geldanamycin derivates was the oral formulation 17-allylaminogeldanamycin (17-AG), the primary long-lived metabolite of IPI-504 and 17-AGG [43] (Table **3**).

- **Radicicol** and derivates are a second group of N-terminal ATPase inhibitors. Radicicol is a macrocyclic antibiotic produced by fungi and recognized as a structurally unique antibiotic that binds to the same N-terminal ATP/ADP binding site on HSP90 as geldanamycin [55] (Fig. **1**). Radicicol will not be developed further for clinical use due to its pharmacological limitations and toxicity [44]. However, derivates of radiciciol, including NVP-AUY922 and AT13387, are currently under clinical investigation [43, 56, 57] (Table **3**).

- **Several Synthetic Drugs** have been obtained by rational design from the crystal structures of the binding pocket of HSP90 [58-60] (Table **3**). These small molecule inhibitors are often derivates from purine, isoxazole or benzamide [43]. Several of them have shown promising preclinical results and some have entered clinical trials [61-73] (Table **3**).

- **Inhibition of C-Terminal ATPase.** Studies have suggested that the C-terminal half of the HSP90 as an equally important regulator of chaperone activity [74]. Novobiocin was first identified as an inhibitor that targeted the ATP binding site of DNA gyrase, but in addition it binds at the second ATP binding site in the C-terminal end of HSP90 [75]. Cisplatin binds to an adjacent sequence at the C-terminal [76].

- **Inhibition of Client Binding to HSP90.** Although inhibition of the ATPase activity offers the most direct route to therapeutic manipulation of HSP90, blocking of interactions between HSP90 and its cochaperones or client molecules is an alternative molecular approach. Although this strategy is technically more difficult, it is facilitated by the availability of crystal structures from which lead compounds might be identified. Inhibition of client-protein interactions with HSP90 seems attractive, but a further development of this strategy is difficult because it is not known where in the binding pocket these interactions occur and whether they are specific or generic. Shepherdin was designed to inhibit the interaction between HSP90 and survivin, an apoptosis inhibitor associated with unfavorable prognosis in AML [77]. Although shepherdin inhibit the N-terminal ATPase activity of HSP90, Gyoroska *et al.* have demonstrated that shepherdin has an additional effect compared to 17-AGG [78]. Shepherdin more rapidly degenerated client proteins and induced cell death without any compensatory increase in HSP70 levels, in contrast to 17-AAG. Inhibition of cochaperones and client proteins are an emerging research field that may contribute to development of more specific HSP90 inhibiting.

- **Molecular Modulation of HSP90.** Histone deacetylases (HDAC) are now emerging as molecular targets in AML therapy [79]. Several studies have documented that HSP90 can be acetylated both by the p300 and PCAF acetyltransferases [80]. HSP90 is affected by HDACs especially HDAC6, and the pan-HDAC inhibitors LAQ824 and LBH589 induce HSP90 acetylation and thereby inhibition of its chaperone functions with depletion of pro-growth and pro-survival client proteins [81] (Fig. **4**). Thus, the functional consequence of increased acetylation is similar although not identical to that of direct pharmacological HSP90 inhibition [80]. The HSP90 cochaperones p23 and HSP72 are also acetylated, but the functional consequences of this are not known [80]. This is discussed more in detail in a separate chapter below.

- **Inhibition of HSP70/HSP90 Interaction.** The interactions between HSP70 and HSP90 are complex and not completely understood. Firstly, HSP70 is a cochaperone for HSP90, which uses HSP70 for recruitment and maturation of client proteins. Interestingly it seems as if HSP90 can use both the "housekeeping" HSC70 and the inducible HSP70 as cochaperone, and only silencing of both these HSP70 isoforms will inhibit HSP90 and lead to degradation of HSP90 clients [82]. Secondly, the interaction between HSP70 and HSP90 is mediated *via* another important cochaperone HOP

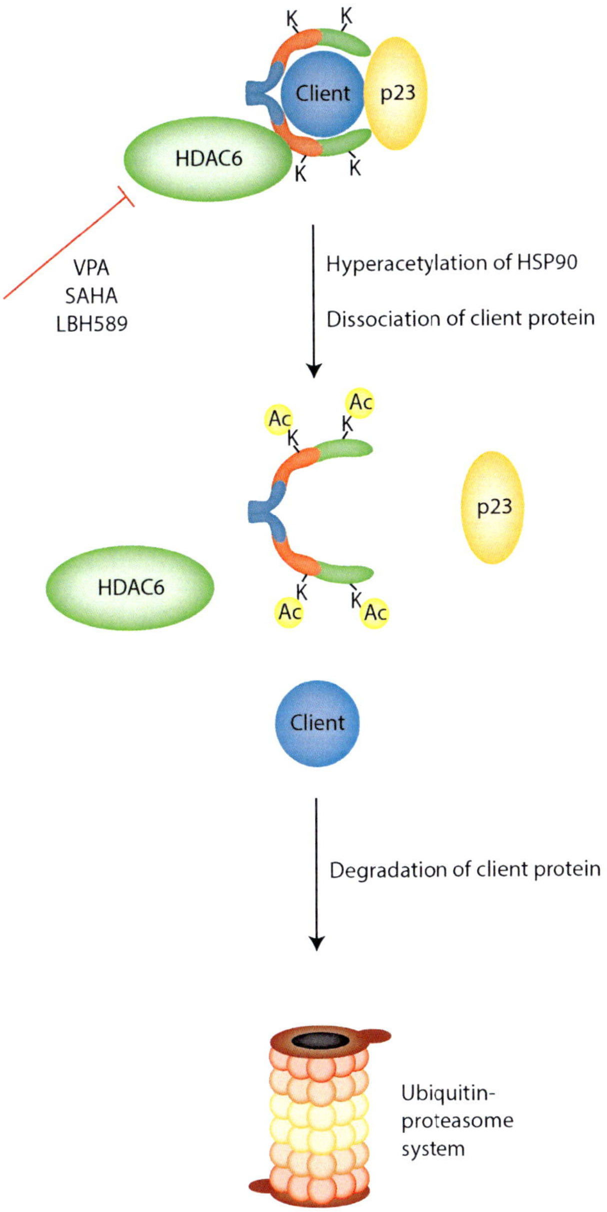

Fig. (4): Histone deacetylase inhibitors destabilize protein folding by HSP90. HSP90 is associated with HDAC6 and co-chaperone p23 to facilitate the correct conformational folding of client proteins. Upon exposure to histone deacetylase inhibitors (*e.g.* VPA, SAHA, LBH589), HDAC6 disassociates, permitting the hyperacetylation of HSP90. This dramatically reduces HSP90 affinity for p23, making it unable to interact with the co-chaperone, and thereby not allowing properly folding of the client protein. The misfolded protein is thereafter targeted for degradation by the ubiquitin-proteasome system.

(Table **2**). Thirdly, HSP70 itself seems to be a client protein of HSP90, *i.e.* HSP70 is dependent of HSP90 for proper maturation and function. Fourthly, HSP90 inhibition leads to compensatory upregulation of HSP70 caused by loss of heat shock transcription factor-1 (HSF-1) repression [83]. Finally, HSP70 inhibition alone seems to disrupt the HSP90 chaperone system, probably because of the earlier mentioned critical HSP70 cochaperone effect for HSP90. HSP70 inhibition leads to degradation of HSP90 client protein [82, 84]. Given these interactions it has been hypotized that combined inhibition of both HSP70 and HSP90 will lead to enhanced efficiency, and recent *in vitro* studies have indicated a potential role for inhibiting both these chaperones in AML [85, 86].

Early Clinical Trials of HSP90 Inhibition; Studies of Dose-Limiting Toxicity and Pharmacokinetics

The pharmacokinetic profile varies between the different HSP90 inhibitors and the newest synthetic drugs seem to have more favorable profiles and less toxicity. The valuable pharmacodynamic advantage of HSP90 inhibitors at the cellular level lies in the fact that the true therapeutic targets, the client proteins, are affected indirectly and for this reason HSP90 inhibition will often have an irreversible effect that last for 12-24 hours until synthesis of new oncoproteins occurs [41].

Tanespimycin/17-AAG is the most widely studied HSP90 inhibitor in cancer patients. The drug is administered intravenously and the drug shows the following pharmacological characteristics:

- The maximal tolerated dose seems to be schedule-dependent; 3-5 doses administered at three weeks intervals seem to have acceptable toxicity although the maximal tolerated dose differs between the regimens, whereas continuous twice-weekly dosing seems unacceptable due to delayed liver toxicity [47]. The dose-limiting toxicities in the early clinical trials have been fatigue, anorexia, abdominal pain, hepatic toxicity, pancreatitis, myalgia, headache and/or thrombocytopenia [45-47, 87]. Reversible increase in liver enzymes seems to be common and was observed in nearly half of the patients in one study [46].

- At 270 mg/m^2/dose (60 minutes intravenous infusion) the mean C_{max} was 5.303 ng/ml and mean area under the plasma concentration curve 13.656 ng/ml/h in pediatric patients; this is similar to adults [88]. Another study of pediatric patients described linear pharmacokinetics with a mean clearance of 21.6 L/h/m^2 and a mean half-life of 2.6 hours [89]. The 17-AAG pharmacokinetics seem to be linear, the peak plasma concentration and area under the curve of the major metabolite 17-AG increases with the administered dose of 17-AAG, but the variation in pharmacokinetics is wider for the metabolite than for the parent drug [87].

- The pharmacokinetics are not altered by coadministration of trastuzumab [45], irinotecan [90] or paclitaxel [91].

Many different regimens have been investigated, and the optimal administration with regard to efficiency and toxicity remains to be established. The most important side effects for HDAC inhibitors are also fatigue, gastrointestinal toxicity, cardiac side effects and thrombocytopenia [92]; this observation suggests that the HSP90 inhibition may contribute to the toxicity of HDAC inhibitors.

Based on these studies it can be concluded that it is possible to achieve pharmacological HSP90 inhibition with acceptable toxicity for a majority of patients with advanced cancer.

Functional Detection of HSP90 Inhibition *In Vitro* and *In Vivo*

The basal expression of HSP90 components does not necessarily correlate with the effect of HSP90 inhibition [93]. Functional evaluation of HSP inhibition is therefore commonly used, and the following strategies are available (see Table **4** for additional references):

- Detection of *reduced client protein levels* is often used as a marker of HSP90 inhibition, including human epidermal growth factor receptor 2 (HER2), serine/threonine kinase/protein kinase B (Akt/PKB) and signal transducer and activator of transcription-3 (STAT3); all these molecules are client proteins of HSP90 (Table **3**).

Table 4: **Categorically List Over Parameters Used to Assay HSP90 Inhibition in Clinical Studies**

Reduced Client Protein Level
v-raf-1 murine leukemia viral oncogene homolog 1 (RAF-1) [47, 100]
Signal transducer and activator of transcription-3 (STAT3) [47]
Serine/threonine kinase/Protein kinase B (Akt/PKB) [100]
Reduced Client Protein Function
Reduced phosphor- Checkpoint kinase (CHK1) [90]
Abrogation of the G2-M cell cycle checkpoint [90]
Loss of HSF1 Repression
Upregulation of HSP70 [45-47, 87, 89]
Upregulation of HSP72 [88, 99]
Evaluation of Cochaperones Dissociation
No reports on its use as biomarker in clinical studies

- Reduction of client proteins can be detected indirectly by *attenuation of receptor signalling* reflected in loss of phosphoreceptors, phospho-S6 or phospho-ERK [94]. However, whether a client protein is affected will probably also depend on whether it is mutated [95].

- Another effect of HSP90 inhibition is *loss of HSF1 repression* with upregulation of HSP70 and HSP27 [96], and this upregulation can be detected even in normal peripheral blood mononuclear cells during *in vivo* therapy [97]. HSP70 has been claimed to have an antiapoptotic effect that may counteract the proapoptotic effect of HSP90 inhibition at least in certain experimental models [82].

- An alternative method of studying the cellular effects of HSP90 inhibitors, which more closely monitors the catalytic cycle of HSP90, is through the evaluation of *disruption of the HSP90 and cochaperones complex* [98], and especially the interactions between HSP90 and cochaperone p23 seem essential for HSP90 activity and client protein stability [98].

These approaches have also been used to document HSP90 inhibition in clinical studies of HSP90 inhibitors in cancer patients, as presented in detail in Table **4**. The evaluation can be performed in cancer cell samples [47, 90, 99]. Alternatively, analysis of peripheral blood mononuclear cells can be used to document that *in vivo* levels of the pharmacological agents are sufficient for

HSP90 inhibition [45-47, 88, 89, 99]. Both detection of reduced client protein levels (Akt, RAF-1), altered signalling downstream to client proteins (phosphor-CHK-1 loss, abrogation of the G2-M cell cycle checkpoint) and loss of HSF1 repression (increased HSP70, HSP72) have then been used to document HSP90 inhibition in clinical studies [45-47, 88-90, 99, 100].

Variation in Cellular Sensitivity to HSP90 Inhibition

Results from *in vitro* studies suggest that the cells most sensitive to HSP90 inhibition are those where the cellular proliferation or survival is supported by mutated oncoproteins that depend on HSP90 for stability or activity; in the case of AML the two most important seem to be the tyrosine kinases FLT3 and KIT [101-103]. This is also consistent with previous observations that mutated molecules are especially dependent on HSP90 to acquire stability and activity.

Differences in binding of HSP90 inhibitors to the target molecule seem to influence the potency of the therapeutic strategy. There seems to be a correlation between biochemical affinity and growth inhibition with a relative activity ranking of isoxazoles derivates (*e.g.* NVP-AUY922) > geldanamycin and derivatives > purine derivates (MPC-3100, BIIB021) (Table **3**) [104]. Furthermore, in contrast to previous studies describing that ansamycines especially bind to HSP90 in cancer cells [40], these authors found that isoxazoles could bind to HSP90 also in normal cells [104]. Taken together these studies thereby suggest that the degree of binding/inhibition depends on both the chemical structure of the inhibitor and the cell type. Whether similar differences contribute to the variations in HSP90 responsiveness between different cancer cells remains to be clarified.

Certain ansamycines are metabolized to hydroquinones that are up to 30 times more potent than the quinine derivatives [105], and some cell lines lack or have only low levels of the enzyme required for this conversion. Such cells may then show decreased susceptibility to those HSP90 inhibitors that depend on this conversion to reach their maximal inhibitory effect [93].

THE IMMUNE SYSTEM AND HSP90 INHIBITION

Adequate adaptive immune responses depend upon proper antigen presentation by antigen presenting cells (APC) like macrophages, dendritic cells and B-cells [106]. The initial step in antigenic processing is the generation of cytosolic peptides that are transported to the endoplasmic reticulum where MHC molecules are loaded with peptides before being transported to the cell surface. The proper loading of MHC class I and class II with peptide seems to depend upon chaperon activity [107, 108]. Studies in murine cell lines demonstrated that HSP90 is directly involved in antigen processing through chaperoning of antigenic peptides, and it has a significant role in cross-priming [107]. Treatment of cells with HSP90 inhibitors (radicocol, geldanamycin or 17-AAG) led to generation of "empty" MHC I due to inhibited loading [107]. Another study demonstrated that geldanamycin inhibited MHC class II restricted peptide presentation by antigen-loaded B cells [108].

Dendritic cells (DC) are regarded as professional antigen-presenting cells. In short, HSP90 inhibition by geldanamycin decreased antigen uptake, processing, and presentation by immature DC, leading to reduced antigen-specific T cell responses [109]. Furthermore, HSP90 inhibition also decreased the ability of mature DC to present antigen, secrete IL-12 and induce IFNγ secretion by alloreactive T cells [109]. In addition, inhibition of HSP90 by geldanamycin directly suppresses both T and B lymphocyte functions [110-113]. This drug directly inhibits the proliferation of mitogen-activated T lymphocytes and is toxic to both resting and activated T cells [112]. Geldanamycin acts probably through effects on the HSP90-dependent and T cell-specific nonreceptor tyrosine kinase Lck. Geldanamycin depleted lck levels in cultured T cells by a slow and dose-dependent process, probably trough degradation of newly synthesized Lck molecules [112]. Another study demonstrated that geldanamycin could alter the expression and phosphorylation of Lck as well as the v-raf-1 murine leukemia viral oncogene homolog 1 (RAF-1) kinase. Moreover, geldanamycin also disrupts the T-cell receptor-mediated activation of nuclear factor of activated T-cells (NF-AT) [111], and it seems to inhibit CD28-initated IL-2 dependent autocrine T-cell proliferation [110]. Thus, immunesuppression should be expected during treatment with HSP90 inhibitors.

IMPORTANT HSP90 CLIENT PROTEINS IN AML

HSP90 Expression by Primary AML Cells

The expression of HSPs by leukemic cells varies between patients [114]. In 98 newly diagnosed AML patients HSP27 was expressed by the leukemia cells for 39%, HSP60 for 26%, HSP70 for 58%, HSP90 for 41%, and HSP110 for 30% of patients. HSP90 and HSP110 expression showed significant correlation with FAB subtype and karyotype [115]. Complete remission rates and overall survival were higher in patients with generally low HSP expression [114, 115]. In another study 65 patients with newly diagnosed AML were examined; HSP90 expression then correlated with the expression of the non-client proteins CD34, p170, and bcl-2 but with no correlations with white cell counts, morphological differentiation (*i.e.* FAB or WHO subclassification) or cytogenetics [116]. A concomitant constitutive activation of the extracellular signal-regulated kinase and Akt pathways was also observed for a majority of samples and this was significantly correlated with HSP90 expression. Finally, this study showed shorter survival for patients with high HSP90 level [116]. All these observations suggest that HSP90 is overexpressed in poor-prognosis AML, and this is similar to the preleukemic MDS where high HSP90 expression is detected in the high-risk subgroups [117].

Intracellular Signalling Involving FMS-Like Tyrosine Kinase 3

Many leukemia-associated oncoproteins are HSP90 clients (Table 5). Approximately 45% of patients with *de novo* AML have normal cytogenetics [6, 118]. Among the most common molecular genetic abnormalities in these patients is mutated FMS-like tyrosine kinase 3 (FLT3) [6], which also has a prognostic impact and is used for therapy guidance [118, 119]. Activating mutations of FLT3 occur in approximately one-third of AML patients and predict a high risk of leukemia relapse [120]. The FLT3-internal tandem duplication (ITD) mutations are most common and consist of in-frame duplications of variable lengths of the juxtamembrane domain of the FLT3 receptor [121]. The FLT3-(tyrosine-kinase domain) TKD mutations consist of single base substitutions, small deletions or insertion in the activation loop of the tyrosine kinase domain [122]. FLT3 is a HSP90 client proteins, and inhibition of HSP90 thereby seems to have an indirect

Table 5: Main HSP90 Client Proteins with Potential Involvement in Leukemogenesis. The Client Proteins are Divided into Four Main Categories and their Functional Importance in Human AML is Briefly Described

Protein Class	Client Proteins	Relevance to Human AML
Chaperones and Relatives	p23	Cochaperone of HSP 90 [98]
	Heat shock protein 70 (HSP70)	Expressed by primary AML cells for more than 50% of the patients [115]
	Nuclear distribution C (NudC)	Important for nuclear migration in cell division, high expression in human AML cells [190]
Transcription Regulation	Peroxisome proliferator-activated receptor-alfa	Involved in the regulation of proliferation in primary human AML cells [191]
	(PPARα)	Upregulated by exposure of HL-60 AML cell to ATRA [192]
	Pregnane X receptor (PXR)	Important for regulation of primary AML cell viability *in vitro* and *in vivo*
	p53	[193]
	Mouse double minute 2 (MDM2)	A p53 inhibitor, the p53-MDM2 complex is a possible therapeutic target in AML therapy [194]
	Signal transducer and activator of transcription-3 (STAT3)	Important intracellular mediator downstream to hematopoietic growth factor receptors [163]
	Calcium-sensing receptor (CAR)	Expressed in HL-60 AML cells and upregulated during monocytic differentiation [195]; calcium is important for intracellular signalling downstream to several chemokine receptors that are expressed by primary human AML cells [124]
	Inhibitor of κB (IκB) kinases α, β, γ, ε; NF-κB-inducing kinase (NIK)	The NF-κB complex is important for proliferation, survival and chemosensitivity in primary human AML cells [125]
	Histone deacetylase 6 (HDAC6)	HDAC inhibitors are now tried in the treatment of AML [92]; these drugs alter
	Histones (H1, H2A, H2B, H3 and H4)	acetylation of several cytoplasmic and nuclear molecules, including histones, and the gene expression in primary human AML cells is thereby altered [92]
Kinases	FMS-like tyrosine kinase 3 (FLT3)	Mutated FLT3 is an adverse prognostic factor in human AML [120], FLT3-ligand is a growth factor for primary human AML cells [142]
	c-Kit	Growth factor receptor in primary human AML cells [142]
	Human epidermal growth factor receptor 2 (HER2)	A possible leukemia-associated antigen in AML [196]
	Insulin receptor	Insulin stimulate primary AML cell proliferation [197]
	Insulin-like growth factor 1 receptor (IGF-1 receptor)	IGF is a growth factor for primary AML cells [197]
	Integrin-linked kinase (ILK)	Interacts with β-integrins and activate several intracellular mediators involved in regulation of AML cell proliferation (STAT3, Akt, ERK1/2) [198]
	Mammalian target or rapamycin (mTOR)	Highly activated in AML, and potential target for pharmacological intervention [199]

(Table 5) contd…..

Protein Class	Client Proteins	Relevance to Human AML
Kinases	Janus kinase 1 (JAK1)	Can be mutated in primary human AML cells and have a disease-modifying effect [200]
	Mitogen-activated protein kinase kinase (ERK/MEK)	Important downstream mediators for hematopoietic growth factor receptors in
	Serine/threonine kinase/Protein kinase B (Akt/PKB)	primary human AML cells [163]
	Bcr-Abl	Involved in malignant transformation in chronic myelogenous leukemia, but also reported in AML [201]
	Cyclin-dependent kinases (Cdk2, Cdk4, Cdk6, Cdk9, Cdk11)	Dysregulation of the cell cycle seems important in leukemogenesis [202]
	Checkpoint kinase (CHK1)	CHK1 phosphorylation correlates with cell cycle arrest in AML [134]
	Cyclin B	Cyclin B1 is a cell cycle regulator expressed in cytoplasm and nucleus of primary human AML cells, a possible cancer-associated antigen [203]
	Death-associated kinases (DAPK, DAPK2, DAPK3)	Dysregulated expression in primary human AML cells [204]
	v-raf-1 murine leukemia viral oncogene homolog 1 (RAF-1)	Overexpressed in erythroleukemias [205]
Others	Matrix metalloprotease 2 and 9 (MMP-2/9)	Expression in primary human AML cells is a possible prognostic parameter [206]
	Survivin	Inhibitor of apoptosis with a possible adverse prognostic impact in AML [77]
	Telomerase	Regulator of proliferation and senescence, it is limiting the growth of primary human AML cells [207]
	Thiopurine S-methyltransferase	Drug-metabolizing enzyme expressed at relatively high levels in AML blasts compared with acute lymphoblastic leukemia cells [208]
	Annexin II	Cell surface coreceptor for tissue plasminogen activator and plasminogen, expressed at relatively high levels in human AML cells [209]
	Human eag-related gene (HERG)	An ion channel that is constitutively activated in primary AML cells and involved in regulation of proliferation [210]
	Mucin-1 (MUC1)	Membrane glycoprotein with increased expression in primary AML cells, possibly involved in regulation of proliferation for the immature fraction of AML cells [211]
	Protease-activated receptor 1 (PAR-1)	Important for regulation of angiogenesis [212]

inhibitory effect on FLT3-dependent intracellular signalling [120]. Mutated FLT3 is constitutively activated and probably mediates signalling that is important for leukemogenesis and chemosensitivity, and the combination of conventional DNA-damaging therapy with direct (tyrosine kinase inhibitors) or indirect (HSP90 inhibitors) FLT3 inhibition may therefore be a therapeutic alternative [123].

Transcriptional Regulation Mediated by NF-κB

The transcription factor NF-κB has a central role in the control of a wide range of genes involved in proliferation and apoptosis, and this is probably true also for primary human AML cells [124]. HSPs can interact with the function of NF-κB through several mechanisms [125]. Firstly, HSPs can bind many of the pro-apoptotic or pro-inflammatory targets of NF-κB and thereby inhibit many of its effects. Secondly, among the client kinases of HSP90 is the NF-κB-inducing kinase (NIK). Under basal conditions, NF-κB is held inactive in the cytoplasm by its inhibitory subunit IκB. Upon receiving relevant stimulation NIK activates IKK that induces phosphorylation and proteolytic processing of NF-κB subunits, and NF-κB together with NIK is thereafter translocated to the nucleus. Thirdly, HSP90 seems important for the stabilization and preservation of the IKK activator of NF-κB [126]. All these observations suggest that pharmacological targeting of chaperones in AML should be further explored [127], and this is also supported by experimental studies suggesting that the role of FLT3 in leukemogenesis involves NF-κB [128].

Cell Cycle Regulation, the Role of Checkpoint Kinases

The two structurally unrelated protein kinases Checkpoint kinases 1 and 2 (CHK1 and CHK2) are emerging as key mediators in several cellular responses to genotoxic stress [129]. Recent studies suggest an important role of both these kinases in the network of genome surveillance pathways that coordinate cell cycle progression with DNA repair and apoptosis regulation. These kinases provide a linkage between upstream sensors of cell cycle checkpoints and cell cycle regulation [130]. DNA damage and replication stress will activate the CHK1 signalling pathway, block S phase progression and thereby participate in G2 arrest. Furthermore, AML cells exposed to cytotoxic agents often show cell cycle arrest at the G2/M checkpoint together with development of chemoresistance [131]. CHK1 inhibition then allows checkpoint exit with induction of chemosensitivity [132]. HSP90 is important for the folding and stabilization of

CHK1 [133], and as expected HSP90 inhibition depletes CHK1, disrupts the S-phase checkpoint and enhances the therapeutic effect of cytarabine in primary AML cells [134].

HSP90 IN THE TREATMENT OF HUMAN AML - EFFECTS OF HSP90 INHIBITION AND SOLUBLE HSP90 AS A POSSIBLE BIOMARKER DURING TREATMENT

The development of chemoresistance in AML appears to be multifactorial [135, 136]. HSP inhibition makes it possible to target several intracellular pathways including oncoprotein-initiated signalling. HSP90 in malignant cells is often present entirely in multichaperone complexes with high ATPase activity, whereas HSP90 in normal tissues is present in a latent, uncomplexed state [137]. All these characteristics make HSP90 a unique target for antileukemic therapy.

The Effect of HSP90 Inhibition in AML Cell Lines

The anti-cancer effect of HSP inhibitors has mainly been demonstrated in solid tumors [138]. Several experimental observations suggest that HSP inhibition should be further investigated as AML therapy. Fiskus *et al.* examined the effect of HSP90 inhibition in the multuresistant HL-60/LR AML cell line [139]. These HL-60/LR variant cells differ from the parent HL-60 cells by having a higher growth fraction and thereby shorter doubling time, and they need a shorter time to generate overt leukemia after xenotransplantation to mice [139]. However, these multiresistant cells were sensitive to the HSP90 inhibitor 17-AAG, and this was observed even though the treatment did not induce HSP70 or deplete known HSP90 client proteins.

The AML cell line Kasumi-1 is characterized by the t(8;21) abnormality, a translocation associated with chemosensitive AML and low relapse risk [140]. The HSP90 inhibitor 17-AAG has an antiproliferative effect with G0/G1 cell cycle blockade and in addition proapoptotic and differentiation-inducing effects associated with reduced KIT protein expression [141]. The effect seems to be synergistic when combining 17-AAG with HDAC inhibitors sodium phenylbutarate and valproic acid [103]. These observations suggest that HSP90 inhibition may further improve the prognosis even for patients with this low-risk disease. Finally, most patients show increased AML cell proliferation in response to KIT ligation [142], and the 17-AAG-induced decrease in KIT expression suggests that HSP90 inhibition will be effective also for other AML patients [141].

The effect of HSP90 inhibition in the APL variant of AML has mainly been investigated in cell lines, and 17-AAG induces apoptosis both in all-trans-retinoic acid (ATRA) sensitive and resistant APL cells [143]. This apoptosis probably differs from ATRA-induced apoptosis because HSP90 inhibition did not induce differentiation prior to cell death. Pharmacodynamic interaction between arsenic trioxide and three HSP90 inhibitors (geldanamycin, 17-AAG and 17-DMAG) also showed synergistic antileukemic effects in APL cell lines [144], and these effects were associated with up-regulation of HSP70 that is regarded as a biomarker of effective HSP90 inhibition [144].

Effects of HSP90 Inhibition in Primary AML Cells

In vitro studies have described a cytotoxic effect of the HSP90 inhibitors in primary AML cells with mutant FLT3 [101, 102]. Combination of 17-AAG with cytarabine resulted in a synergistic or additive effect for approximately half of the patients [102]. These observations suggest that combining HSP90 inhibition with conventional therapy may be beneficial for AML patients with high-risk FLT3 mutations.

The possibility of combining 17-AAG with the FLT3-inhibitory tyrosine kinase inhibitor PKC412 has also been investigated for the FLT3-ITD positive cell line MV4-11 [145]. PKC412 inhibits the FLT3-associated receptor tyrosine kinase, and additional HSP90 inhibition caused downregulation of FLT3 as well as other oncoproteins together with a synergistic proapoptotic effect. Importantly, the proapoptotic synergism was stronger for FLT3-ITD positive than wildtype FLT3 cells [145]. It is known from studies of other malignancies that mutated oncoproteins are relatively unstable and more dependent on chaperones than their normal counterparts [146], and this may explain the stronger proapoptotic effect for AML cells with mutated FLT3.

Observations in other malignant cells have demonstrated that HSP90 acetylations have functional similarities with HSP90 inhibition [147]. The HDAC inhibitor MS-275, an inhibitor of both Class 1 and 2 HDACs [148], induced acetylation of HSP90 and at the same time ubiquitination and degradation of FLT3 in AML cells. This effect was antagonized by the proteasome inhibitor bortezomib, an observation strongly suggesting that FLT3 was degraded *via* the ubiquitin/proteasome pathway [149].

HSP90 Inhibition of Human Endothelial Cells

The endothelium functions as a barrier between different compartments and plays a key role in several physiological processes such as vessel permeability, immune cell trafficking, inflammation and angiogenesis. HSP90 is an important coordinator of signalling in endothelial cells and HSP inhibitors have been shown to suppress angiogenesis in clinical trials, however their specific effects on endothelial cells have not been well characterized. A few studies have reported that inhibitors of HSP90, including SNX-2112, NVP-AUY922, 17-AAG and 17-DMAG, can inhibit endothelial cell motility, invasion and/or tubule formation *in vitro* [56, 150, 151], with concomitant downregulation of HSP90 client proteins such as Akt, vascular endothelial growth factor receptor 2 (VEGFR2) and c-Raf. One mechanism by which HSP inhibitors may exert their antiangiogenic effects is through downregulation of Akt and endothelial nitric oxide synthase (eNOS) signalling [66, 152]. HSP90 associates with eNOS in endothelial cells, which increases eNOS activity [153], and nitric oxide (NO) generated by this enzyme is important in the regulation of endothelial proliferation, migration and cell permeability [154]. VEGF is a strong promoter of NO production in endothelial cells by facilitating recruitment of HSP90 to eNOS, and VEGF-induced *in vitro* angiogenesis can be inhibited by means of a dominant-negative HSP90 through inhibition of Akt/eNOS [152]. Binding of VEGF to VEGFR2 has also been reported to recruit HSP90 to VEGFR2 which initiates a signalling cascade promoting endothelial cell migration [155], and endothelial cells have been shown to have reduced expression of VEGFRs *in vitro* as well as reduced levels in human xenograft models *in vivo* in response to HSP90 inhibitors [56, 150].

HSP90 functions as a chaperon to several proteins involved in angiogenesis, including hypoxia inducible factor (HIF)-1α, VEGFR, NF-κB, insulin-like growth factor receptor (IGFR), c-MET and Akt [156] and HSP90 inhibitors can thus destabilize several key regulators of angiogenesis; although it has not been clarified whether the specific mechanisms of HSP90 inhibition are the same in cancer cells as in normal/tumor endothelial cells.

HSP90 inhibitors can inhibit proliferation and induce apoptosis in primary microvascular and macrovascular endothelial cells *in vitro* [101, 150, 151], though the inhibitory effect seems to be stronger on proliferating endothelial cells rather than contact-inhibited cells [150]. Collectively, HSP90 inhibitors have the potential to impair several endothelial cell functions either by affecting endothelial cells directly and/or indirectly through their actions on other cell types. HSP90 inhibitors will have an apoptotic effect on endothelial cells through their effect on apoptotic signalling proteins [151], but the main effect of HSP90 inhibitors will most likely be through their ability to suppress angiogenesis both by direct effects on endothelial function and indirectly through effects on cancer cells. Thus, the available evidence suggests that HSP90 inhibitors can inhibit endothelial cell function and angiogenesis, and this therapeutic strategy may thereby have indirect antileukemic effects through reversal of the increased microvascular density in AML bone marrow. An additional indirect effect could be inhibition of the stem cell supporting function of endothelial cells in the vascular stem cell niche, but this possibility has not been investigated.

HSP90 Inhibition, Mesenchymal Stem Cells and Differentiated Mesenchymanl Cells

Mesenchymal stem cells (MSCs) have the potential to differentiate into a variety of mature cells such as osteoblasts, chondrocytes, adipocytes, fibroblasts and muscle cells [157]. Endogenous MSCs circulate to inflammatory sites [158] but they are also attracted by malignant cells and contribute to the microenvironment that is important for disease progression and drug resistance [157].

HSP90 family proteins are constitutively expressed in MSCs but the level depends on factors like localization and cell density. MSCs from the umbilical cord express more HSP90 than MSCs derived from bone marrow, resulting in a reduced predisposition towards differentiation into osteoblasts of the former [159]. HSP90 and other chaperones are also more highly expressed in cultures with low cell density (1000 cells/mm^2), an effect possibly caused by the regulator role of HSPs mediated *via* several transcription factors [160]. Experimental studies suggest that the HSP90α protein is a survival factor for MSCs during hypoxia and serum deprivation [161].

High HSP90 expression is also coupled with hematological malignancies. HSP90α and HSP90β are expressed to a higher degree in MSCs from MDS patients compared to healthy controls [162]. HSP90 proteins seem to increase MSC proliferation rates [159, 162] and activate the Akt and ERK pathways [161] which both are linked to cancer development and progression [163]. One would therefore expect HSP90 inhibition to have effects on MSCs.

HSP90 inhibition also seems to affect more differentiated mesenchymal cells. The cytostatic S06 binds to HSP90α in stromal fibroblasts and disrupts the secretion of several important cytokines and chemokines, inhibiting tumour invasion and eventually leading to apoptosis [164]. Both 17-AAG and U0126 abrogate the anti-apoptotic effect of fibroblasts [161], whereas HSP90 inhibitors in general prevent angiogenesis and osteoclastogenesis [165].

Modulation of HSP90 Acetylation by HDAC Inhibitors

Histone deacetylases (HDAC) have also been suggested as therapeutic targets in AML [79]. HSP90 activity is regulated through reversible acetylation [80], and HSP90 chaperone activities are thereby affected by HDACs (Fig. **4**). Initially, only HDAC6 was believed to deacetylate HSP90 [81], but HDAC1 also seems to have a similar function [149]. Several HDAC inhibitors with specificity towards HDAC6, including the pan-inhibitors LAQ824 and LBH589 (panobinostat), induce hyperacetylation of HSP90 with subsequent loss of its chaperone activity [81], and depletion of pro-growth and pro-survival client proteins [81]. HDAC inhibitors also induce/increase the acetylation of the two HSP90 co-chaperones p23 and HSP70, but the functional consequences of these modifications are not known [80]. Observations in solid tumours suggest that HSP90 acetylation has functional similarities with HSP90 inhibition [147], but despite these similarities it should be emphasized that the effects of increased acetylation and direct pharmacological inhibition are not identical [80].

MS-275 inhibits both Class 1 and 2 HDACs [148], induces acetylation of HSP90 and causes ubiquitination and degradation of FLT3 in AML cells. The proteasome inhibitor bortezomib antagonized this effect; this observation suggest that the ubiquitin/proteasome pathway was involved in the FLT3 degradation [149]. Another adverse prognostic factor in human AML is increased CXCR4 protein levels [166]; panobinostat reduces the chaperon association between CXCR4 and HSP90 and thereby causes degradation and depletion of CXCR4 especially in primary AML cells [167]. Finally, synergistic antiproliferative and proapoptotic effects by combining HDAC inhibitors (valproic acid, sodium phenylbutyrate) and the HSP90 inhibitor 17-AAG have also been observed in experimental studies of the Kasumi-1 cells that harbor a mutation in the HSP90 client protein KIT [103].

LAQ834 is a hydroxamate HDAC inhibitor with a HSP90 inhibitory profile. It has been investigated in a phase I trial in patients with advanced malignancies; it was then administered as a 3 hours intravenous infusion for three consecutive days every third weeks [99], and the doses were 6, 12, 24, 48, 72 and 100 mg/m^2. The dose-limiting toxicities were liver toxicity (increased liver transaminases, hyperbilirubinemia), fatigue, atrial fibrillation and renal failure with raised serum creatinine; several of these toxic effects are also seen with the HSP90 inhibitor 17-AAG (see above). The area under the curve increased proportionally with increasing dose, and the median terminal half-life ranged from 8 to 14 hours. HSP90 inhibition was documented for the higher doses by changes in client proteins and increased HSP72.

Valproic acid is the HDAC inhibitor that is most extensively studied in human AML [168]. The toxicity of this drug has been extensively reviewed recently [92], the most common side effects being CNS (including fatigue) and gastrointenstinal toxicity (nausea, vomiting). In one study the daily doses of valproic acid were gradually increased until side effects [4], and the most common and dose-dependent side effect was fatigue but nausea was also common. These side effects were reversible with dose reduction. Previous clinical studies of HDAC inhibitors in cancer patients have described electrolyte disturbances, heart arrhythmia, liver toxicity and metabolic disturbances as side effects for other HDAC inhibitors [92], but this has not been observed in previous studies of valproic acid in AML patients [4]. Even though the target serum level of valproic acid in other clinical AML studies has been 310-690 μM (higher then the levels reached in [4]), treatment responses with improvement of thrombocytopenia lasting for several weeks have been observed in several studies even with serum levels below <200 μM [4, 92, 169]. However, it should be emphasized that the clinical improvement during treatment with HDAC inhibitors is probably caused by different mechanisms and not only HSP90 inhibition.

In a recent AML study valproic acid was shown to decrease the levels of soluble serum HSP90 in 22 patients, and HSP90 was further reduced after additional treatment with all-*trans* retinoic acid (ATRA) and low-dose cytarabine [170]. Furthermore, low levels of HSP90 prior to therapy was associated with prolonged survival in patients treated with valproic acid, ATRA and theophylline, suggesting serum HSP90 levels to be a potential prognostic marker in AML [170]. However, these observations were seen in relatively small clinical studies and need further confirmation.

HSP90 Inhibitors - Is Combination with Other Antileukemic Agents Possible?

The large majority of patients included in the initial clinical studies of HSP90 inhibitors in cancer patients have had advanced solid tumours. Initial conclusion can be summarized as follow:

- Thrombocytopenia can be a side effect in patients treated with HSP90 inhibitors (see above), and this observation suggests that the *in vivo* drug concentrations reached in the human bone marrow compartment are sufficient to affect hematopoietic cells.

- The growth factor receptors KIT and FLT3 are both HSP90 client proteins (see above), they are important growth factors for primary human AML cells [142], and the receptor tyrosine kinases for both these receptors are inhibited by the pharmacological inhibitors SU11248 [171] and SU5416 [172]. Thus, inhibition of growth factor-initiated signalling by HSP90 inhibition may have similar antileukemic effects as the pharmacological inhibition.

- Akt is another client protein of HSP90, and clinical studies in patients with relapsed or refractory AML have demonstrated that inhibition of the PI3K/Akt/mTOR pathway has antileukemic effects [173-175].

- MDM2 is a HSP90 client protein and a p53 inhibitor. Inhibition of the MDM2-p53 interaction induces apoptosis in human AML cells, and this pharmacological strategy is therefore considered in the treatment of human AML [176, 177]. Results from a recent clinical study suggest that p53 is important for chemosensitivity in human AML, and targeting MDM2 through HSP90 inhibition may therefore have additive or synergistic effects with conventional chemotherapy [178].

All these clinical observations strongly suggest that direct pharmacological targeting of various HSP90 client proteins has antileukemic effects *in vivo*, and the observations thereby suggest that HSP90 inhibition should be further investigated in clinical AML studies.

Soluble HSP90 in Human AML

HSP90 can be released by primary human AML cells during *in vitro* culture [179]. *In vitro* studies have then demonstrated that (i) there is a wide variation between patients in AML cell release of HSP70 and HSP90; (ii) this difference is not dependent on drug-induced or spontaneous stress-induced *in vitro* apoptosis; (iii) there is a significant correlation between HSP70 and HSP90 *in vitro* release; and (iv) the release does not differ for cells collected before and during ATRA+ valproic acid based anti-leukemic treatment. Furthermore, HSP70 and HSP90 release was significantly correlated during *in vitro* culture, but these levels showed no correlation with calreticulin exposure [179]. Thus, it seems likely that HSP70 and HSP90 release is at least partly dependent on the same regulatory mechanisms, whereas HSP release and calreticulin exposure seem to be independent phenotypic characteristics during stress-induced *in vitro* apoptosis of primary human AML cells.

HSP90 can also be detected in human serum and plasma both in healthy individuals and AML patients. A recent study described that HSP90 serum levels were dependent on several factors, including patient age (inverse correlation), AML cell morphology/FAB classification (higher levels with neutrophil or monocytic differentiation), peripheral blood blast counts and serum LDH levels; but the strongest association was to expression of the CD34 stem cell marker (inverse correlation) [170]. HSP90 serum levels do not differ between relapse and newly diagnosed AML or between *de novo* and secondary AML either, and no significant correlation between intracellular AML cell levels and serum levels of HSP90 could be detected [170]. These observations demonstrate that the biological characteristics of the AML cells are a major determinant for the serum HSP90 level. Furthermore, although the leukemia cell burden cannot be estimated accurately in AML patients it is probably reflected at least partly in the percentage of bone marrow blasts as well as the degree of peripheral blood leukemization, serum LDH and bone marrow failure. However, serum HSP90 levels show a significant correlation with serum LDH levels and degree of peripheral blood leukemization but not with the bone marrow blast percentage or degree of bone marrow failure. Taken together our observations suggest that the most important determinants for the variation in HSP90 serum levels are qualitative (*i.e.* the biological characteristics of the AML cells) rather than quantitative differences in AML cell burden.

Early Clinical Trials of HSP90 Inhibitors in AML

Four recent clinical studies illustrate the possibility of using HSP90 inhibitors in the treatment of human AML (Table **6**). Kaufmann *et al.* investigated the HSP90 inhibitor tanespimycin/17-AAG in combination with cytarabine 400 mg/m^2/day continuously for 5 days and tanespimycin/17-AGG infusions was given at escalating doses on days 3 and 6 in 26 patients with refractory or relapsed acute leukemia [50]. The maximum tolerated doses were cytarabine 400 mg/m^2/day for 5 days along with tanespimycin/17-AGG 300 mg/m^2 on days 3 and 6. Treatment-related adverse

Table 6: Combination of HSP90 Inhibition with Other Antileukemic Agents. A Summary of the Clinical and Experimental Evidence Supporting the Use of Combined Therapy and Comparison with Clinical Studies of HSP90 Inhibition Alone

Treatment [Reference]	Effect of the Treatment
Clinical Studies of HSP90 Inhibition Alone	
HSP90 Inhibition alone Phase I study [67]	HSP90 inhibitor: PF-04929113 (SNX-5422) Patients: 25 patients with various resistant/relapsed hematologic malignancies. Observations: The most common toxicities were prolonged QTc interval, diarrhea, pruritus, thrombocytopenia, fatigue and nausea. No clinical AML responses.
Phase I study [69]	HSP90 inhibitor: STA-9090 Patients: 18 patients, median age 65 years, including 13 AML patients. Observations: Adverse events reported in >25% of patients were diarrhea, fatigue, decreased appetite, febrile neutropenia, nausea, and anemia; the majority of the adverse effects were mild to moderate in severity. No formal responses, but one AML patient with 10 weeks disease stabilization.
Phase I study [52]	HSP90 inhibitor: alvespimycin (KOS-1022,17-DMAG). Patients: Advanced AML, n=24 Observations: Generally well tolerated; common toxicities being neutropenic fever, fatigue, nausea and diarrhea, elevated troponin and myocardial infarction. Complete remission with incomplete blood count recovery occurred in 3 of 17 evaluable patients.
Clinical and Experimental Studies - HSP90 Inhibition in Combined Treatment	
HSP70 inhibition - VER-155008 Experimental study [85]	HSP90 inhibitor: 17-dimetylaminoethylamino-17-demethoxygeldanamycin (17-DMAG) Cells: Primary human AML cells from unselected patients Observations: Additive antiproliferative and proapoptotic effects without compensatory increases in other HSPs.
KIT inhibition Experimental study [141]	HSP90 inhibitor: 17-allylamino-17-demethoxygeldanamycin (17-AAG) Cells: KIT mutated and AML-ETO expressing Kasumi-1 cell line Observation: Disruption of downstream signalling from mutated KIT.
Inhibition of PI3K-Akt-mTOR signalling Experimental study [175]	HSP90 inhibitor: NVP-AUY922AG Cells: Human AML cell lines and primary AML cells. Observation: Depletion of AKT as well as IKKα and IKKβ
NF-κB inhibition Experimental study [126]	HSP90 inhibitor: 17-allylamino-17-demethoxygeldanamycin (17-AAG) Cells: The NB4 AML cell line Observation: HSP90 inhibition has proapoptotic effects through inhibition of NFκB signalling.
Proteasomal inhibition **Bortezomib** Phase I study [49]	HSP90 inhibitor: 17-allyamino-17-demethoxygeldanamycin (17-AAG) Patients: 11 patients with refractory or relapsed AML Observations: Maximal tolerated doses were 17-AAG 150 mg/m2 and bortezomib 0.7 mg/m2, hepatic and cardiac toxicity were dose limiting. None of the patients responded to the treatment.

(Table 6) contd.....

Treatment [Reference]	Effect of the Treatment
HDAC inhibition, CXCR4 inhibition, Experimental study [167]	Drug: The pan-HDAC inhibitor panobinostat Cells: Primary human AML cells. Observations: The HDAC inhibitor increased HSP90-acetylation and thereby reduced the chaperone association with CXCR4 and directing this chemokine receptor to proteasomal degradation. The combined treatment of HDAC inhibition (*i.e.* increased HSP90 acetylation) and CXCR4 inhibition had synergistic effects.
Experimental study [147]	HSP90 inhibition: 17-allyamino-17-demethoxygeldanamycin (17-AAG) Observation: Hyperacetylation increase 17-AAG binding and increase its HSP90 inhibitory effect. 17-AAG binding also decreases HDAC binding to HSP90 and thereby increases acetylation. Cotreatment with 17-AAG and HDAC6 inhibition had synergistic HSP90 inhibitory effects.
Experimental study [149]	HDAC inhibitor: MS-275 As described in detail in these two articles MS275 has the following effects: • HSP90 is a chaperon for mutated but not for wild-type FLT3. • The drug reduces both the total and the phosphorylated form of FLT3 in FLT3-ITD$^+$ AML cell lines; the result is inactivation of downstream signalling through PI3K-Akt, RAS/RAF/MEK/ERK, JAK/STAT and STAT5. • At the same time MS-275 induce HSP90 acetylation as well as ubiquitination followed by proteasomal degradation of FLT3. • MS-275 induces growth arrest in FLT3-ITD$^+$ human AML cell lines. These observations may then explain why the antiproliferative effect of HSP90 is strongest for FLT3-ITD$^+$ AML cells [101].
Cytarabine Phase I study [50]	HSP90 inhibitor: 17-allylamino-17-demethoxygeldanamycin (17-AAG) Patients: Relapsed or refractory acute leukemia, n=26 Observations: Treatment-related adverse events included disseminated intravascular coagulation, acute respiratory distress syndrome, and myocardial infarction. Among 21 evaluable patients, there were two complete and four partial remissions.
Experimental study [175]	HSP90 inhibitor: NVP-AUY922AG Cells: AML cell lines and primary human AML cells Observations: Synergistic killing of AML cell lines as well as primary AML cells. No correlation between the effect of HSP90 inhibition and cytarabine.

events included disseminated intravascular coagulation, acute respiratory distress syndrome, and myocardial infarction associated with prolonged exposure to tanespimycin/17-AGG and its active metabolite 17-AG. Among 21 evaluable patients, there were two complete and four partial remissions. Increased HSP70 levels as a marker of effective HSP90 inhibition was observed in more than 80% of samples harvested 24 hours after tanespimycin/17-AGG administration, but reduction of client proteins was modest. However, despite the short exposure to potentially effective HSP90 inhibitor drug concentrations clinically relevant responses were seen when using this combination treatment.

The second study by Reddy *et al.* undertook a phase I trial of the oral HSP90 inhibitor PF-04929113 (SNX-5422) in patients with various relapsed or refractory hematologic malignancies [67]. The drug was administered orally every other day for 21 days of a 28-day cycle. Twenty-five patients were treated. The most common toxicities included prolonged QTc interval, diarrhea, pruritus, thrombocytopenia, fatigue, and nausea and 28% of the patients experienced grade 3/4 adverse events and thrombocytopenia being most common. Partial response was experienced by a patient with transformed lymphoma and prolonged stabilization of disease was observed in a patient with multiple myeloma. The authors concluded that the drug was generally well tolerated.

A third phase I study investigated 17-AAG in combination with bortezomib in 11 patients with relapsed or refractory AML [49]. The maximal tolerated doses were 17-AAG 150 mg/m^2 and bortezomib 0.7 mg/m^2 with hepatic and cardiac toxicity being dose-limiting. Co-administration led to a decrease in the clearance of the metabolite 17-amino-17-demethoxygeldanamycin, and the combination led to toxicity without clinically relevant responses in any patients.

The last phase I study the use of 17-DMAG as monotherapy in 24 patients with advanced AML [52]. Patients received escalating doses of intravenous 17-DMAG twice weekly for 2 of 3 weeks. The drug was well tolerated and common toxicities included neutropenic fever, fatigue, nausea and diarrhea. Cardiac dose-limiting toxicity occurred at 32 mg/m^2 (elevated troponin and myocardial infarction). Only minor accumulation was seen upon repeated doses. Pharmacodynamic analyses on day 15 revealed increased apoptosis and HSP70 levels when compared with baseline within marrow blasts. Antileukemic activity occurred in 3 of 17 evaluable patients (complete remission with incomplete blood count recovery).

Taken together these observations suggest that (i) the use of HSP90 inhibition in combination with conventional chemotherapy should be further investigated; (ii) pharmacokinetic studies will be important when investigating new drug combinations and (iii) especially the risk of severe bone marrow toxicity has to be carefully addressed in future clinical studies; but antileukemic responses have been observed with different agents and this therapeutic strategy should be further investigated in future clinical studies.

CONCLUDING COMMENTS

Direct *Versus* Indirect Effects of HSP90 Inhibition

HSP90 can show high expression in AML cells as well as in other malignant cells, and for this reason HSP90 is regarded as a possible therapeutic target in human AML [10, 11, 101]. However, leukemogenesis is not only dependent on the biological characteristics of the transformed cell, the proliferation and survival of the leukemia cells are supported by the nonleukemic stromal cells [25, 180-183]. As described in this review HSP90 is important also for mesenchymal and endothelial cells. The possible use of HSP90 inhibition in leukemia therapy may thus induce both direct antileukemic effects on the AML cells, but also indirect effects mediated by pharmacological effects on AML supporting stromal elements.

HSP90 Inhibition as Monotherapy

The conventional chemotherapy of AML is based on combination therapy [119], and in our opinion it would be surprising if targeted therapy should be more effective as monotherapy. One exception might be the use of HSP90 inhibition as maintenance therapy or if one could identify subsets of patients where HSP90 inhibition would be expected to be particularly effective. However, the initial results from clinical studies of HSP90 monotherapy are not convincing, and in our opinion future clinical studies should focus on combination therapy.

HSP90 Inhibition in Combination with Other Targeted Therapies

As described above both experimental and clinical studies suggest that HSP90 inhibition can be combined with other therapeutic agents, including both conventional chemotherapy as well as in targeted therapies. However, based on the available clinical data it is not possible to decide whether the optimal use of HSP90 inhibition is as (i) simultaneous or sequential therapy; (ii) induction or consolidation treatment; or (iii) whether it should be used as maintenance therapy to prevent late AML relapse.

Both clinical and experimental studies suggest that the combination of HSP90 inhibition and NF-κB inhibition is possible; NF-κB inhibition can then be achieved either by specific inhibition [124], or through proteasomal inhibition [125, 184]. This combination has synergistic effects at least in some of these studies. Furthermore, NF-κB inhibition seems to affect the leukemic stem cells [185], and the combination may then be particularly useful in postremission therapy to prevent late leukemic relapse.

HSP90 Inhibition and Allogeneic Stem Cell Transplantation

Allogeneic stem cell transplantation requires immunosuppressive treatment as a prophylaxis against graft *versus* host disease (GVHD) [186]. However, at the same time this nonspecific reactivity as well as specific graft *versus* leukemia reactivity are important for the antileukemic effects of allotransplantation [187]. HSP90 inhibition is an antileukemic strategy with immunosuppressive effects; this treatment may therefore become useful in allotransplant recipients as a prophylaxis/treatment of GVHD but with an additional antileukemic reactivity that may compensate for the suppression of antileukemic immune reactivity during this treatment [187]. PI3K-Akt-mTOR inhibitors have similar immunosuppressive and antileukemic effects and combination between HSP90 inhibition and inhibition of this pathway should therefore be considered.

Low-Toxicity Treatment

Low-toxicity treatment is now tried in the treatment of AML, one alternative being HDAC inhibition by valproic acid in combination with ATRA, demethylating agents or low-toxicity conventional chemotherapy [168, 188]. As reviewed above HSP90 inhibition can be a mechanism behind the effect of this treatment. HSP90 inhibition may thus become useful in such treatment of elderly or unfit patients. It should be emphasized that prolonged survival not necessarily depends on remission induction [168, 188]. A second alternative could be as a part of prolonged and low-toxicity consolidation therapy. However, it should be emphasized that the toxicity of the various HSP90 inhibitors have to be better characterized, especially the risk of severe bone marrow toxicity.

Final Conclusion

AML is a very heterogeneous disorder caused by a wide range of cytogenetic and molecular genetic abnormalities. Thus, new therapeutic strategies should target several and not only single molecules or signalling pathways. HSP90 has a wide range of client proteins, and HSP90 inhibition will thereby target several intracellular signalling pathways. Furthermore, studies in experimental models suggest that HSP90 inhibition, leading to degradation of client proteins, has multiple antileukemic effects. Initial clinical trials of HSP90 inhibition in AML have been carried out, although further clinical trials should be carried out to fully evaluate the effect of such approaches in AML.

ACKNOWLEDGEMENTS

The study received financial support from the Norwegian Cancer Society.

CONFLICT OF INTEREST

The authors confirm that this chapter contents have no conflict of interest.

DISCLOSURE

The chapter submitted for the eBook Series entitled **"Advances in Cancer Drug Targets, Volume 2"** is an update of our article in **Current Cancer Drug Targets, Volume 9, Issue 6, 2009, pp. 761-776,** with additional text and references.

REFERENCES

[1] Ferrara F, Schiffer CA. Acute myeloid leukemia in adults. Lancet 2013 Feb 9;381(9865):484-95.

[2] Wang ZY, Chen Z. Acute promyelocytic leukemia: from highly fatal to highly curable. Blood 2008 Mar 1;111(5):2505-15. eng.

[3] Latagliata R, Bongarzoni V, Carmosino I, Mengarelli A, Breccia M, Borza PA, *et al.* Acute myelogenous leukemia in elderly patients not eligible for intensive chemotherapy: the dark side of the moon. Ann Oncol 2006 Feb;17(2):281-5.

[4] Ryningen A, Stapnes C, Lassalle P, Corbascio M, Gjertsen BT, Bruserud O. A subset of patients with high-risk acute myelogenous leukemia shows improved peripheral blood cell counts when treated with the combination of valproic acid, theophylline and all-trans retinoic acid. Leuk Res 2009 Jun;33(6):779-87.

[5] Valk PJ, Verhaak RG, Beijen MA, Erpelinck CA, Barjesteh van Waalwijk van Doorn-Khosrovani S, Boer JM, *et al.* Prognostically useful gene-expression profiles in acute myeloid leukemia. N Engl J Med 2004 Apr 15;350(16):1617-28.

[6] Network CGAR. Genomic and epigenomic landscapes of adult *de novo* acute myeloid leukemia. New Engl J Med 2013 May 30;368(22):2059-74.

[7] Saibil HR. Chaperone machines in action. Curr Opin Struct Biol 2008 Feb;18(1):35-42.

[8] Lanneau D, Brunet M, Frisan E, Solary E, Fontenay M, Garrido C. Heat shock proteins: essential proteins for apoptosis regulation. J Cell Mol Med 2008 Jun;12(3):743-61.

[9] Barginear MF, Van Poznak C, Rosen N, Modi S, Hudis CA, Budman DR. The heat shock protein 90 chaperone complex: an evolving therapeutic target. Curr Cancer Drug Targets 2008 Sep;8(6):522-32.

[10] Bruserud O, Reikvam H. Heat shock protein 90 (HSP90) inhibition--from experimental to clinical studies. Leuk Res 2010 Nov;34(11):1422-3.

[11] Bruserud O, Hatfield KJ, Reikvam H. Heat shock protein 90 (HSP90) inhibition in acute myeloid leukemia-Targeting of disease heterogeneity through direct and indirect antileukemic effects. Leuk Res 2011 Sep;35(9):1156-8.

[12] Trepel J, Mollapour M, Giaccone G, Neckers L. Targeting the dynamic HSP90 complex in cancer. Nat Rev Cancer 2010 Aug;10(8):537-49.

[13] Shamovsky I, Nudler E. New insights into the mechanism of heat shock response activation. Cell Mol Life Sci 2008 Mar;65(6):855-61.

[14] Dezwaan DC, Freeman BC. HSP90: the Rosetta stone for cellular protein dynamics? Cell Cycle 2008 Apr 15;7(8):1006-12.

[15] Burger AM, Seth AK. The ubiquitin-mediated protein degradation pathway in cancer: therapeutic implications. Eur J Cancer 2004 Oct;40(15):2217-29. eng.

[16] Caplan AJ, Mandal AK, Theodoraki MA. Molecular chaperones and protein kinase quality control. Trends Cell Biol 2007 Feb;17(2):87-92.

[17] Lindquist S, Craig EA. The heat-shock proteins. Annu Rev Genet 1988;22:631-77.

[18] Mathew A, Mathur SK, Jolly C, Fox SG, Kim S, Morimoto RI. Stress-specific activation and repression of heat shock factors 1 and 2. Mol Cell Biol 2001 Nov;21(21):7163-71.

[19] Morimoto RI. Cells in stress: transcriptional activation of heat shock genes. Science 1993 Mar 5;259(5100):1409-10.

[20] Zou J, Guo Y, Guettouche T, Smith DF, Voellmy R. Repression of heat shock transcription factor HSF1 activation by HSP90 (HSP90 complex) that forms a stress-sensitive complex with HSF1. Cell 1998 Aug 21;94(4):471-80.

[21] Guettouche T, Boellmann F, Lane WS, Voellmy R. Analysis of phosphorylation of human heat shock factor 1 in cells experiencing a stress. BMC Biochem 2005;6:4.

[22] Jolly C, Morimoto R, Robert-Nicoud M, Vourc'h C. HSF1 transcription factor concentrates in nuclear foci during heat shock: relationship with transcription sites. J Cell Sci 1997 Dec;110 (Pt 23):2935-41.

[23] Voellmy R. On mechanisms that control heat shock transcription factor activity in metazoan cells. Cell Stress Chaperones 2004 Summer;9(2):122-33.

[24] Tang D, Khaleque MA, Jones EL, Theriault JR, Li C, Wong WH, *et al.* Expression of heat shock proteins and heat shock protein messenger ribonucleic acid in human prostate carcinoma *in vitro* and in tumors *in vivo*. Cell Stress Chaperones 2005 Spring;10(1):46-58.

[25] Hatfield K, Ryningen A, Corbascio M, Bruserud O. Microvascular endothelial cells increase proliferation and inhibit apoptosis of native human acute myelogenous leukemia blasts. Int J Cancer 2006 Nov 15;119(10):2313-21.

[26] Huston A, Leleu X, Jia X, Moreau AS, Ngo HT, Runnels J, *et al.* Targeting Akt and heat shock protein 90 produces synergistic multiple myeloma cell cytotoxicity in the bone marrow microenvironment. Clin Cancer Res 2008 Feb 1;14(3):865-74.

[27] Francis LK, Alsayed Y, Leleu X, Jia X, Singha UK, Anderson J, *et al.* Combination mammalian target of rapamycin inhibitor rapamycin and HSP90 inhibitor 17-allylamino-17-demethoxygeldanamycin has synergistic activity in multiple myeloma. Clin Cancer Res 2006 Nov 15;12(22):6826-35.

[28] Shih TT, Hou HA, Liu CY, Chen BB, Tang JL, Chen HY, *et al.* Bone marrow angiogenesis magnetic resonance imaging in patients with acute myeloid leukemia: peak enhancement ratio is an independent predictor for overall survival. Blood 2009 Apr 2;113(14):3161-7.

[29] Smith M, Barnett M, Bassan R, Gatta G, Tondini C, Kern W. Adult acute myeloid leukemia. Crit Rev Oncol Hematol 2004 Jun;50(3):197-222.

[30] Schuler D, Szende B. Apoptosis in acute leukemia. Leuk Res 2004 Jul;28(7):661-6.

[31] Del Principe MI, Del Poeta G, Venditti A, Buccisano F, Maurillo L, Mazzone C, *et al.* Apoptosis and immaturity in acute myeloid leukemia. Hematology 2005 Feb;10(1):25-34.

[32] Solary E, Droin N, Bettaieb A, Corcos L, Dimanche-Boitrel MT, Garrido C. Positive and negative regulation of apoptotic pathways by cytotoxic agents in hematological malignancies. Leukemia 2000 Oct;14(10):1833-49. eng.

[33] Mosser DD, Morimoto RI. Molecular chaperones and the stress of oncogenesis. Oncogene 2004 Apr 12;23(16):2907-18. eng.

[34] Samali A, Cotter TG. Heat shock proteins increase resistance to apoptosis. Exp Cell Res 1996 Feb 25;223(1):163-70.

[35] Galea-Lauri J, Richardson AJ, Latchman DS, Katz DR. Increased heat shock protein 90 (hsp90) expression leads to increased apoptosis in the monoblastoid cell line U937 following induction with TNF-alpha and cycloheximide: a possible role in immunopathology. J Immunol 1996 Nov 1;157(9):4109-18.

[36] Kondo Y, Kondo S. Autophagy and cancer therapy. Autophagy 2006 Apr-Jun;2(2):85-90. eng.

[37] Agarraberes FA, Dice JF. A molecular chaperone complex at the lysosomal membrane is required for protein translocation. J Cell Sci 2001 Jul;114(Pt 13):2491-9. eng.

[38] Qing G, Yan P, Xiao G. Hsp90 inhibition results in autophagy-mediated proteasome-independent degradation of IkappaB kinase (IKK). Cell Res 2006 Nov;16(11):895-901. eng.

[39] Scheibel T, Weikl T, Buchner J. Two chaperone sites in Hsp90 differing in substrate specificity and ATP dependence. Proc Natl Acad Sci USA 1998 Feb 17;95(4):1495-9.

[40] Workman P, Burrows F, Neckers L, Rosen N. Drugging the cancer chaperone HSP90: combinatorial therapeutic exploitation of oncogene addiction and tumor stress. Ann N Y Acad Sci 2007 Oct;1113:202-16.

[41] Zhang H, Burrows F. Targeting multiple signal transduction pathways through inhibition of Hsp90. J Mol Med 2004 Aug;82(8):488-99.

[42] Whitesell L, Mimnaugh EG, De Costa B, Myers CE, Neckers LM. Inhibition of heat shock protein HSP90-pp60v-src heteroprotein complex formation by benzoquinone ansamycins: essential role for stress proteins in oncogenic transformation. Proc Natl Acad Sci USA 1994 Aug 30;91(18):8324-8.

[43] Neckers L, Workman P. Hsp90 molecular chaperone inhibitors: are we there yet? Clin Cancer Res 2012 Jan 1;18(1):64-76.

[44] Solit DB, Chiosis G. Development and application of Hsp90 inhibitors. Drug Discov Today 2008 Jan;13(1-2):38-43.

[45] Modi S, Stopeck AT, Gordon MS, Mendelson D, Solit DB, Bagatell R, *et al.* Combination of trastuzumab and tanespimycin (17-AAG, KOS-953) is safe and active in trastuzumab-refractory HER-2 overexpressing breast cancer: a phase I dose-escalation study. J Clin Oncol 2007 Dec 1;25(34):5410-7.

[46] Ramanathan RK, Egorin MJ, Eiseman JL, Ramalingam S, Friedland D, Agarwala SS, *et al.* Phase I and pharmacodynamic study of 17-(allylamino)-17-demethoxygeldanamycin in adult patients with refractory advanced cancers. Clin Cancer Res 2007 Mar 15;13(6):1769-74.

[47] Solit DB, Osman I, Polsky D, Panageas KS, Daud A, Goydos JS, *et al.* Phase II trial of 17-allylamino-17-demethoxygeldanamycin in patients with metastatic melanoma. Clin Cancer Res 2008 Dec 15;14(24):8302-7.

[48] Richardson PG, Chanan-Khan AA, Alsina M, Albitar M, Berman D, Messina M, *et al.* Tanespimycin monotherapy in relapsed multiple myeloma: results of a phase 1 dose-escalation study. Br J Haematol 2010 Aug;150(4):438-45.

[49] Walker AR, Klisovic R, Johnston JS, Jiang Y, Geyer S, Kefauver C, *et al.* Pharmacokinetics and dose escalation of the heat shock protein inhibitor 17-allyamino-17-demethoxygeldanamycin in combination with bortezomib in relapsed or refractory acute myeloid leukemia. Leuk Lymphoma 2013 Sep;54(9):1996-2002.

[50] Kaufmann SH, Karp JE, Litzow MR, Mesa RA, Hogan W, Steensma DP, *et al.* Phase I and pharmacological study of cytarabine and tanespimycin in relapsed and refractory acute leukemia. Haematologica 2011 November 1, 2011;96(11):1619-26.

[51] Smith V, Sausville EA, Camalier RF, Fiebig HH, Burger AM. Comparison of 17-dimethylaminoethylamino-17-demethoxy-geldanamycin (17DMAG) and 17-allylamino-17-demethoxygeldanamycin (17AAG) *in vitro*: effects on Hsp90 and client proteins in melanoma models. Cancer Chemother Pharmacol 2005 Aug;56(2):126-37.

[52] Lancet JE, Gojo I, Burton M, Quinn M, Tighe SM, Kersey K, *et al.* Phase I study of the heat shock protein 90 inhibitor alvespimycin (KOS-1022, 17-DMAG) administered intravenously twice weekly to patients with acute myeloid leukemia. Leukemia 2010 Apr;24(4):699-705.

[53] Sydor JR, Normant E, Pien CS, Porter JR, Ge J, Grenier L, *et al.* Development of 17-allylamino-17-demethoxygeldanamycin hydroquinone hydrochloride (IPI-504), an anti-cancer agent directed against Hsp90. Proc Natl Acad Sci USA 2006 Nov 14;103(46):17408-13.

[54] Wagner AJ, Chugh R, Rosen LS, Morgan JA, George MDS, Gordon M, *et al.* A phase 1 study of the heat shock protein 90 inhibitor retaspimycin hydrochloride (IPI-504) in patients with gastrointestinal stromal tumors or soft tissue sarcomas. Clin Cancer Res 2013 Sep 17.

[55] Kwon HJ, Yoshida M, Abe K, Horinouchi S, Beppu T. Radicicol, an agent inducing the reversal of transformed phenotypes of src-transformed fibroblasts. Biosci Biotechnol Biochem 1992 Mar;56(3):538-9.

[56] Eccles SA, Massey A, Raynaud FI, Sharp SY, Box G, Valenti M, *et al.* NVP-AUY922: a novel heat shock protein 90 inhibitor active against xenograft tumor growth, angiogenesis, and metastasis. Cancer Res 2008 Apr 15;68(8):2850-60.

[57] Kang MH, Reynolds CP, Houghton PJ, Alexander D, Morton CL, Kolb EA, *et al.* Initial testing (Stage 1) of AT13387, an HSP90 inhibitor, by the pediatric preclinical testing program. Pediatr Blood Cancer 2012 Jul 15;59(1):185-8.

[58] Taldone T, Gozman A, Maharaj R, Chiosis G. Targeting Hsp90: small-molecule inhibitors and their clinical development. Curr Opin Pharmacol 2008 Aug;8(4):370-4.

[59] Pearl LH, Prodromou C, Workman P. The Hsp90 molecular chaperone: an open and shut case for treatment. Biochem J 2008 Mar 15;410(3):439-53.

[60] Drysdale MJ, Brough PA. Medicinal chemistry of Hsp90 inhibitors. Curr Top Med Chem 2008;8(10):859-68.

[61] Kim SH, Bajji A, Tangallapally R, Markovitz B, Trovato R, Shenderovich M, *et al.* Discovery of (2S)-1-[4-(2-{6-amino-8-[(6-bromo-1,3-benzodioxol-5-yl)sulfanyl]-9H-purin-9-yl}et hyl)piperidin-1-yl]-2-hydroxypropan-1-one (MPC-3100), a purine-based Hsp90 inhibitor. J Med Chem 2012 Sep 13;55(17):7480-501.

[62] Dickson MA, Okuno SH, Keohan ML, Maki RG, D'Adamo DR, Akhurst TJ, *et al.* Phase II study of the HSP90-inhibitor BIIB021 in gastrointestinal stromal tumors. Ann Oncol 2013 Jan;24(1):252-7.

[63] Lundgren K, Zhang H, Brekken J, Huser N, Powell RE, Timple N, *et al.* BIIB021, an orally available, fully synthetic small-molecule inhibitor of the heat shock protein Hsp90. Mol Cancer Ther 2009 Apr;8(4):921-9.

[64] Bao R, Lai CJ, Qu H, Wang D, Yin L, Zifcak B, *et al.* CUDC-305, a novel synthetic HSP90 inhibitor with unique pharmacologic properties for cancer therapy. Clin Cancer Res 2009 Jun 15;15(12):4046-57.

[65] Cerchietti LC, Lopes EC, Yang SN, Hatzi K, Bunting KL, Tsikitas LA, *et al.* A purine scaffold Hsp90 inhibitor destabilizes BCL-6 and has specific antitumor activity in BCL-6-dependent B cell lymphomas. Nat Med 2009 Dec;15(12):1369-76.

[66] Okawa Y, Hideshima T, Steed P, Vallet S, Hall S, Huang K, *et al.* SNX-2112, a selective Hsp90 inhibitor, potently inhibits tumor cell growth, angiogenesis, and osteoclastogenesis in multiple myeloma and other hematologic tumors by abrogating signaling *via* Akt and ERK. Blood 2009 Jan 22;113(4):846-55.

[67] Reddy N, Voorhees PM, Houk BE, Brega N, Hinson JM, Jr., Jillela A. Phase I trial of the HSP90 inhibitor PF-04929113 (SNX5422) in adult patients with recurrent, refractory hematologic malignancies. Clin Lymphoma Myeloma Leuk 2013 Aug;13(4):385-91.

[68] Goldman JW, Raju RN, Gordon GA, El-Hariry I, Teofilivici F, Vukovic VM, *et al.* A first in human, safety, pharmacokinetics, and clinical activity phase I study of once weekly administration of the Hsp90 inhibitor ganetespib (STA-9090) in patients with solid malignancies. BMC Cancer 2013;13:152.

[69] Lancet JE, Smith BD, Bradley R, Komrokji RS, Teofilovici F, Rizzieri DA. A phase I/II trial of the potent Hsp90 inhibitor STA-9090 administered once weekly in patients with advanced hematologic malignancies. ASH Annual Meeting Abstracts 2010 November 19, 2010;116(21):Abstract no 3294.

[70] Shimamura T, Perera SA, Foley KP, Sang J, Rodig SJ, Inoue T, *et al.* Ganetespib (STA-9090), a nongeldanamycin HSP90 inhibitor, has potent antitumor activity in *in vitro* and *in vivo* models of non-small cell lung cancer. Clin Cancer Res 2012 Sep 15;18(18):4973-85.

[71] Bussenius J, Blazey CM, Aay N, Anand NK, Arcalas A, Baik T, *et al.* Discovery of XL888: a novel tropane-derived small molecule inhibitor of HSP90. Bioorg Med Chem Lett 2012 Sep 1;22(17):5396-404.

[72] Massey AJ, Schoepfer J, Brough PA, Brueggen J, Chene P, Drysdale MJ, *et al.* Preclinical antitumor activity of the orally available heat shock protein 90 inhibitor NVP-BEP800. Mol Cancer Ther 2010 Apr;9(4):906-19.

[73] Nakashima T, Ishii T, Tagaya H, Seike T, Nakagawa H, Kanda Y, *et al.* New molecular and biological mechanism of antitumor activities of KW-2478, a novel nonansamycin heat shock protein 90 inhibitor, in multiple myeloma cells. Clin Cancer Res 2010 May 15;16(10):2792-802.

[74] Marcu MG, Neckers LM. The C-terminal half of heat shock protein 90 represents a second site for pharmacologic intervention in chaperone function. Curr Cancer Drug Targets 2003 Oct;3(5):343-7.

[75] Marcu MG, Chadli A, Bouhouche I, Catelli M, Neckers LM. The heat shock protein 90 antagonist novobiocin interacts with a previously unrecognized ATP-binding domain in the carboxyl terminus of the chaperone. J Biol Chem 2000 Nov 24;275(47):37181-6.

[76] Itoh H, Ogura M, Komatsuda A, Wakui H, Miura AB, Tashima Y. A novel chaperone-activity-reducing mechanism of the 90-kDa molecular chaperone HSP90. Biochem J 1999 Nov 1;343 Pt 3:697-703.

[77] Adida C, Recher C, Raffoux E, Daniel MT, Taksin AL, Rousselot P, *et al.* Expression and prognostic significance of survivin in *de novo* acute myeloid leukemia. Br J Haematol 2000 Oct;111(1):196-203.

[78] Gyurkocza B, Plescia J, Raskett CM, Garlick DS, Lowry PA, Carter BZ, *et al.* Antileukemic activity of shepherdin and molecular diversity of hsp90 inhibitors. J Natl Cancer Inst 2006 Aug 2;98(15):1068-77.

[79] Stapnes C, Gjertsen BT, Reikvam H, Bruserud O. Targeted therapy in acute myeloid leukemia: current status and future directions. Expert Opin Investig Drugs 2009 Apr;18(4):433-55.

[80] Reynald K, Rowlands M, Hardcastle A, Stimson L, A. B, Workman P, *et al.* Acetylation of molecular chaperones by histone deactylase inhibitors (HDACI). Eur J Cancer 2008 October 2008;supl, 6(12):48.

[81] Bali P, Pranpat M, Bradner J, Balasis M, Fiskus W, Guo F, *et al.* Inhibition of histone deacetylase 6 acetylates and disrupts the chaperone function of heat shock protein 90: a novel basis for antileukemia activity of histone deacetylase inhibitors. J Biol Chem 2005 Jul 22;280(29):26729-34.

[82] Powers MV, Clarke PA, Workman P. Dual targeting of HSC70 and HSP72 inhibits HSP90 function and induces tumor-specific apoptosis. Cancer Cell 2008 Sep 9;14(3):250-62.

[83] Reikvam H, Ersvaer E, Bruserud O. Heat shock protein 90 - a potential target in the treatment of human acute myelogenous leukemia. Curr Cancer Drug Targets 2009 Sep;9(6):761-76.

[84] Massey AJ, Williamson DS, Browne H, Murray JB, Dokurno P, Shaw T, *et al.* A novel, small molecule inhibitor of Hsc70/Hsp70 potentiates Hsp90 inhibitor induced apoptosis in HCT116 colon carcinoma cells. Cancer Chemother Pharmacol 2010 Aug;66(3):535-45.

[85] Reikvam H, Nepstad I, Sulen A, Gjertsen BT, Hatfield KJ, Bruserud O. Increased antileukemic effects in human acute myeloid leukemia by combining HSP70 and HSP90 inhibitors. Expert Opin Investig Drugs 2013 May;22(5):551-63.

[86] Kaiser M, Kuhnl A, Reins J, Fischer S, Ortiz-Tanchez J, Schlee C, *et al.* Antileukemic activity of the HSP70 inhibitor pifithrin-mu in acute leukemia. Blood Cancer J 2011 Jul;1(7):e28.

[87] Ramanathan RK, Trump DL, Eiseman JL, Belani CP, Agarwala SS, Zuhowski EG, *et al.* Phase I pharmacokinetic-pharmacodynamic study of 17-(allylamino)-17-demethoxygeldanamycin (17AAG, NSC 330507), a novel inhibitor of heat shock protein 90, in patients with refractory advanced cancers. Clin Cancer Res 2005 May 1;11(9):3385-91.

[88] Weigel BJ, Blaney SM, Reid JM, Safgren SL, Bagatell R, Kersey J, *et al.* A phase I study of 17-allylaminogeldanamycin in relapsed/refractory pediatric patients with solid tumors: a Children's Oncology Group study. Clin Cancer Res 2007 Mar 15;13(6):1789-93.

[89] Bagatell R, Gore L, Egorin MJ, Ho R, Heller G, Boucher N, *et al.* Phase I pharmacokinetic and pharmacodynamic study of 17-N-allylamino-17-demethoxygeldanamycin in pediatric patients with recurrent or refractory solid tumors: a pediatric oncology experimental therapeutics investigators consortium study. Clin Cancer Res 2007 Mar 15;13(6):1783-8.

[90] Tse AN, Klimstra DS, Gonen M, Shah M, Sheikh T, Sikorski R, *et al.* A phase 1 dose-escalation study of irinotecan in combination with 17-allylamino-17-demethoxygeldanamycin in patients with solid tumors. Clin Cancer Res 2008 Oct 15;14(20):6704-11.

[91] Ramalingam SS, Egorin MJ, Ramanathan RK, Remick SC, Sikorski RP, Lagattuta TF, *et al.* A phase I study of 17-allylamino-17-demethoxygeldanamycin combined with paclitaxel in patients with advanced solid malignancies. Clin Cancer Res 2008 Jun 1;14(11):3456-61.

[92] Bruserud O, Stapnes C, Ersvaer E, Gjertsen BT, Ryningen A. Histone deacetylase inhibitors in cancer treatment: a review of the clinical toxicity and the modulation of gene expression in cancer cell. Curr Pharm Biotechnol 2007 Dec;8(6):388-400.

[93] Clarke PA, Welsh L, Valenti M, Eccles SA, Workman P. Hsp90 inhibitors target addiction to mutant oncoproteins in colorectal cancer. Eur J Cancer 2008;supl, 6(12):47.

[94] Chatterjee M, Jain S, Stuhmer T, Andrulis M, Ungethum U, Kuban RJ, *et al.* STAT3 and MAPK signaling maintain overexpression of heat shock proteins 90alpha and beta in multiple myeloma cells, which critically contribute to tumor-cell survival. Blood 2007 Jan 15;109(2):720-8.

[95] Lin K, Rockliffe N, Johnson GG, Sherrington PD, Pettitt AR. Hsp90 inhibition has opposing effects on wild-type and mutant p53 and induces p21 expression and cytotoxicity irrespective of p53/ATM status in chronic lymphocytic leukemia cells. Oncogene 2008 Apr 10;27(17):2445-55.

[96] Bao R, Lai CJ, Qu H, Wang D, Yin L, Zifcak B, *et al.* CUDC-305, a Novel Synthetic HSP90 Inhibitor with Unique Pharmacologic Properties for Cancer Therapy. Clin Cancer Res 2009 Jun 9.

[97] Jensen MR, Ide S, Brueggen J, Schoepfer J, Motwani M, Wang X, *et al.* Pharmakokinetic/pharmacodynamic relationship in human xenograft models and PBMC's treated with the Hsp90 inhibitor NVP-AUY922. Eur J Cancer 2008;supl, 6(12):50.

[98] Sullivan WP, Owen BA, Toft DO. The influence of ATP and p23 on the conformation of hsp90. J Biol Chem 2002 Nov 29;277(48):45942-8.

[99] de Bono JS, Kristeleit R, Tolcher A, Fong P, Pacey S, Karavasilis V, *et al.* Phase I pharmacokinetic and pharmacodynamic study of LAQ824, a hydroxamate histone deacetylase inhibitor with a heat shock protein-90 inhibitory profile, in patients with advanced solid tumors. Clin Cancer Res 2008 Oct 15;14(20):6663-73.

[100] Solit DB, Ivy SP, Kopil C, Sikorski R, Morris MJ, Slovin SF, *et al.* Phase I trial of 17-allylamino-17-demethoxygeldanamycin in patients with advanced cancer. Clin Cancer Res 2007 Mar 15;13(6):1775-82.

[101] Reikvam H, Hatfield KJ, Ersvaer E, Hovland R, Skavland J, Gjertsen BT, *et al.* Expression profile of heat shock proteins in acute myeloid leukemia patients reveals a distinct signature strongly associated with FLT3 mutation status - consequences and potentials for pharmacological intervention. Br J Haematol 2012 Feb;156(4):468-80.

[102] Al Shaer L, Walsby E, Gilkes A, Tonks A, Walsh V, Mills K, *et al.* Heat shock protein 90 inhibition is cytotoxic to primary AML cells expressing mutant FLT3 and results in altered downstream signalling. Br J Haematol 2008 May;141(4):483-93.

[103] Yu W, Wang J, Jin J, Qian W, Qian J, Cheng Y, *et al.* Heat shock protein 90 inhibition results in altered downstream signaling of mutant KIT and exerts synergistic effects on Kasumi-1 cells when combining with histone deacetylase inhibitor. Leuk Res 2011 Sep;35(9):1212-8.

[104] Fritz C, Tillotson B, Ge J, Normant E, Depew K, Basuki J, *et al.* Comparison of the cellular and biochemical properties of ansamycin and non-ansamycin based Hsp90 inhibitors. Eur J Cancer 2008; 6(Suppl 12): 48.

[105] Guo W, Reigan P, Siegel D, Zirrolli J, Gustafson D, Ross D. The bioreduction of a series of benzoquinone ansamycins by NAD(P)H:quinone oxidoreductase 1 to more potent heat shock protein 90 inhibitors, the hydroquinone ansamycins. Mol Pharmacol 2006 Oct;70(4):1194-203.

[106] Germain RN, Jenkins MK. *In vivo* antigen presentation. Curr Opin Immunol 2004 Feb;16(1):120-5.

[107] Callahan MK, Garg M, Srivastava PK. Heat-shock protein 90 associates with N-terminal extended peptides and is required for direct and indirect antigen presentation. Proc Natl Acad Sci USA 2008 Feb 5;105(5):1662-7.

[108] Rajagopal D, Bal V, Mayor S, George A, Rath S. A role for the Hsp90 molecular chaperone family in antigen presentation to T lymphocytes *via* major histocompatibility complex class II molecules. Eur J Immunol 2006 Apr;36(4):828-41.

[109] Bae J, Mitsiades C, Tai YT, Bertheau R, Shammas M, Batchu RB, *et al.* Phenotypic and functional effects of heat shock protein 90 inhibition on dendritic cell. J Immunol 2007 Jun 15;178(12):7730-7.

[110] Schnaider T, Somogyi J, Csermely P, Szamel M. The Hsp90-specific inhibitor, geldanamycin, blocks CD28-mediated activation of human T lymphocytes. Life Sci 1998;63(11):949-54.

[111] Schnaider T, Somogyi J, Csermely P, Szamel M. The Hsp90-specific inhibitor geldanamycin selectively disrupts kinase-mediated signaling events of T-lymphocyte activation. Cell Stress Chaperones 2000 Jan;5(1):52-61.

[112] Yorgin PD, Hartson SD, Fellah AM, Scroggins BT, Huang W, Katsanis E, *et al.* Effects of geldanamycin, a heat-shock protein 90-binding agent, on T cell function and T cell nonreceptor protein tyrosine kinases. J Immunol 2000 Mar 15;164(6):2915-23.

[113] Piatelli MJ, Doughty C, Chiles TC. Requirement for a hsp90 chaperone-dependent MEK1/2-ERK pathway for B cell antigen receptor-induced cyclin D2 expression in mature B lymphocytes. J Biol Chem 2002 Apr 5;277(14):12144-50.

[114] Chant ID, Rose PE, Morris AG. Analysis of heat-shock protein expression in myeloid leukemia cells by flow cytometry. Br J Haematol 1995 May;90(1):163-8.

[115] Thomas X, Campos L, Mounier C, Cornillon J, Flandrin P, Le QH, *et al.* Expression of heat-shock proteins is associated with major adverse prognostic factors in acute myeloid leukemia. Leuk Res 2005 Sep;29(9):1049-58.

[116] Flandrin P, Guyotat D, Duval A, Cornillon J, Tavernier E, Nadal N, *et al.* Significance of heat-shock protein (HSP:) 90 expression in acute myeloid leukemia cells. Cell Stress Chaperones 2008 Autumn;13(3):357-64.

[117] Duval A, Olaru D, Campos L, Flandrin P, Nadal N, Guyotat D. Expression and prognostic significance of heat-shock proteins in myelodysplastic syndromes. Haematologica 2006 May;91(5):713-4.

[118] Schlenk RF, Dohner K, Krauter J, Frohling S, Corbacioglu A, Bullinger L, *et al.* Mutations and treatment outcome in cytogenetically normal acute myeloid leukemia. N Engl J Med 2008 May 1;358(18):1909-18. eng.

[119] Döhner H, Estey EH, Amadori S, Appelbaum FR, Buchner T, Burnett AK, *et al.* Diagnosis and management of acute myeloid leukemia in adults: recommendations from an international expert panel, on behalf of the European LeukemiaNet. Blood 2010 Jan 21;115(3):453-74.

[120] Knapper S. FLT3 inhibition in acute myeloid leukemia. Br J Haematol 2007 Sep;138(6):687-99.

[121] Nakao M, Yokota S, Iwai T, Kaneko H, Horiike S, Kashima K, *et al.* Internal tandem duplication of the flt3 gene found in acute myeloid leukemia. Leukemia 1996 Dec;10(12):1911-8.

[122] Yamamoto Y, Kiyoi H, Nakano Y, Suzuki R, Kodera Y, Miyawaki S, *et al.* Activating mutation of D835 within the activation loop of FLT3 in human hematologic malignancies. Blood 2001 Apr 15;97(8):2434-9.

[123] Yao Q, Weigel B, Kersey J. Synergism between etoposide and 17-AAG in leukemia cells: critical roles for Hsp90, FLT3, topoisomerase II, Chk1, and Rad51. Clin Cancer Res 2007 Mar 1;13(5):1591-600.

[124] Bruserud O, Ryningen A, Olsnes AM, Stordrange L, Oyan AM, Kalland KH, *et al.* Subclassification of patients with acute myelogenous leukemia based on chemokine responsiveness and constitutive chemokine release by their leukemic cells. Haematologica 2007 Mar;92(3):332-41.

[125] Reikvam H, Olsnes AM, Gjertsen BT, Ersvar E, Bruserud O. Nuclear factor-kappaB signaling: a contributor in leukemogenesis and a target for pharmacological intervention in human acute myelogenous leukemia. Crit Rev Oncog 2009;15(1-2):1-41.

[126] Jiang Q, Wang Y, Li T, Shi K, Li Z, Ma Y, *et al.* Heat shock protein 90-mediated inactivation of nuclear factor-kappaB switches autophagy to apoptosis through becn1 transcriptional inhibition in selenite-induced NB4 cells. Mol Biol Cell 2011 Apr 15;22(8):1167-80.

[127] Citri A, Harari D, Shohat G, Ramakrishnan P, Gan J, Lavi S, *et al.* Hsp90 recognizes a common surface on client kinases. J Biol Chem 2006 May 19;281(20):14361-9.

[128] Grosjean-Raillard J, Ades L, Boehrer S, Tailler M, Fabre C, Braun T, *et al.* Flt3 receptor inhibition reduces constitutive NFkappaB activation in high-risk myelodysplastic syndrome and acute myeloid leukemia. Apoptosis 2008 Sep;13(9):1148-61.

[129] Shimada M, Nakanishi M. DNA damage checkpoints and cancer. J Mol Histol 2006 Sep;37(5-7):253-60.

[130] Chen Y, Poon RY. The multiple checkpoint functions of CHK1 and CHK2 in maintenance of genome stability. Front Biosci 2008;13:5016-29.

[131] Amico D, Barbui AM, Erba E, Rambaldi A, Introna M, Golay J. Differential response of human acute myeloid leukemia cells to gemtuzumab ozogamicin *in vitro*: role of Chk1 and Chk2 phosphorylation and caspase 3. Blood 2003 Jun 1;101(11):4589-97.

[132] Didier C, Cavelier C, Quaranta M, Galcera MO, Demur C, Laurent G, *et al.* G2/M checkpoint stringency is a key parameter in the sensitivity of AML cells to genotoxic stress. Oncogene 2008 Jun 19;27(27):3811-20.

[133] Arlander SJ, Eapen AK, Vroman BT, McDonald RJ, Toft DO, Karnitz LM. Hsp90 inhibition depletes Chk1 and sensitizes tumor cells to replication stress. J Biol Chem 2003 Dec 26;278(52):52572-7.

[134] Mesa RA, Loegering D, Powell HL, Flatten K, Arlander SJ, Dai NT, *et al.* Heat shock protein 90 inhibition sensitizes acute myelogenous leukemia cells to cytarabine. Blood 2005 Jul 1;106(1):318-27.

[135] Izquierdo MA, Shoemaker RH, Flens MJ, Scheffer GL, Wu L, Prather TR, *et al.* Overlapping phenotypes of multidrug resistance among panels of human cancer-cell lines. Int J Cancer 1996 Jan 17;65(2):230-7.

[136] Kasimir-Bauer S, Beelen D, Flasshove M, Noppeney R, Seeber S, Scheulen ME. Impact of the expression of P glycoprotein, the multidrug resistance-related protein, bcl-2, mutant p53, and heat shock protein 27 on response to induction therapy and long-term survival in patients with *de novo* acute myeloid leukemia. Exp Hematol 2002 Nov;30(11):1302-8.

[137] Kamal A, Thao L, Sensintaffar J, Zhang L, Boehm MF, Fritz LC, *et al.* A high-affinity conformation of Hsp90 confers tumour selectivity on Hsp90 inhibitors. Nature 2003 Sep 25;425(6956):407-10.

[138] Munster PN, Marchion DC, Basso AD, Rosen N. Degradation of HER2 by ansamycins induces growth arrest and apoptosis in cells with HER2 overexpression *via* a HER3, phosphatidylinositol 3'-kinase-AKT-dependent pathway. Cancer Res 2002 Jun 1;62(11):3132-7.

[139] Fiskus W, Rao R, Fernandez P, Herger B, Yang Y, Chen J, *et al.* Molecular and biologic characterization and drug sensitivity of pan-histone deacetylase inhibitor-resistant acute myeloid leukemia cells. Blood 2008 Oct 1;112(7):2896-905.

[140] Reikvam H, Hatfield KJ, Kittang AO, Hovland R, Bruserud O. Acute Myeloid Leukemia with the t(8;21) Translocation: Clinical Consequences and Biological Implications. J Biomed Biotechnol 2011;2011:104631.

[141] Yu W, Rao Q, Wang M, Tian Z, Lin D, Liu X, *et al.* The Hsp90 inhibitor 17-allylamide-17-demethoxygeldanamycin induces apoptosis and differentiation of Kasumi-1 harboring the Asn822Lys KIT mutation and down-regulates KIT protein level. Leuk Res 2006 May;30(5):575-82. eng.

[142] Bruserud O, Hovland R, Wergeland L, Huang TS, Gjertsen BT. Flt3-mediated signaling in human acute myelogenous leukemia (AML) blasts: a functional characterization of Flt3-

ligand effects in AML cell populations with and without genetic Flt3 abnormalities. Haematologica 2003 Apr;88(4):416-28.
[143] Meyer PN, Roychowdhury S, Kini AR, Alkan S. HSP90 inhibitor 17AAG causes apoptosis in ATRA-resistant acute promyelocytic leukemia cells. Leuk Res 2008 Jan;32(1):143-9.
[144] Wetzler M, Earp JC, Brady MT, Keng MK, Jusko WJ. Synergism between arsenic trioxide and heat shock protein 90 inhibitors on signal transducer and activator of transcription protein 3 activity--pharmacodynamic drug-drug interaction modeling. Clin Cancer Res 2007 Apr 1;13(7):2261-70.
[145] George P, Bali P, Cohen P, Tao J, Guo F, Sigua C, *et al.* Cotreatment with 17-allylamino-demethoxygeldanamycin and FLT-3 kinase inhibitor PKC412 is highly effective against human acute myelogenous leukemia cells with mutant FLT-3. Cancer Res 2004 May 15;64(10):3645-52.
[146] Kamynina E, Kauppinen K, Duan F, Muakkassa N, Manor D. Regulation of proto-oncogenic dbl by chaperone-controlled, ubiquitin-mediated degradation. Mol Cell Biol 2007 Mar;27(5):1809-22.
[147] Rao R, Fiskus W, Yang Y, Lee P, Joshi R, Fernandez P, *et al.* HDAC6 inhibition enhances 17-AAG--mediated abrogation of hsp90 chaperone function in human leukemia cells. Blood 2008 Sep 1;112(5):1886-93.
[148] Inoue S, Mai A, Dyer MJ, Cohen GM. Inhibition of histone deacetylase class I but not class II is critical for the sensitization of leukemic cells to tumor necrosis factor-related apoptosis-inducing ligand-induced apoptosis. Cancer Res 2006 Jul 1;66(13):6785-92.
[149] Nishioka C, Ikezoe T, Yang J, Takeuchi S, Koeffler HP, Yokoyama A. MS-275, a novel histone deacetylase inhibitor with selectivity against HDAC1, induces degradation of FLT3 *via* inhibition of chaperone function of heat shock protein 90 in AML cells. Leuk Res 2008 Sep;32(9):1382-92.
[150] Sanderson S, Valenti M, Gowan S, Patterson L, Ahmad Z, Workman P, *et al.* Benzoquinone ansamycin heat shock protein 90 inhibitors modulate multiple functions required for tumor angiogenesis. Mol Cancer Ther 2006 Mar;5(3):522-32.
[151] Kaur G, Belotti D, Burger AM, Fisher-Nielson K, Borsotti P, Riccardi E, *et al.* Antiangiogenic properties of 17-(dimethylaminoethylamino)-17-demethoxygeldanamycin: an orally bioavailable heat shock protein 90 modulator. Clin Cancer Res 2004 Jul 15;10(14):4813-21.
[152] Miao RQ, Fontana J, Fulton D, Lin MI, Harrison KD, Sessa WC. Dominant-negative Hsp90 reduces VEGF-stimulated nitric oxide release and migration in endothelial cells. Arterioscler Thromb Vasc Biol 2008 Jan;28(1):105-11.
[153] Garcia-Cardena G, Fan R, Shah V, Sorrentino R, Cirino G, Papapetropoulos A, *et al.* Dynamic activation of endothelial nitric oxide synthase by Hsp90. Nature 1998 Apr 23;392(6678):821-4.
[154] Van Buren G, 2nd, Camp ER, Yang AD, Gray MJ, Fan F, Somcio R, *et al.* The role of nitric oxide in mediating tumour blood flow. Expert Opin Ther Targets 2006 Oct;10(5):689-701.
[155] Lamalice L, Le Boeuf F, Huot J. Endothelial cell migration during angiogenesis. Circ Res 2007 Mar 30;100(6):782-94.
[156] Bohonowych JE, Gopal U, Isaacs JS. Hsp90 as a gatekeeper of tumor angiogenesis: clinical promise and potential pitfalls. J Oncol 2010;2010:412985.

[157] Bergfeld SA, DeClerck YA. Bone marrow-derived mesenchymal stem cells and the tumor microenvironment. Cancer Metast Rev 2010 Jun;29(2):249-61.

[158] Xiang X, Zhao J, Xu G, Li Y, Zhang W. mTOR and the differentiation of mesenchymal stem cells. Acta Biochimica Et Biophysica Sinica 2011 Jul;43(7):501-10.

[159] Kuo HC, Chiu CC, Chang WC, Sheen JM, Ou CY, Kuo HC, *et al.* Use of proteomic differential displays to assess functional discrepancies and adjustments of human bone marrow- and Wharton jelly-derived mesenchymal stem cells. J Proteome Res 2011 Mar 4;10(3):1305-15.

[160] Inberg A, Bogoch Y, Bledi Y, Linial M. Cellular processes underlying maturation of P19 neurons: Changes in protein folding regimen and cytoskeleton organization. Proteomics 2007 Mar;7(6):910-20.

[161] Gao F, Hu XY, Xie XJ, Xu QY, Wang YP, Liu XB, *et al.* Heat shock protein 90 protects rat mesenchymal stem cells against hypoxia and serum deprivation-induced apoptosis *via* the PI3K/Akt and ERK1/2 pathways. J Zhejiang Univ Sci B 2010 Aug;11(8):608-17.

[162] Aanei CM, Eloae FZ, Flandrin-Gresta P, Tavernier E, Carasevici E, Guyotat D, *et al.* Focal adhesion protein abnormalities in myelodysplastic mesenchymal stromal cells. Exp Cell Res 2011 Nov 1;317(18):2616-29.

[163] Irish JM, Hovland R, Krutzik PO, Perez OD, Bruserud O, Gjertsen BT, *et al.* Single cell profiling of potentiated phospho-protein networks in cancer cells. Cell 2004 Jul 23;118(2):217-28.

[164] Jung DW, Kim J, Che ZM, Oh ES, Kim G, Eom SH, *et al.* A triazine compound S06 inhibits proinvasive crosstalk between carcinoma cells and stromal fibroblasts *via* binding to heat shock protein 90. Chem Biol 2011 Dec 23;18(12):1581-90.

[165] Richardson PG, Mitsiades CS, Laubach JP, Lonial S, Chanan-Khan AA, Anderson KC. Inhibition of heat shock protein 90 (HSP90) as a therapeutic strategy for the treatment of myeloma and other cancers. Br J Haematol 2011 Feb;152(4):367-79.

[166] Spoo AC, Lubbert M, Wierda WG, Burger JA. CXCR4 is a prognostic marker in acute myelogenous leukemia. Blood 2007 Jan 15;109(2):786-91.

[167] Mandawat A, Fiskus W, Buckley KM, Robbins K, Rao R, Balusu R, *et al.* Pan-histone deacetylase inhibitor panobinostat depletes CXCR4 levels and signaling and exerts synergistic antimyeloid activity in combination with CXCR4 antagonists. Blood 2010 Dec 9;116(24):5306-15.

[168] Fredly H, Gjertsen BT, Bruserud O. Histone deacetylase inhibition in the treatment of acute myeloid leukemia: the effects of valproic acid on leukemic cells, and the clinical and experimental evidence for combining valproic acid with other antileukemic agents. Clin Epigenetics 2013;5(1):12.

[169] Bug G, Ritter M, Wassmann B, Schoch C, Heinzel T, Schwarz K, *et al.* Clinical trial of valproic acid and all-trans retinoic acid in patients with poor-risk acute myeloid leukemia. Cancer 2005 Dec 15;104(12):2717-25.

[170] Fredly H, Reikvam H, Gjertsen BT, Bruserud O. Disease-stabilizing treatment with all-trans retinoic acid and valproic acid in acute myeloid leukemia: serum hsp70 and hsp90 levels and serum cytokine profiles are determined by the disease, patient age, and anti-leukemic treatment. Am J Hematol 2012 Apr;87(4):368-76.

[171] Fiedler W, Serve H, Dohner H, Schwittay M, Ottmann OG, O'Farrell AM, *et al.* A phase 1 study of SU11248 in the treatment of patients with refractory or resistant acute myeloid

leukemia (AML) or not amenable to conventional therapy for the disease. Blood 2005 Feb 1;105(3):986-93.

[172] Fiedler W, Mesters R, Tinnefeld H, Loges S, Staib P, Duhrsen U, *et al.* A phase 2 clinical study of SU5416 in patients with refractory acute myeloid leukemia. Blood 2003 Oct 15;102(8):2763-7.

[173] Rizzieri DA, Feldman E, Dipersio JF, Gabrail N, Stock W, Strair R, *et al.* A phase 2 clinical trial of deforolimus (AP23573, MK-8669), a novel mammalian target of rapamycin inhibitor, in patients with relapsed or refractory hematologic malignancies. Clin Cancer Res 2008 May 1;14(9):2756-62.

[174] Yee KW, Zeng Z, Konopleva M, Verstovsek S, Ravandi F, Ferrajoli A, *et al.* Phase I/II study of the mammalian target of rapamycin inhibitor everolimus (RAD001) in patients with relapsed or refractory hematologic malignancies. Clin Cancer Res 2006 Sep 1;12(17):5165-73.

[175] Walsby EJ, Lazenby M, Pepper CJ, Knapper S, Burnett AK. The HSP90 inhibitor NVP-AUY922-AG inhibits the PI3K and IKK signalling pathways and synergizes with cytarabine in acute myeloid leukemia cells. Br J Haematol 2013 Apr;161(1):57-67.

[176] Kojima K, Shimanuki M, Shikami M, Samudio IJ, Ruvolo V, Corn P, *et al.* The dual PI3 kinase/mTOR inhibitor PI-103 prevents p53 induction by Mdm2 inhibition but enhances p53-mediated mitochondrial apoptosis in p53 wild-type AML. Leukemia 2008 Sep;22(9):1728-36.

[177] Kojima K, Shimanuki M, Shikami M, Andreeff M, Nakakuma H. Cyclin-dependent kinase 1 inhibitor RO-3306 enhances p53-mediated Bax activation and mitochondrial apoptosis in AML. Cancer Sci 2009 Jun;100(6):1128-36.

[178] Oyan AM, Anensen N, Bo TH, Stordrange L, Jonassen I, Bruserud O, *et al.* Genes of cell-cell interactions, chemotherapy detoxification and apoptosis are induced during chemotherapy of acute myeloid leukemia. BMC Cancer 2009;9:77.

[179] Fredly H, Ersvaer E, Gjertsen BT, Bruserud O. Immunogenic apoptosis in human acute myeloid leukemia (AML): primary human AML cells expose calreticulin and release heat shock protein (HSP) 70 and HSP90 during apoptosis. Oncol Rep 2011 Jun;25(6):1549-56.

[180] Bruserud O, Ryningen A, Wergeland L, Glenjen NI, Gjertsen BT. Osteoblasts increase proliferation and release of pro-angiogenic interleukin 8 by native human acute myelogenous leukemia blasts. Haematologica 2004 Apr;89(4):391-402.

[181] Glenjen NI, Hatfield K, Bruserud O. Coculture of native human acute myelogenous leukemia blasts with fibroblasts and osteoblasts results in an increase of vascular endothelial growth factor levels. Eur J Haematol 2005 Jan;74(1):24-34.

[182] Hatfield K, Oyan AM, Ersvaer E, Kalland KH, Lassalle P, Gjertsen BT, *et al.* Primary human acute myeloid leukemia cells increase the proliferation of microvascular endothelial cells through the release of soluble mediators. Br J Haematol 2009 Jan;144(1):53-68.

[183] Reikvam H, Nepstad I, Bruserud O, Hatfield KJ. Pharmacological targeting of the PI3K/mTOR pathway alters the release of angioregulatory mediators both from primary human acute myeloid leukemia cells and their neighboring stromal cells. Oncotarget 2013 Jun;4(6):830-43.

[184] Stapnes C, Doskeland AP, Hatfield K, Ersvaer E, Ryningen A, Lorens JB, *et al.* The proteasome inhibitors bortezomib and PR-171 have antiproliferative and proapoptotic effects on primary human acute myeloid leukemia cells. Br J Haematol 2007 Mar;136(6):814-28.

[185] Guzman ML, Neering SJ, Upchurch D, Grimes B, Howard DS, Rizzieri DA, *et al.* Nuclear factor-kappaB is constitutively activated in primitive human acute myelogenous leukemia cells. Blood 2001 Oct 15;98(8):2301-7.

[186] Cornelissen JJ, Gratwohl A, Schlenk RF, Sierra J, Bornhauser M, Juliusson G, *et al.* The European LeukemiaNet AML Working Party consensus statement on allogeneic HSCT for patients with AML in remission: an integrated-risk adapted approach. Nat Rev Clin Oncol 2012 Oct;9(10):579-90.

[187] Reikvam H, Kittang AO, Melve G, Mosevoll KA, Bentsen PT, Ersvaer E, *et al.* Targeted anti-leukemic therapy as disease-stabilizing treatment for acute myeloid leukemia relapse after allogeneic stem cell transplantation: Will it be possible to combine these strategies with retransplantation or donor lymphocyte infusions? Curr Cancer Drug Targets 2013 Jan;13(1):30-47.

[188] Fredly H, Ersvaer E, Kittang AO, Tsykunova G, Gjertsen BT, Bruserud O. The combination of valproic acid, all-trans retinoic acid and low-dose cytarabine as disease-stabilizing treatment in acute myeloid leukemia. Clin Epigenetics 2013;5(1):13.

[189] Lee J, Greiner L, Holson E, Slocum K, Ge J, Normant E, *et al.* IPI-493, a potent bioaviable Hsp90 inhibitor of the ansamycins class. Eur J Cancer 2008; 6(Suppl 12):Abstract no 153.

[190] Gocke CD, Reaman GH, Stine C, Zhang MY, Osmani SA, Miller BA. The nuclear migration gene NudC and human hematopoiesis. Leuk Lymphoma 2000 Nov;39(5-6):447-54.

[191] Tronstad KJ, Bruserud O, Berge K, Berge RK. Antiproliferative effects of a non-beta-oxidizable fatty acid, tetradecylthioacetic acid, in native human acute myelogenous leukemia blast cultures. Leukemia 2002 Nov;16(11):2292-301.

[192] Kawai M, Chen J, Cheung CY, Chang TK. Transcript profiling of cytochrome P450 genes in HL-60 human leukemic cells: upregulation of CYP1B1 by all-trans-retinoic acid. Mol Cell Biochem 2003 Jun;248(1-2):57-65.

[193] Anensen N, Oyan AM, Bourdon JC, Kalland KH, Bruserud O, Gjertsen BT. A distinct p53 protein isoform signature reflects the onset of induction chemotherapy for acute myeloid leukemia. Clin Cancer Res 2006 Jul 1;12(13):3985-92.

[194] McCormack E, Haaland I, Venas G, Forthun RB, Huseby S, Gausdal G, *et al.* Synergistic induction of p53 mediated apoptosis by valproic acid and nutlin-3 in acute myeloid leukemia. Leukemia 2012 May;26(5):910-7.

[195] Yamaguchi T, Ye C, Chattopadhyay N, Sanders JL, Vassilev PM, Brown EM. Enhanced expression of extracellular calcium sensing receptor in monocyte-differentiated *versus* undifferentiated HL-60 cells: potential role in regulation of a nonselective cation channel. Calcif Tissue Int 2000 May;66(5):375-82.

[196] Wenandy L, Kollgaard T, Letsch A, Andersen RS, Stather D, Seremet T, *et al.* The 1170 A-P single-nucleotide polymorphism (SNP) in the Her-2/neu protein (HER2) as a minor histocompatibility antigen (mHag). Leukemia 2009 Oct; 23(10): 1926-9.

[197] Frostad S, Bruserud O. *In vitro* effects of insulin-like growth factor-1 (IGF-1) on proliferation and constitutive cytokine secretion by acute myelogenous leukemia blasts. Eur J Haematol 1999 Mar;62(3):191-8.

[198] Tabe Y, Jin L, Tsutsumi-Ishii Y, Xu Y, McQueen T, Priebe W, *et al.* Activation of integrin-linked kinase is a critical prosurvival pathway induced in leukemic cells by bone marrow-derived stromal cells. Cancer Res 2007 Jan 15;67(2):684-94.

[199] Reikvam H, Tamburini J, Skrede S, Holdhus R, Poulain L, Ersvaer E, *et al.* Antileukaemic effect of PI3K-mTOR inhibitors in acute myeloid leukemia-gene expression profiles reveal CDC25B expression as determinate of pharmacological effect. Br J Haematol 2014 Jan;164(2):200-11.

[200] Xiang Z, Zhao Y, Mitaksov V, Fremont DH, Kasai Y, Molitoris A, *et al.* Identification of somatic JAK1 mutations in patients with acute myeloid leukemia. Blood 2008 May 1;111(9):4809-12.

[201] Soupir CP, Vergilio JA, Dal Cin P, Muzikansky A, Kantarjian H, Jones D, *et al.* Philadelphia chromosome-positive acute myeloid leukemia: a rare aggressive leukemia with clinicopathologic features distinct from chronic myeloid leukemia in myeloid blast crisis. Am J Clin Pathol 2007 Apr;127(4):642-50.

[202] Chim CS, Wong AS, Kwong YL. Epigenetic inactivation of INK4/CDK/RB cell cycle pathway in acute leukemias. Ann Hematol 2003 Dec;82(12):738-42.

[203] Ersvaer E, Zhang JY, McCormack E, Olsnes A, Anensen N, Tan EM, *et al.* Cyclin B1 is commonly expressed in the cytoplasm of primary human acute myelogenous leukemia cells and serves as a leukemia-associated antigen associated with autoantibody response in a subset of patients. Eur J Haematol 2007 Sep;79(3):210-25.

[204] Aggerholm A, Hokland P. DAP-kinase CpG island methylation in acute myeloid leukemia: methodology *versus* biology? Blood 2000 May 1;95(9):2997-9.

[205] Schmidt CA, Oettle H, Ludwig WD, Serke S, Pawlaczyk-Peter B, Wilborn F, *et al.* Overexpression of the Raf-1 proto-oncogene in human myeloid leukemia. Leuk Res 1994 Jun;18(6):409-13.

[206] Reikvam H, Hatfield KJ, Oyan AM, Kalland KH, Kittang AO, Bruserud O. Primary human acute myelogenous leukemia cells release matrix metalloproteases and their inhibitors: release profile and pharmacological modulation. Eur J Haematol 2010 Mar;84(3):239-51.

[207] Roth A, Vercauteren S, Sutherland HJ, Lansdorp PM. Telomerase is limiting the growth of acute myeloid leukemia cells. Leukemia 2003 Dec;17(12):2410-7.

[208] Coulthard SA, Howell C, Robson J, Hall AG. The relationship between thiopurine methyltransferase activity and genotype in blasts from patients with acute leukemia. Blood 1998 Oct 15;92(8):2856-62.

[209] Olwill SA, McGlynn H, Gilmore WS, Alexander HD. Annexin II cell surface and mRNA expression in human acute myeloid leukemia cell lines. Thromb Res 2005;115(1-2):109-14.

[210] Pillozzi S, Brizzi MF, Balzi M, Crociani O, Cherubini A, Guasti L, *et al.* HERG potassium channels are constitutively expressed in primary human acute myeloid leukemias and regulate cell proliferation of normal and leukemic hemopoietic progenitors. Leukemia 2002 Sep;16(9):1791-8.

[211] Fatrai S, Schepers H, Tadema H, Vellenga E, Daenen SM, Schuringa JJ. Mucin1 expression is enriched in the human stem cell fraction of cord blood and is upregulated in majority of the AML cases. Exp Hematol 2008 Oct;36(10):1254-65.

[212] Smadja DM, Laurendeau I, Avignon C, Vidaud M, Aiach M, Gaussem P. The angiopoietin pathway is modulated by PAR-1 activation on human endothelial progenitor cells. J Thromb Haemost 2006 Sep;4(9):2051-8.

CHAPTER 2

Spindle Assembly Checkpoint (SAC): More New Targets for Anti-Cancer Drug Therapies

Maria Kapanidou and Victor M. Bolanos-Garcia*

Faculty of Health and Life Sciences, Department of Biological and Medical Sciences; Oxford Brookes University, Oxford, England, OX3 0BP, UK

Abstract: The spindle assembly checkpoint (SAC) is an essential control system of the eukaryotic cell cycle that ensures genome stability. The essence of this evolutionarily conserved mechanism is to delay mitosis progression until proper chromosome bi-orientation and attachment is achieved. Mutations in the genes encoding for diverse checkpoint proteins lead to the impairment of the mitotic checkpoint mechanism, thus resulting in the premature separation of sister chromatids and aneuploidy, a condition that is associated with various classes of cancer. The understanding of the organisation, structure and function of SAC components is essential for the molecular understanding of the process and to identify and evaluate new targets for cancer drug therapy.

Keywords: Cancer, chromosome segregation, genome instability, kinetochore-microtubule, mitosis, spindle assembly checkpoint (SAC).

INTRODUCTION

The spindle assembly checkpoint (SAC) is an essential internal control mechanism of higher organisms that ensures that all chromosomes have stably attached to microtubules during the process of cell division. Once all sister chromatids have achieved bipolar attachment from two opposing centrosomes and their kinetochores are under tension, the anaphase-promoting complex/cyclosome (APC/C) in association with its pseudo-substrate Cdc20 ubiquitinates the protein securin. The macromolecular assembly APC/C-Cdc20 plays a crucial role in checkpoint silencing and mitotic progression: degradation of polyubiquitinated securin activates the protease separase, which in turn degrades a subunit of the

***Corresponding Author Victor M. Bolanos-Garcia:** Department of Biological and Medical Sciences, Oxford Brookes University. Gipsy Lane, Headington, Oxford, England. OX3 0BP, UK; Tel: 44 (0) 1865 482778; Fax: 44 (0) 1865 483242; E-mail: vbolanos-garcia@brookes.ac.uk

Atta-ur-Rahman (Ed)

cohesin complex, Scc1. These events, together with the APC/C-mediated degradation of Cyclin B, trigger the destruction of cohesion between sister chromatids thus defining the exit from metaphase and the initiation of anaphase. The main series of events involved in the activation and silencing of the SAC are depicted in Fig. (**1**). Regulation of the SAC is mediated by a complex network of molecular interactions often involving proteins that are organized in multiple domains Fig. (**2**). If the formation of the spindle assembly is unsatisfied, the spindle assembly checkpoint delays the onset of anaphase, preventing chromosomal instability (CIN) and aneuploidy. The latter condition is a hallmark of cancer cells, as Theodor Boveri first proposed about 100 years ago [1].

Mutations in genes encoding essential mitotic spindle assembly (SAC) components such as *BUB1, BUBR1, MAD1, MAD2, MPS1, CDC20, ZW10, ROD and ZWILCH* have been associated with aneuploidy and tumorigenesis [2-7]. Also, changes in the expression profiles of SAC proteins are related to the accumulation of chromosome aberrations, resulting in the impairment of mitotic checkpoint function.

Earlier promising observations showing that the weakening of SAC proteins inhibited tumour cell growth suggest that this signalling pathway may constitute a good target for the treatment of cancer [8-12]. Targeting SAC components either individually or when forming part of the macromolecular subcomplexes that mediate SAC function with small-molecules in order to impair catalytic activity and/or protein assembly into larger complexes seems attractive. For instance, small-size drugs can be advantageous over modern alternative strategies in the clinic such as therapeutic antibodies as the latter are expensive, present limited cell-permeability and are often administrated intravenously [13,14]. Protein-protein interfaces of multiprotein complexes are widely represented in most metabolic and signalling pathways underpinning cell division, growth and survival [15-19]. The design of small-molecules that target protein-protein interfaces of SAC subcomplexes seems particularly attractive because the structural and chemical features of the interfaces are far more diverse than the substrate binding and catalytic sites of protein kinases and proteases for instance, two protein superfamilies that for many years have been considered *ad hoc* targets

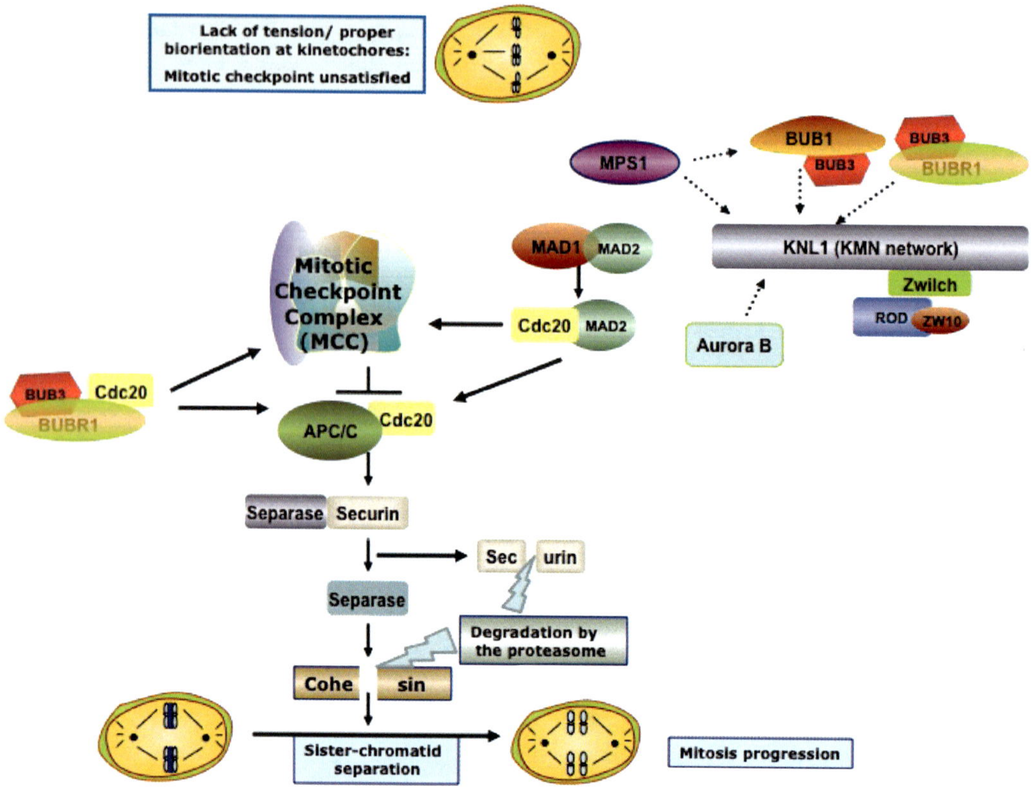

Fig. (1): Schematic representation of some of the interactions underpinning SAC signalling.

represents an opportunity to affect specific interactions mediated by pleiotropic proteins -such as growth factor receptors- and those underlying protein misfolding and aggregation -such as Huntington's and Alzheimer's diseases- [20, 21]. Modern methods in X-ray crystallography when combined with nuclear magnetic resonance (NMR), isothermal titration calorimetry (ITC), surface plasmon resonance (SPR), thermal shift analysis and microscale thermophoresis (MST) among other biophysical techniques provide unprecedented insight into the molecular interactions that mediate the assembly of SAC components to form larger assemblies and facilitates the selection of drug candidates from high-throughput screenings of libraries of small size compounds. Given the preponderant role of SAC signalling to control proper chromosome segregation and the dramatic, deleterious effect of mutations of SAC components on genome stability, here we discuss the current understanding of the structure and function of core components of the spindle assembly checkpoint and discuss their potential as novel molecular targets for the development of anti-cancer drugs.

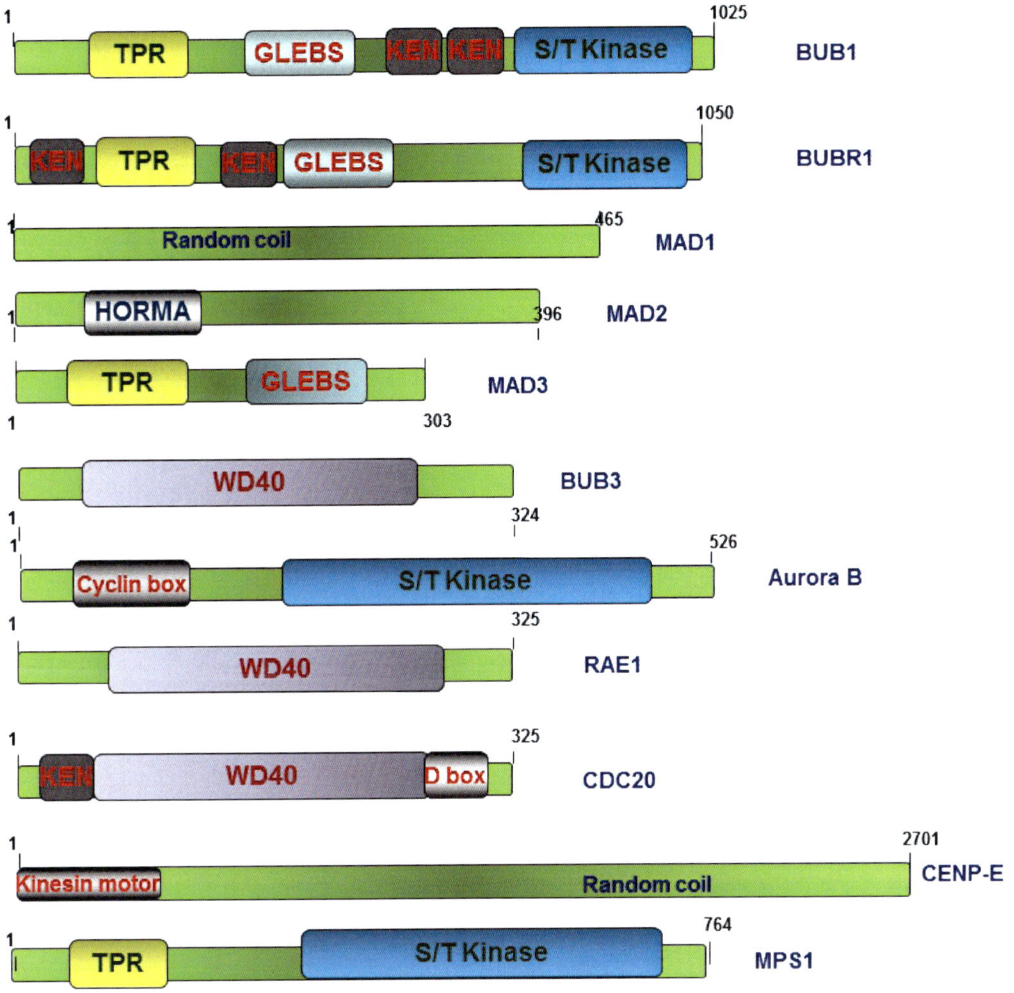

Fig. (2): Domain organisation of central SAC components.

Aurora B

Aurora B is expressed in normal proliferating cells with protein concentration levels peaking at the G_2/M phase of the cell cycle. Aurora B associates with the inner centromere protein (INCENP), survivin and borealin to form a "chromosomal passenger complex" (CPC), the protein assembly that is required to localize Aurora B to the centromere and the mitotic spindle [22-24]. The CPC first localizes along the chromosome during prophase, become concentrated at the inner centromere region during prometaphase, leaves the chromosome and relocalizes to the central region of the mitotic spindle and in telophase to the site of the contractile ring [25, 26]. These features confirmed that Aurora B is an important regulator of kinetochore function, that it is required for correct chromosomal alignment and segregation and that it plays roles in cytokinesis and the spindle assembly checkpoint [27]. Moreover, phosphorylation of kinetochore proteins by Aurora B during early mitosis increases kinetochore-microtubule (MT) turnover and prevents premature stabilization of kinetochore-MT attachments. For instance, the kinetochore protein KNL1 recruits the mitotic checkpoint kinases Bub1 and BubR1 as well as protein phosphatases -such as PP1 and PP2A- that counteract Aurora B function [28].

Normal cells treated with a small molecule inhibitor that affects only the catalytic function of Aurora B show miss-oriented chromosomes at anaphase, a defective spindle assembly checkpoint and the inhibition of cytokinesis [29]. Similarly, abrogation of Aurora B by gene knockdown or RNAi disrupts the CPC.

The crystal structure of Aurora B bound to INCENP [30] provided light into the activation of Aurora B by the latter protein. Full activation requires phosphorylation of a conserved Threonine-Serine-Serine motif near the C-terminal of INCENP [23]. In the Aurora B-INCENP complex the latter forms a molecular 'crown' extending across the N-terminal and the C-terminal domain of Aurora B (pdb 2BFY). This complex represents an intermediate state of activation in relation to the fully active state show by the Aurora A-TPX2 complex [31]. A comparative analysis of the structure of the Aurora B-INCENP-hesperadin ternary complex with that of the Aurora A-TPX2 binary complex shows that Aurora B undergoes little conformational changes in the free and the ligand-bound states. An exception is the glycine-rich loop which shows a more ordered conformation in the Aurora B-INCENP complex upon hesperadin binding [30].

Several pharma groups have developed a series of novel and potent small molecule inhibitors of Aurora B that compete for the ATP-binding site. Such inhibitors function as effective anti-proliferative agents (Table **1**) Fig. (**3**). The study of the specificity, efficacy and potency of these novel compounds has been carried out in cell-based assays, mouse xenograft models of cancer and *in vitro* kinase assays [32, 33]. These series of tests have shown that the disruption of the enzymatic activity of Aurora kinases with small size compounds that selectively target the ATP binding site such as ZM447439 [34], VX-680 (Vertex [35, 36]) and hesperadin (Boehringer Ingelheim [35]), is satisfactory to proceed towards the clinic.

Table 1: Physicochemical Properties of Small Size Inhibitors of Aurora Kinases

Compound	Selectivity	MW (Da)	References
Hesperadin	Aurora A, Aurora B	516.6	[37]
MLN8054	Aurora A >> Aurora B	476.8	[38]
VX-680	Aurora A, Aurora B	464.5	[35,36]
Pyrimido-oxazepine	Aurora A, Aurora B	468.2	[39]
ZM447439	Aurora A, Aurora B	513.6	[34]
AZD1152-HQPA	Aurora A, Aurora B	507.5	[40]
PHA-680632	Aurora A > Aurora B	513.7	[41]
MP235	Aurora A > Aurora B	605.6	[42]
JNJ-7706621	Aurora A, Aurora B	394.3	[43]
GSK1070916	Aurora B, Aurora C	507.6	[44]
CCT129202	Aurora A, Aurora B, Aurora C	497.0	[45]

Bub1 and BubR1

Bub1 (budding uninhibited by benzimidazole 1) and BubR1 (budding uninhibited by benzimidazole-related 1) also known as Mad3 (for mitotic-arrest deficient) in yeast, worms and plants, are essential for recruiting mitotic checkpoint proteins to the kinetochore and play a central role in the mitotic checkpoint response [46]. Bub1 and BubR1 share a similar organization with a conserved N-terminal domain, a middle non-conserved domain that mediates the physical interaction with the spindle assembly component Bub3 and a C-terminal serine/threonine kinase domain. The N-terminal regions of Bub1 and BubR1 are important for the

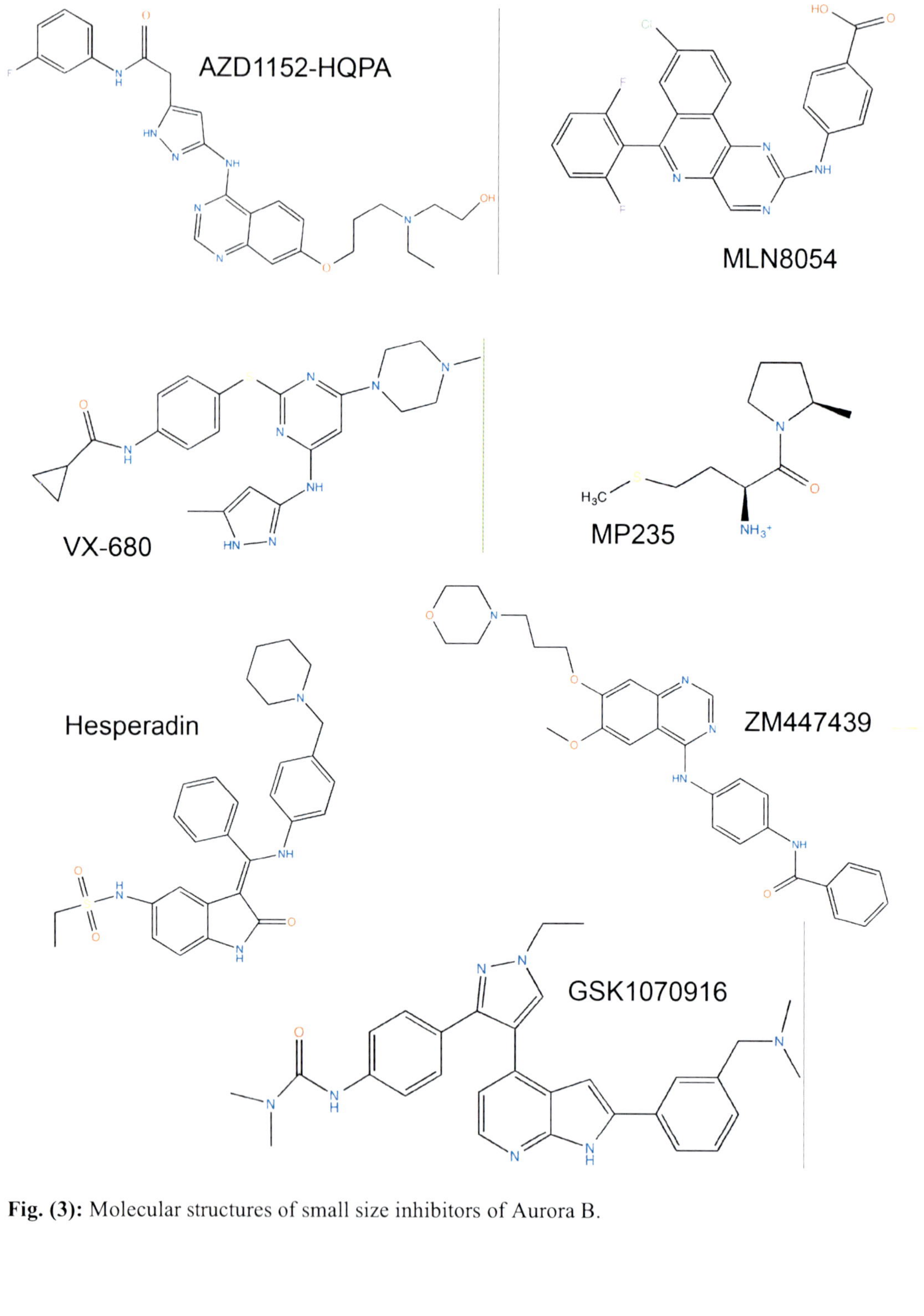

Fig. (3): Molecular structures of small size inhibitors of Aurora B.

accumulation of these proteins to the kinetochore [47]. In both cases, the N-terminal domain of Bub1 and BubR1 are organized as tandem arrangements of the tetratricopeptide repeat (TPR) motif. Bub1 and BubR1 TPRs are required for productive interactions with KNL1 in a process involving two short conserved motifs (commonly referred to as the KI motifs) of the latter protein [48-50]. BubR1 presents additional distinguishing structural and functional features: it contains a conserved sequence in the N-terminal domain that closely resembles the KEN box. This motif has been reported to act as Cdh1-dependent APC/C recognition signal [51]. Also, BubR1 but not Bub1 forms part of the mitotic checkpoint complex (MCC). The MCC -which in addition to BubR1 includes Bub3, Mad2 and Cdc20- is a pseudo-substrate inhibitor of APC/C [52-55].

Bub1 regulates the recruitment of components of the outer and inner kinetochore including Mad2, BubR1, and centromere-associated proteins CenpE and CenpF in cells with unsatisfied mitotic checkpoint [56] (Table **3**). BubR1 is also required for proper chromosome congression and for the establishment of efficient bipolar attachment to spindle microtubules [57-59]. BubR1 stabilizes kinetochore-microtubules attachments through regulation of Aurora B [59-62]. Recent studies have shown that Bub1, BubR1 and a newly identified mitotic checkpoint protein BuGZ (Bub3-interacting GLEBS-motif-containing ZNF207 protein) bind to Bub3 through a middle domain that contains the GLEBS (Gle2-binding-sequence) motif. The interaction is required for the kinetochore recruitment of Bub1 and BubR1 [63-65]. The small compound inhibitor 2OH-BNPP1, initially designed to inhibit mutant kinases with glycine gatekeeper residues, has been reported as a potent Bub1 kinase inhibitor with an IC_{50} around 250 nM [66]. The crystal structure of the Bub1 kinase domain in complex with 2OH-BNPP1 [66] provides the structural framework that is required to design more potent inhibitors of Bub1 kinase activity.

Mps1

In recent years Mps1 (monopolar-spindle 1) has emerged as a mitotic checkpoint kinase with prominent roles in SAC signalling. Mps1 is a protein organised in two domains, a N-terminal domain that adopt a triple tandem array of the TPR motif and a C-terminal region containing a catalytically active kinase domain, Fig. (**6**).

The recruitment of Mps1 to the kinetochore depends on its N-terminal domain [67]. In humans and yeast cells, the mitotic checkpoint response involves the Mps1-dependent phosphorylation of KNL1/Spc105 MELT motifs [68]. The MELT motif shows the sequence consensus (M/I/L/V)-(E/D)-(L/M/I/V)-(T/S). Phosphorylation of the Threonine residue in position 4 of the MELT motif located in N-terminal KNL1 is the target of Mps1. Because inhibition of Mps1 kinase activity preferentially impairs mitotic checkpoint signalling in tumour cells [69] this SAC component has been considered a promising target to treat cancer. Some of the small molecules that have been reported as inhibitors of Mps1 are presented in Table **2** and Figs. (**4** and **6**).

Table 2: Physicochemical Properties of Small Molecule Inhibitors of Mps1

Compound	Selectivity	Mol. Mass (Da)	References
NMS-P715	Mps1	676.3	[70]
1H-pyrrolo[3,2-c]pyridine	Mps1	118.1	[71]
MPS1-IN-3	Mps1	535.6	[72]
AZ 3146	Mps1	452.5	[73]
MPI-0479605	Mps1	328.4	[74]

Bub3

As mentioned above, the mitotic checkpoint protein Bub3 associates with Bub1 and BubR1 to form heterocomplexes. The requirement of Bub3 and the phosphorylation of Cdc20 by Bub1 are important for the inhibition of the anaphase-promoting complex or cyclosome (APC/C) in cells with the spindle assembly checkpoint unsatisfied [75,76]. Moreover, the association of Bub3 with Bub1 and BubR1 is essential for the targeting of Bub1 and BubR1 to the kinetochore and to promote correct kinetochore-microtubule attachment and chromosome alignment. Kinetochore recruitment of Bub1 and BubR1 is accomplished through the binding of Bub3 to phosphorylated MELT repeat motifs in KNL1 [50, 77]. Phosphorylation of the MELT motif by Mps1 is an important requirement for the recruitment of Bub1, BubR1 and Bub3 to the kinetochore [68, 77, 78]. A bioinformatics study showed that the Methionine

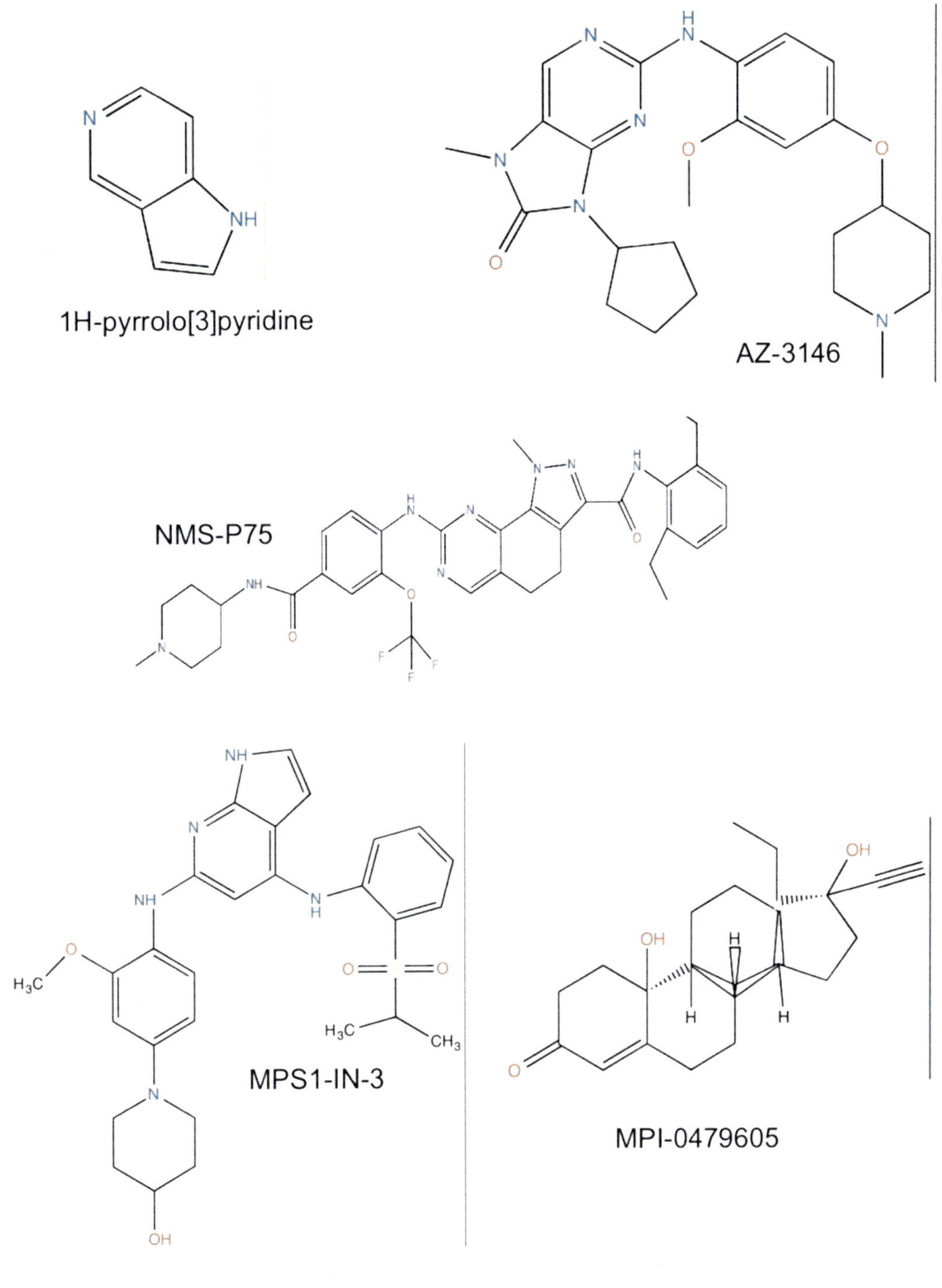

Fig. (4): Molecular structures of small size Mps1 inhibitors.

residue of the MELT motif is highly conserved across species whereas Leucine and Threonine are often substituted by acidic residues [79]. The bioinformatics analysis also showed that repeating MELT motifs are often flanked on the N-terminal side by the sequence TΦΦ-(F/Y)-(ST)-(DE), where Φ denotes a hydrophobic residue, and by the sequence SHT at the C-terminal end. Both flanking sequences seem to be important for the recruitment of human Bub1 to the kinetochore [79]. Interestingly, the various MELT motifs seem to unevenly contribute to KNL1 function to recruit Bub1 and BubR1 to the kinetochore [79]. Such differential requirements vary in different organisms thus suggesting that the number, location, and specific sequences flanking the MELT motifs may constitute a layer of regulation to exquisitely control chromosome congression and mitotic checkpoint signalling.

The crystal structures of Bub3 in complex with Bub1 GLEBS motif (pdb 2I3S) and Bub3 in complex with BubR1(Mad3) GLEBS motif (pdb 2I3T) revealed a similar interaction in both cases, with the Bub1 and BubR1 GLEBS motifs binding to the top surface of the Bub3 β-propeller [80]. Earlier reports of the crystal structures of yeast Bub3 alone (pdb 1YFQ) showed that this protein consists of a canonical WD40 repeat fold [81, 82]. Structure superposition of the crystal structure of Bub3 alone with that of the Bub3/Bub1 GLEBS motif (pdb 2I3S) and Bub3/BubR1(Mad3) GLEBS motif (pdb 2I3T) complexes indicate that Bub3 is a rigid scaffold as little conformational changes occur upon ligand (*i.e.*, GLEBS and MELT repeat motifs) binding, Fig. (**5**). More recently, the crystal structure of a ternary complex formed between Bub3, a synthetic MELT phosphopeptide and the Bub3-binding domain of Bub1, showed that a Bub3 region that appears well conserved in the canonical WD40 repeat structure acts as the binding site of a phosphomimetic peptide of the MELT motif [77].

The newly discovered protein BuGZ (Bub3-interacting GLEBS-motif-containing ZNF207 protein) promotes kinetochore targeting of the Bub1/Bub3 and BubR1/Bub3 heterodimer complexes. BuGZ consists of a N-terminal zinc finger domain and a GLEBS motif that is conserved from yeast to human and acts as Bub3 binding site [63, 64].

Heterozygous mutations in Bub3 and Bub1 had been linked with colorectal cancer (CRC). The patients affected by these mutations presented an aneuploidy profile in multiple tissues [83]. Interestingly, suppression of Bub3, Mad2 and BubR1 expression also promoted tumorigenesis and induced aneuploidy and hyperplasia in a *Drosophila melanogaster* tumorigenesis model [84].

Mad1 and Mad2

Mad1 (Mitotic arrest-deficient protein 1) is a coiled coil protein of 718 amino acid residues in humans that interacts with Mad2 (Mitotic arrest-deficient protein 2) (Table **3**). The interaction leads to the activation of Mad2 in a process that involves a conformational transition from a Mad2 open (inactive) to a close (active) state [85]. The Mad2-dependent inhibition of Cdc20 and the assembly of the mitotic checkpoint complex occur in cells with the mitotic checkpoint unsatisfied in a process that is promoted by Mps1 [86, 87]. The C-terminal region of Mad1, a α-helix rich domain (pdb 4DZO), is required for its kinetochore recruitment [88]. The crystal structure of Mad2 in complex with Mad1 residues 485 to 584 (pdb 1GO4) and Fig. (**5**) shows that Mad2 consists of a single α/β domain organised in three layers: a central layer formed by three α-helices, a large six- stranded β-sheet on one side, and a short β-hairpin on the other side whereas the Mad1 fragment is predominantly α-helical [89]. Recent evidence support the early observation that Mad1 interacts directly with Bub1 [90] while others have reported that mutation of the Bub1 region that interacts with Mad1 displayed mitotic assembly checkpoint defects and impaired the recruitment of Mad1 and Mad2 to kinetochores [85, 91-93]. It has been suggested that the interaction recruits Mad1 to kinetochores and facilitates phosphorylation of Mad1 by Mps1 [94]. Changes in Mad1 and Mad2 levels or in the stoichiometry of a Mad1:Mad2 complex have been observed in human cancers presumably as a result of impairment of the mitotic checkpoint [95]. Heterozygous deletion of Mad1 causes aneuploidy and promotes tumours in mice [96] while Mad1 overexpression has been reported in human cancers resistant to microtubule drugs [97]. Mad2 plays major roles in the activation of APC/C^{Cdc20} and the proper switch between APC/C^{Cdc20} and APC/C^{Cdh1} [98]. Similar to the case of Mad1, the overexpression of Mad2 leads to various types of tumours in transgenic mice [99] and has been associated with the ovarian cancer cells that are resistant to chemotherapy [100].

Bub1 and Mad2 expression have been proposed as prognostic factor in endometrial cancer [101]. In a recent comprehensive study based on genetic arrays in yeast, the protein phosphatase 2 (PP2) was proposed as a cancer drug target in tumours overexpressing Mad2 [102] because reduced levels of Mad2 and viability of tumour cells overexpressing Mad2 were achieved after PP2 depletion and/or inhibition [102].

Since the disruption of specific protein-protein interfaces (PPI) is a strategy that is gaining momentum in drug discovery [17, 18], it would be interesting to study if the targeting of the Mad1-Mad2 interface can represent a new therapeutic window.

Cdc20 and Cdh1

The Cdc20 (Cell division cycle homologue 20) is the activator of the APC/C. The inhibition of APC/C, which normally targets Cyclin B and Securin for degradation, thus preventing cell cycle exit from mitosis, is the major event during insufficient or improper kinetochore-microtubule attachment [53, 103]. BubR1 contains two Cdc20-binding regions, one located in N-terminal domain and the other in the centre of the protein. However, only the first Cdc20-binding site seems to be required for the productive interaction with Cdc20 [53,54,104,105]. Studies conducted in HeLa cells have proved that BubR1 N-terminal fragment is sufficient for binding to APC/C^{Cdc20} [54,106]. The crystal structures of Cdc20 alone (pdb 4GGA) and in complex with a BubR1 KEN-box surrogate peptide (pdb 4GGD) revealed a disorder N-terminal region in Cdc20 and a C-terminal WD40 fold β-propeller in which the KEN-box and D-box binding regions are located on the top face of the WD40 fold [107]. Cdc20 degradation involves Cdh1, a Cdc20 homologue, in a process mediated by the protein motifs CRY and KEN boxes. The two motifs are specifically recognized by APC/C^{Cdc20} in human cells and by two N-termini destruction (D)-boxes in yeast cells [108-110]. The significance of Cdh1 in mitotic checkpoint signalling is evidenced by the abnormal low concentration of this protein observed in metastatic tumour tissues [111]. In a similar fashion to other mitotic checkpoint proteins, overexpression of Cdc20 has been observed in certain tumours. For example, increased expression of Cdc20 has been reported in oral squamous cell carcinoma (OSCC) [112], carcinoma of the human bladder (UCB) [113], pancreatic ductal adenocarcinoma [114], colorectal cancer [115] and cell lung cancer [116]. Recent *in vitro* studies in Cdc20 knockdowns claimed to have achieved inhibition of growth of human pancreatic carcinoma cells after delivering intravenous, liposome encapsulated Cdc20siRNA [117]. These results suggest the use of siRNA methods as a potential effective therapeutic strategy for the inhibition of tumour growth [117].

OTHER SAC PROTEINS

Skp1

Skp1(S-phase kinase-associated protein 1) is essential for the assembly of a functional kinetochore [118]. Skp1 forms part of the invariant core of the multisubunit SCF [Skp1/Cullin/F-box] E3 ligase complex. The interaction of the kinetochore protein CenpE with Skp1 plays a critical role in midbody dynamics. Elimination of Skp1 disrupts proteolysis of CenpE at the midbody, abrogates cytokinetic checkpoint arrest, and induces prolonged mid- body cross-bridges in HeLa cells that exit cytokinesis prematurely [119]. Skp1 is a protein organised as the BTB/POZ fold with a C-terminal helical extension. The later region was identified as to mediate the binding of Bub1 in yeast two-hybrid screenings. The interaction *in vitro* has been observed in binding assays of recombinant proteins. These findings suggest that Skp1 is required for the recruitment of yeast Bub1 to kinetochores [118, 120]. However, whether Skp1 plays a role in the recruitment of Bub1 to kinetochores in mammalian cells is an aspect that remains to be clarified.

Rae1

Rae1 exists in a large ribonucleoprotein complex that requires RNA for its activity to control microtubule dynamics *in vitro*. It has been reported that Rae1 binds to Bub1 but not to BubR1 [121] and that suppression of Rae1 expression severely inhibits the mitotic checkpoint [122]. Studies conducted in *D. melanogaster* have shown that Rae1 is required for proper cell proliferation and progression through the G1 phase of the cell cycle. Because the amino acid sequence of Rae1 from flies closely resembles that of its human counterpart [123], it is possible that human Rae1 exhibits a similar function during the cell cycle.

Table 3: Functions and Established Interactions of Central Protein Components of the SAC

Protein	Interacting Partners	Function	References
Mad1	Mad2, Bub1/Bub3 complex	Recruitment of Mad2 to kinetochores; phosphorylated by Mps1 and Bub1 in cells with the SAC unsatisfied	[90-92]
Mad2	Mad1, Cdc20, Bub3	binds to Cdc20 leading to APC/C inhibition.	[86,87]
BubR1 (Mad3)	Cdc20, Bub3, BuGZ, Blinkin, Mad2	APC/C inhibition	[53-55]
Bub1	Bub3, BuGZ, Blinkin	Mad1 binding and phosphorylation;	[63,65]
Bub3	Bub1, BubR1(Mad3), BuGZ, Mad2	Recruits Bub1 and BubR1 to kinetochores	[50,63-65]
BuGZ	Bub1, BubR1 (Mad3), Bub3	Promotes kinetochore targeting of Bub1-Bub3 and BubR1-Bub3 complexes	[63,65]
Mps1	Mad2, BubR1	Phosphorylates the kinetochore hub KNL1	[94]
Aurora B	INCENP, Cenp-A, Histone H3, Borealin, Ndc80	Involved in the bipolar attachment of spindle microtubules to kinetochores; regulates the onset of cytokinesis	[22-24,28]
Cdc20	Mad2, BubR1 (Mad3)	Activates APC/C to target securin and mitotic cycling for degradation; substrate of Cdk1 in mammals	[54, 103]
Cenp-E	BubR1 (Mad3), MAP kinase	Recruits BubR1(Mad3), Mad1 and Mad2 to kinetochores; regulates kinetochore microtubule attachments	[133]
Rae1	Bub1	Binds the nuclear pore complex through a GLEBS motif that closely resembles that of Bub1 and BubR1	[121]
Skp1	Cenp-E, Bub1	Recruitment of Bub1 to kinetochores	[118, 119]
ZW10	Rod10, Zwint1	Required for the assembly of dynein/dynein and Mad1-Mad2 into the kinetochores	[130,132]

Rae1 binds the nuclear pore complex through the GLEBS motif [124] (Table **3**). While Bub3 binding appears to be specific for Mad3 and Bub1 GLEBS motifs, Rae1 appears to be less specific as it binds Bub1 and the nuclear pore complex. Interestingly, Bub3 and Rae1 haplo-insufficiency have similar phenotypes exhibiting spindle checkpoint and chromosome segregation defects [125]. Rae1 and Bub3 have 26% identity and 42% similarity in yeast, and 34% identity and 52% similarity in humans. The sequence alignment of Rae1 with Bub3 shows conserved residues located along the top surface of the β-propeller and the lateral surface spanning blades 5-6 (particularly in the region separating WD repeats 3 and 4) [82], including the Bub3 region that binds the MELT motif of the central kinetochore protein component KNL1 [77].

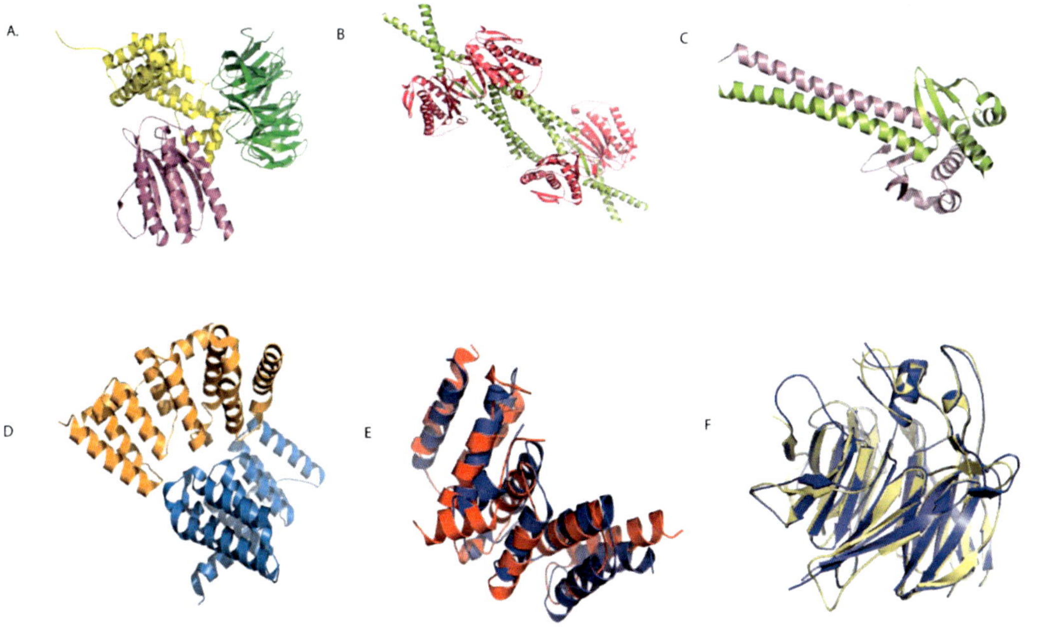

Fig. (5): A) Crystal structure of the Mitotic Checkpoint Complex, which consists of Mad2, Mad3 and APC/C pseudo-inhibitor Cdc20 (pdb 4AEZ). **B)** Crystal structure of the tetrameric Mad1-Mad2 complex. The Mad1 is presented with green and Mad2 with pink colour (pdb 1GO4). **C)** Crystal structure of human Mad1 C-terminal domain (pdb 4DZO). **D)** Crystal structure of Bub1 N-terminal domain contains the TPR motif (pdb 3ESL). **E)** Superposition of crystal structures of human Bub1 and BubR1 TPR domains in complex with KI motifs of KNL1 (pdb 4A1 and 3SI5, respectively). **F)** Superposition of the crystal structures of Bub3 with Mad3 (pdb 2I3T) and Bub1 (pdb (2I3S). Figures generated with Pymol [134].

ZW10, *ROD* and *ZWILCH*

The genes *zeste-white 10* (*ZW10*) and *rough deal* (*ROD*), originally identified in *D. melanogaster*, are conserved among multicellular eukaryotes [126-129]. Null mutations in either gene lead to chromosome segregation defects, such as lagging chromatids, anaphase bridges and nondisjunction. These classes of chromosome aberrations cause extensive aneuploidy in mitotic and meiotic cells with disastrous consequences.

ZW10 and Rod seem to be *bona fide* checkpoint components in fly, frog and human cells [130]. In their absence, cells no longer arrest in M phase in response to spindle damage, but go on to separate sister chromatids, degrade cyclin B and exit from mitosis. Interestingly, in *C. elegans* and vertebrate cells depletion of *ZW10* and Rod homologs showed comparatively similar mitotic defects.

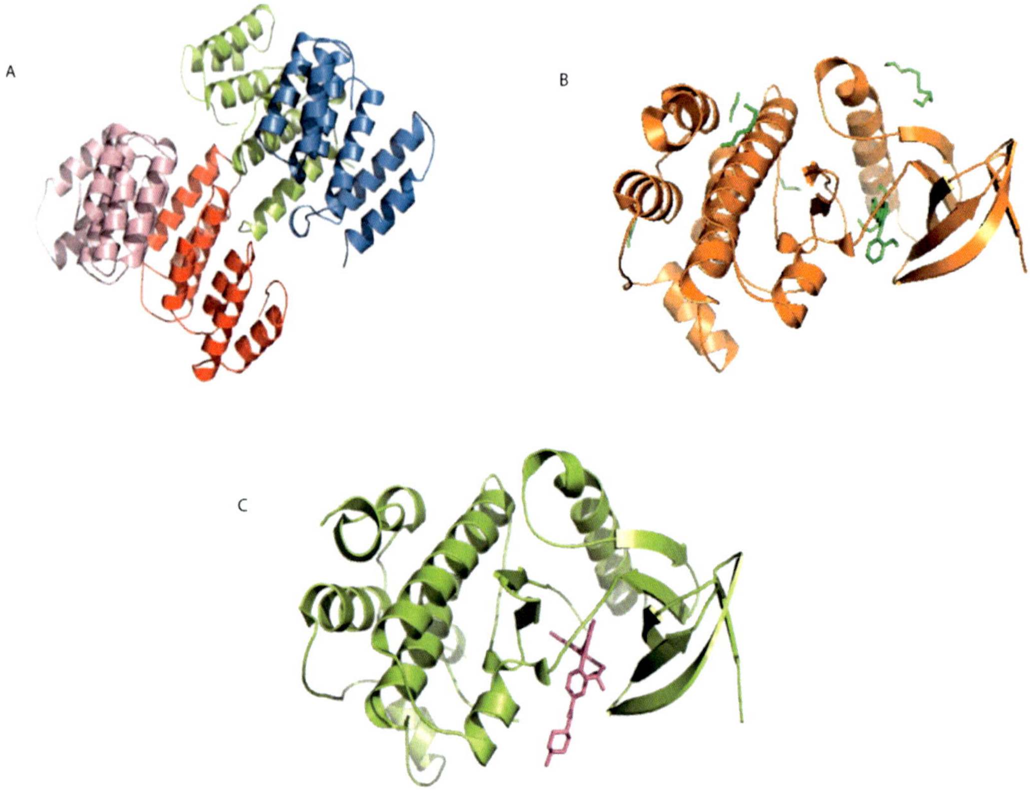

Fig. (6): A) Crystal structure of human Mps1 TPR domain (pdb 4B94). **B**) Crystal structure of Mps1 kinase domain in complex with a 1H-pyrrolo[3,2-c]pyridine compound (pdb 4C4F). **C**) Crystal structure of Mps1 kinase domain in complex with NMS-P715 inhibitor (pdb 2X9E). Figures generated with Pymol [134].

The *in vivo* immunostaining of *ZW10* [126] and Rod [127] in mitotic cells and their co-immunoprecipitation in fly and human cell extracts [128] suggested an interdependence of each other for their recruitment to the kinetochore. Analytical gel permeation chromatography showed that Rod and *ZW10* co-elute in a complex of approximately 800 kDa. A third component of the complex of an approximate molecular mass of 75kDa has been identified by immune affinity chromatography and named *ZWILCH* [131]. Remarkably, *ZWILCH* mutations produce the same mitotic phenotype as *rod* and *ZW10*, thus confirming a role of this protein in the process. *ZWILCH*, *Rod* and *ZW10* from human extracts were isolated by affinity chromatography using *ZW10* as bait [132], strongly suggesting that the three proteins form a stable complex.

The combined mass of the single polypeptide chain of Rod, *ZW10* and *ZWILCH* (240, 85, 75kDa, respectively) is about half the apparent mass of the complex. This suggests that the complex contains two copies of each protein. Further studies of the complex in solution, for example using small angle X-ray scattering (SAXS) and/or non-dissociative mass spectrometry, should provide clues of the oligomerization state of the complex which in turn should provide clues about the potential to interfere with the assembly of these proteins using small size compounds.

CLOSING REMARKS

Numerous studies of the molecular mechanism underpinning SAC signalling and the use of medicinal chemistry and drug development approaches to tackle chromosome segregation defects have been reported in the past few years. The studies have confirmed that the SAC self-monitoring cell system is an important therapeutic target. Indeed, a number of drugs that act upon SAC kinases Aurora B and Mps1 have entered clinical trials. Definition of novel drug targets and small drug compounds to interfere with catalytic activities and the assembly of SAC subcomplexes in parallel with genome-wide characterisation of SAC expression profiles in cancer cell lines should advance our understanding of the SAC pathway and therefore, help to identify the factors that confer chemotherapy drug sensitivity and resistance to human cells, thus contributing to the advancement of novel strategies for the treatment of cancer.

ACKNOWLEDGEMENTS

MK thanks OBU for financial support (Professor Nigel Groome PhD studentship).

CONFLICT OF INTEREST

The authors confirm that this chapter contents have no conflict of interest.

DISCLOSURE

The chapter submitted for the eBook Series entitled **"Advances in Cancer Drug Targets, Volume 2"** is an update of our article in **Current Cancer Drug Targets, Volume 9, Issue 2, 2009, pp. 131-141,** with additional text and references.

REFERENCES

[1] Satzinger H. Theodor and Marcella Boveri: chromosomes and cytoplasm in heredity and development. Nature Reviews Genetics 2008; 68: 231-8.

[2] Pradhan A, Singh TR, Ali AM, Wahengbam K, Meetei AR. Monopolar spindle 1 (MPS1) protein-dependent phosphorylation of RecQ-mediated genome instability protein 2 (RMI2) at serine 112 is essential for BLM-Topo III α-RMI1-RMI2 (BTR) protein complex function upon spindle assembly checkpoint (SAC) activation. J Biol Chem 2013; 288: 33500-8.

[3] Park I, Lee H, Choi E, *et al.* Loss of BubR1 acetylation causes defects in spindle assembly checkpoint signaling and promotes tumor formation. J Cell Biol 2013; 202: 295-309.

[4] Li M, Fang X, Wei Z, York JP, Zhang P. Loss of spindle assembly checkpoint-mediated inhibition of Cdc20 promotes tumorigenesis in mice. J Cell Biol 2009; 185: 983-94.

[5] Hernando E, Orlow I, Liberal V, Nohales G, Benezra R, Cordon-Cardo C. Molecular analyses of the mitotic checkpoint components hsMAD2, hBUB1 and hBUB3 in human cancer. Int J Cancer 2001; 95: 223-7.

[6] Gemma A, Seike M, Seike Y, *et al.* Somatic mutation of the hBUB1 mitotic checkpoint gene in primary lung cancer. Genes Chromosomes Cancer 2000; 29: 213-8.

[7] Ohshima K, Haraoka S, Yoshioka S, *et al.* Mutation analysis of mitotic checkpoint genes (hBUB1 and hBUBR1) and microsatellite instability in adult T-cell leukemia/lymphoma. Cancer Lett 2000; 158: 141-50.

[8] Gemoll T, Habermann JK, Becker S, *et al.* Chromosomal aneuploidy affects the global proteome equilibrium of colorectal cancer cells. Anal Cell Pathol (Amst) 2014; [Epub ahead of print].

[9] Gemoll T, Roblick UJ, Szymczak S, *et al.* HDAC2 and TXNL1 distinguish aneuploid from diploid colorectal cancers. Cell Mol Life Sci 2011; 68: 3261-74.

[10] Sudo T, Nitta M, Saya H, Ueno NT. Dependence of Paclitaxel Sensitivity on a Functional Spindle Assembly Checkpoint Dependence of Paclitaxel Sensitivity on a Functional Spindle Assembly Checkpoint. Cancer Res 2004; 64: 2502-8.

[11] Kops GJ, Weaver BA, Cleveland DW. On the road to cancer: aneuploidy and the mitotic checkpoint. Nat Rev Cancer. 2005; 5: 773-85.

[12] Kops GJ, Foltz DR, Cleveland DW. Lethality to human cancer cells through massive chromosome loss by inhibition of the mitotic checkpoint. Proc Natl Acad Sci USA 2004; 101: 8699-704.

[13] Collins I, Workman P. New approaches to molecular cancer therapeutics. Nat Chem Biol 2006; 2: 689-700.

[14] Arkin MR, Wells JA. Small-molecule inhibitors of protein-protein interactions: progressing towards the dream. Nat Rev Drug Discov 2004; 3: 301-17.

[15] White AW, Westwell AD, Brahemi G. Protein-protein interactions as targets for small-molecule therapeutics in cancer. Expert Rev Mol Med 2008; 10: e8.

[16] Wells JA, McClendon CL. Reaching for high-hanging fruit in drug discovery at protein-protein interfaces. Nature 2007; 450: 1001-9.

[17] Higueruelo AP, Jubb H, Blundell TL. Protein-protein interactions as druggable targets: recent technological advances. Curr Opin Pharmacol 2013; 13: 791-6.

[18] Surade S, Blundell TL. Structural biology and drug discovery of difficult targets: the limits of ligandability. Chem Biol 2012; 19: 42-50.

[19] Venkatesan K, Rual J, Vazquez A, *et al.* An empirical framework for binary interactome mapping. Nat Methods 2009; 6: 83-90.

[20] Young AB. Huntingtin in health and disease. J Clin Invest 2003; 111: 299-302.

[21] Bonda DJ, Lee H, Lee H, *et al.* Novel therapeutics for Alzheimer ' s disease : An update. Curr Opin Drug Discov Devel 2011; 13: 235-46.

[22] Bolton MA, Lan W, Powers SE, Mccleland ML, Kuang J, Stukenberg PT. Aurora B kinase exists in a complex with survivin and INCENP and its kinase activity is stimulated by survivin binding and phosphorylation. Mol Biol Cell 2002; 13: 3064-77.

[23] Honda R, Korner R, Nigg EA, Synchronization C. Exploring the Functional Interactions between Aurora B, INCENP, and Survivin in Mitosis. Mol Biol Cell 2003;14: 3325-41.

[24] Gassmann R, Carvalho A, Henzing AJ, *et al.* Borealin: a novel chromosomal passenger required for stability of the bipolar mitotic spindle. J Cell Biol 2004; 166: 179-91.

[25] Carmena M, Wheelock M, Funabiki H, Earnshaw WC. The chromosomal passenger complex (CPC): from easy rider to the godfather of mitosis. Nat Rev Mol Cell Biol 2012; 13: 789-803.

[26] Van der Horst A, Lens SM. Cell division: control of the chromosomal passenger complex in time and space. Chromosoma 2013; [Epub ahead of print].

[27] Hegyi K, Méhes G. Mitotic failures in cancer: Aurora B kinase and its potential role in the development of aneuploidy. Pathol Oncol Res 2012; 18: 761-9.

[28] Caldas GV, DeLuca KF, DeLuca JG. KNL1 facilitates phosphorylation of outer kinetochore proteins by promoting Aurora B kinase activity. J Cell Biol 2013; 203: 957-69.

[29] Ditchfield C, Johnson VL, Tighe A, *et al.* Aurora B couples chromosome alignment with anaphase by targeting BubR1, Mad2, and Cenp-E to kinetochores. J Cell Biol 2003; 161: 267-80.

[30] Sessa F, Mapelli M, Ciferri C, *et al.* Mechanism of Aurora B activation by INCENP and inhibition by hesperadin. Mol Cell 2005; 18: 379-91.

[31] Bayliss R, Sardon T, Vernos I, Conti E. Structural basis of Aurora-A activation by TPX2 at the mitotic spindle. Mol Cell 2003; 12: 851-62.

[32] Warner SL, Bashyam S, Vankayalapati H, *et al.* Identification of a lead small-molecule inhibitor of the Aurora kinases using a structure-assisted, fragment-based approach. Mol Cancer Ther 2006; 5: 1764-73.

[33] Gautschi O, Mack PC, Davies AM, Lara PN, Gandara DR. Aurora kinase inhibitors: a new class of targeted drugs in cancer. Clin Lung Cancer 2006; 8: 93-8.

[34] Girdler F, Gascoigne KE, Eyers P, Hartmuth S, Crafter C, Foote K M, Keen NJ, Taylor SS. Validating Aurora B as an anti-cancer drug target. J Cell Sci 2006; 119, 3664-75.

[35] Harrington E, Bebbington D, Moore J, *et al.* VX-680, a potent and selective small-molecule inhibitor of the Aurora kinases, suppresses tumor growth *in vivo*. Nat Med 2004; 10: 262-7.

[36] Cheetham, GMT, Charlton P, Golec JMC, Pollard JR. Structural basis for potent inhibition of the Aurora kinases and a T315I multi-drug resistant mutant form of Abl kinase by VX-680. Cancer Lett 2007; 251, 323-9.

[37] Hauf S, Cole RW, LaTerra S, *et al.* The small molecule Hesperadin reveals a role for Aurora B in correcting kinetochore-microtubule attachment and in maintaining the spindle assembly checkpoint. J Cell Biol 2003; 161: 281-94.

[38] Hoar K, Chakravarty A, Rabino C, Wysong D, Bowman D, Roy N, Ecsedy J. MLN8054, a small-molecule inhibitor of Aurora A, causes spindle pole and chromosome congression defects leading to aneuploidy. Mol Cell Biol 2007; 27 4513-25.

[39] Pan W, Liu H, Xu Y-J, *et al.* Pyrimido-oxazepine as a versatile template for the development of inhibitors of specific kinases. Bioorg Med Chem Lett 2005; 15: 5474-7.

[40] Wilkinson RW, Odedra R, Heaton SP, *et al.* AZD1152, a selective inhibitor of Aurora B kinase, inhibits human tumor xenograft growth by inducing apoptosis. Clinical Cancer Res 2007; 13: 3682-8.

[41] Soncini C, Carpinelli P, Gianellini L, *et al.* PHA-680632, a novel Aurora kinase inhibitor with potent antitumoral activity. Clin Cancer Res 2006; 12: 4080-9.

[42] Warner SL, Bashyam S, Vankayalapati H, Bearss DJ, Han H, Von Hoff DD, Hurley LH. Identification of a lead small-molecule inhibitor of the Aurora kinases using a structure-assisted, fragment-based approach. Mol Cancer Ther 2006; 5: 1764-73.

[43] Emanuel S, Rugg C, Gruninger RH, *et al.* The *in vitro* and *in vivo* effects of JNJ-7706621: a dual inhibitor of cyclin-dependent kinases and aurora kinases. Cancer Res 2005; 65: 9038-46.

[44] Moy C, Oleykowski C, Plant R, *et al.* High chromosome number in hematological cancer cell lines is a negative predictor of response to the inhibition of Aurora B and C by GSK1070916. J Transl Med 2011; 9: 110.

[45] Cheng C, Liu Z-G, Zhang H, *et al.* Enhancing Chemosensitivity in ABCB1- and ABCG2-Overexpressing Cells and Cancer Stem-like Cells by An Aurora Kinase Inhibitor CCT129202. Mol Pharm 2012; 9: 1971-82.

[46] Musacchio A. Spindle assembly checkpoint: the third decade. Philos Trans R Soc Lond B Biol Sci 2011; 366: 3595-604.

[47] Kiyomitsu T, Obuse C, Yanagida M. Human Blinkin/AF15q14 is required for chromosome alignment and the mitotic checkpoint through direct interaction with Bub1 and BubR1. Dev Cell 2007; 13: 663-76.

[48] Bolanos-Garcia VM, Lischetti T, Matak-Vinković D, *et al.* Structure of a Blinkin-BUBR1 Complex Reveals an Interaction Crucial for Kinetochore-Mitotic Checkpoint Regulation *via* an Unanticipated Binding Site. Structure 2011; 19: 1691-700.

[49] Bolanos-Garcia VM, Kiyomitsu T, D'Arcy S, *et al.* The crystal structure of the N-terminal region of BUB1 provides insight into the mechanism of BUB1 recruitment to kinetochores. Structure 2009; 17: 105-16.

[50] Krenn V, Overlack K, Primorac I, van Gerwen S, Musacchio A. KI Motifs of Human Knl1 Enhance Assembly of Comprehensive Spindle Checkpoint Complexes around MELT Repeats. Curr Biol 2014; 24: 29-39.

[51] Pfleger CM, Kirschner MW. The KEN box: an APC recognition signal distinct from the D box targeted by Cdh1. Genes Dev. 2000; 14: 655-65.

[52] Reddy SK, Rape M, Margansky W, Kirschner MW. Ubiquitination by the anaphase-promoting complex drives spindle checkpoint inactivation. Nature 2007; 446: 921-5.

[53] Nilsson J, Yekezare M, Minshull J, Pines J. The APC/C maintains the spindle assembly checkpoint by targeting Cdc20 for destruction. Nat Cell Biol 2009; 10: 1411-20.

[54] Han JS, Holland AJ, Fachinetti D, Kulukian A, Cetin B, Cleveland DW. Catalytic assembly of the mitotic checkpoint inhibitor BubR1-Cdc20 by a Mad2-induced functional switch in Cdc20. Mol Cell 2013; 51: 92-104.

[55] Caldas GV, Deluca JG. Mad2 "opens" Cdc20 for BubR1 binding. Mol Cell 2013; 51: 3-4.

[56] Johnson VL, Scott MIF, Holt S V, Hussein D, Taylor SS. Bub1 is required for kinetochore localization of BubR1, Cenp-E, Cenp-F and Mad2, and chromosome congression. J Cell Sci 2004;117: 1577-89.

[57] Meraldi P, Sorger PK. A dual role for Bub1 in the spindle checkpoint and chromosome congression. EMBO J. 2005; 24: 1621-33.

[58] McGuinness BE, Anger M, Kouznetsova A, *et al.* Regulation of APC/C activity in oocytes by a Bub1-dependent spindle assembly checkpoint. Curr Biol 2009; 19: 369-80.

[59] Elowe S. Bub1 and BubR1: at the interface between chromosome attachment and the spindle checkpoint. Mol Cell Biol 2011; 31: 3085-93.

[60] Klebig C, Korinth D, Meraldi P. Bub1 regulates chromosome segregation in a kinetochore-independent manner. J Cell Biol 2009; 185: 841-58.

[61] Boyarchuk Y, Salic A, Dasso M, Arnaoutov A. Bub1 is essential for assembly of the functional inner centromere. J Cell Biol 2007; 176: 919-28.

[62] Lampson M, Kapoor TM. The human mitotic checkpoint protein BubR1 regulates chromosome-spindle attachments. Nat Cell Biol 2005; 7: 93-8.

[63] Jiang H, He X, Wang S, *et al.* A Microtubule-Associated Zinc Finger Protein, BuGZ, Regulates Mitotic Chromosome Alignment by Ensuring Bub3 Stability and Kinetochore Targeting. Dev Cell 2014; 28: 268-81.

[64] Toledo CM, Herman JA, Olsen JB, *et al.* BuGZ Is Required for Bub3 Stability, Bub1 Kinetochore Function, and Chromosome Alignment. Dev Cell 2014; 28: 282-94.

[65] Ji Z, Yu H. A protective chaperone for the kinetochore adaptor bub3. Dev Cell 2014; 28: 223-4.

[66] Kang J, Yang M, Li B, Qi W, Zhang C, Shokat KM, Tomchick DR, Machius M, Yu H. Structure and substrate recruitment of the human spindle checkpoint kinase Bub1. Mol Cell 2008; 32: 394-405.

[67] Lee S, Thebault P, Freschi L, *et al.* Characterization of spindle checkpoint kinase Mps1 reveals domain with functional and structural similarities to tetratricopeptide repeat motifs of Bub1 and BubR1 checkpoint kinases. J Biol Chem 2012; 287: 5988-6001.

[68] London N, Ceto S, Ranish J a, Biggins S. Phosphoregulation of Spc105 by Mps1 and PP1 regulates Bub1 localization to kinetochores. Curr Biol 2012; 22: 900-6.

[69] Sliedrecht T, Zhang C, Shokat KM, Kops GJPL. Chemical Genetic Inhibition of Mps1 in Stable Human Cell Lines Reveals Novel Aspects of Mps1 Function in Mitosis. PLoS One 2010; 5: e10251.

[70] Slee RB, Grimes BR, Bansal R, *et al.* Selective Inhibition of Pancreatic Ductal Adenocarcinoma Cell Growth by the Mitotic MPS1 Kinase Inhibitor NMS-P715. Mol Cancer Ther 2014; 13: 307-15.

[71] Naud S, Westwood IM, Faisal A, *et al.* Structure-based design of orally bioavailable 1H-pyrrolo[3,2-c]pyridine inhibitors of mitotic kinase monopolar spindle 1 (MPS1). J Med Chem 2013; 56 :10045-65.

[72] Tannous B, Kerami M, Van der Stoop PM, *et al.* Effects of the selective MPS1 inhibitor MPS1-IN-3 on glioblastoma sensitivity to antimitotic drugs. J Natl Cancer Inst 2013; 105: 1322-31.

[73] Tipton AR, Ji W, Sturt-Gillespie B, *et al.* Monopolar Spindle 1 (MPS1) Kinase Promotes Production of Closed MAD2 (C-MAD2) Conformer and Assembly of the Mitotic Checkpoint Complex. J Biol Chem 2013; 288: 35149-58.

[74] Tardif KD, Rogers A, Cassiano J, *et al.* Characterization of the cellular and antitumor effects of MPI-0479605, a small-molecule inhibitor of the mitotic kinase Mps1. Mol Cancer Ther 2011; 10: 2267-75.

[75] Logarinho E, Resende T, Bousbaa H. The Human Spindle Assembly Checkpoint Protein Bub3 Is Required for the Establishment of Efficient Kinetochore - Microtubule Attachments. Mol Biol Cell 2008; 19: 1798-813.

[76] Tang Z, Shu H, Oncel D, Chen S, Yu H. Phosphorylation of Cdc20 by Bub1 provides a catalytic mechanism for APC/C inhibition by the spindle checkpoint. Mol Cell 2004; 16: 387-97.

[77] Primorac I, Weir JR, Chiroli E, *et al.* Bub3 reads phosphorylated MELT repeats to promote spindle assembly checkpoint signaling. Elife 2013; 2:e01030.

[78] Shepperd LA, Meadows JC, Sochaj AM, *et al.* Phospho-dependent recruitment of Bub1 and Bub3 to Spc7 / KNL1 by Mph1 kinase maintains the spindle checkpoint. Curr Biol 2012; 22: 891-9.

[79] Vleugel M, Tromer E, Omerzu M, *et al.* Arrayed BUB recruitment modules in the kinetochore scaffold KNL1 promote accurate chromosome segregation. J Cell Biol 2013; 203: 943-55.

[80] Larsen NA, Al-Bassam J, Wei RR, Harrison SC. Structural analysis of Bub3 interactions in the mitotic spindle checkpoint. Proc Natl Acad Sci USA 2007; 104: 1201-6.

[81] Wilson DK, Cerna D, Chew E. The 1.1-angstrom structure of the spindle checkpoint protein Bub3p reveals functional regions. J Biol Chem 2005; 280: 13944-51.

[82] Larsen NA, Harrison SC. Crystal structure of the spindle assembly checkpoint protein Bub3. J Mol Biol 2004; 344: 885-92.

[83] de Voer RM, van Kessel AG, *et al.* Germline mutations in the spindle assembly checkpoint genes BUB1 and BUB3 are risk factors for colorectal cancer. Gastroenterology 2013; 145: 544-7.

[84] Morais da Silva S, Moutinho-Santos T, Sunkel CE. A tumor suppressor role of the Bub3 spindle checkpoint protein after apoptosis inhibition. J Cell Biol 2013; 201: 385-93.

[85] Kruse T, Larsen MSY, Sedgwick GG, *et al.* A direct role of Mad1 in the spindle assembly checkpoint beyond Mad2 kinetochore recruitment. EMBO Rep 2014; 1-9.

[86] Tipton AR, Ji W, Sturt-Gillespie B, *et al.* Monopolar spindle 1 (MPS1) kinase promotes production of closed MAD2 (C-MAD2) conformer and assembly of the mitotic checkpoint complex. J Biol Chem 2013; 288: 35149-58.

[87] Luo X, Tang Z, Rizo J, Yu H. The Mad2 spindle checkpoint protein undergoes similar major conformational changes upon binding to either Mad1 or Cdc20. Mol Cell 2002; 9: 59-71.

[88] Kim S, Sun H, Tomchick DR, Yu H, Luo X. Structure of human Mad1 C-terminal domain reveals its involvement in kinetochore targeting. Proc Natl Acad Sci USA 2012; 109: 6549-54.

[89] Sironi L, Mapelli M, Knapp S, De Antoni A, Jeang K-T, Musacchio A. Crystal structure of the tetrameric Mad1-Mad2 core complex: implications of a "safety belt" binding mechanism for the spindle checkpoint. EMBO J 2002; 21: 2496-506.
[90] Zich J, Sochaj AM, Syred HM, *et al.* Kinase activity of fission yeast Mph1 is required for Mad2 and Mad3 to stably bind the anaphase promoting complex. Curr Biol 2012; 22: 296-301.
[91] Kim S, Sun H, Tomchick DR, Yu H, Luo X. Structure of human Mad1 C-terminal domain reveals its involvement in kinetochore targeting. Proc Natl Acad Sci USA. 2012; 109: 6549-54.
[92] Heinrich S, Sewart K, Windecker H, *et al.* Mad1 contribution to spindle assembly checkpoint signalling goes beyond presenting Mad2 at kinetochores. EMBO Rep 2014; 15: 291-8.
[93] Moyle MW, Kim T, Hattersley N, *et al.* A Bub1-Mad1 interaction targets the Mad1-Mad2 complex to unattached kinetochores to initiate the spindle checkpoint. J Cell Biol 2014; 204: 647-57.
[94] London N, Biggins S. Mad1 kinetochore recruitment by Mps1-mediated phosphorylation of Bub1 signals the spindle checkpoint. Genes Dev 2014; 28: 140-52.
[95] Schuyler SC, Wu Y-F, Kuan VJ-W. The Mad1-Mad2 balancing act - a damaged spindle checkpoint in chromosome instability and cancer. J Cell Sci 2012; 125: 4197-206.
[96] Iwanaga Y, Chi Y-H, Miyazato A, *et al.* Heterozygous deletion of mitotic arrest-deficient protein 1 (MAD1) increases the incidence of tumors in mice. Cancer Res 2007; 67: 160-6.
[97] Ryan SD, Britigan EMC, Zasadil LM, *et al.* Up-regulation of the mitotic checkpoint component Mad1 causes chromosomal instability and resistance to microtubule poisons. Proc Natl Acad Sci USA 2012; 109: E2205-14.
[98] Listovsky T, Sale JE. Sequestration of CDH1 by MAD2L2 prevents premature APC/C activation prior to anaphase onset. J Cell Biol 2013; 203: 87-100.
[99] Yu L, Liu S, Guo W, Zhang B, Liang Y, Feng Q. Upregulation of Mad2 facilitates *in vivo* and *in vitro* osteosarcoma progression. Oncol Rep 2012; 28: 2170-6.
[100] Park PE, Jeong JY, Kim SZ, Park JY. MAD2 Expression in Ovarian Carcinoma: Different Expression Patterns and Levels among Various Types of Ovarian Carcinoma and Its Prognostic Significance in High-Grade Serous Carcinoma. Korean J Pathol 2013; 47: 418-25.
[101] Li L, Xu D-B, Zhao X-L, Hao T-Y. Combination analysis of Bub1 and Mad2 expression in endometrial cancer: act as a prognostic factor in endometrial cancer. Arch Gynecol Obstet 2013; 288: 155-65.
[102] Bian Y, Kitagawa R, Bansal PK, Fujii Y, Stepanov A, Kitagawa K. Synthetic genetic array screen identifies PP2A as a therapeutic target in Mad2-overexpressing tumors. Proc Natl Acad Sci USA 2014; 111: 1628-33.
[103] Hein JB, Nilsson J. Stable MCC binding to the APC/C is required for a functional spindle assembly checkpoint. EMBO Rep. 2014; 15: 264-72.
[104] Davenport J, Harris LD, Goorha R. Spindle checkpoint function requires Mad2-dependent Cdc20 binding to the Mad3 homology domain of BubR1. Exp Cell Res 2006; 312: 1831-42.
[105] Kulukian A, Han JS, Cleveland DW. Unattached kinetochores catalyze production of an anaphase inhibitor that requires a Mad2 template to prime Cdc20 for BubR1 binding. Dev Cell 2009; 16: 105-17.

[106] Jia L, Kim S, Yu H. Tracking spindle checkpoint signals from kinetochores to APC/C. Trends Biochem Sci 2013; 38: 302-11.
[107] Tian W, Li B, Warrington R, Tomchick DR, Yu H, Luo X. Structural analysis of human Cdc20 supports multisite degron recognition by APC/C. Proc Natl Acad Sci USA. 2012; 109: 18419-24.
[108] Reis A, Levasseur M, Chang H, Elliott DJ, Jones KT. EMBO Rep 2006;7: 1040-5.
[109] Huang JN. Activity of the APCCdh1 form of the anaphase-promoting complex persists until S phase and prevents the premature expression of Cdc20p. J Cell Biol 2001; 154: 85-94.
[110] Izawa D, Pines J. Mad2 and the APC/C compete for the same site on Cdc20 to ensure proper chromosome segregation. J Cell Biol 2012; 199: 27-37.
[111] Cheng L, Yang T, Kuang Y, *et al.* MicroRNA-23a promotes neuroblastoma cell metastasis by targeting CDH1. Oncol Lett 2014; 7: 839-45.
[112] Moura IM, Delgado ML, Silva PM, Lopes CA, do Amaral JB, Monteiro LS, Bousbaa H. High CDC20 expression is associated with poor prognosis in oral squamous cell carcinoma. J Oral Pathol Med 2014; 43(3): 225-31.
[113] Choi J-W, Kim Y, Lee J-H, Kim Y-S. High expression of spindle assembly checkpoint proteins CDC20 and MAD2 is associated with poor prognosis in urothelial bladder cancer. Virchows Arch 2013; 463: 681-7.
[114] Chang DZ, Ma Y, Ji B, *et al.* Increased CDC20 expression is associated with pancreatic ductal adenocarcinoma differentiation and progression. J Hematol Oncol 2012; 5: 15.
[115] Wu W, Hu K, Wang D, *et al.* CDC20 overexpression predicts a poor prognosis for patients with colorectal cancer. J Transl Med 2013; 11: 142.
[116] Kato T, Daigo Y, Aragaki M, Ishikawa K, Sato M, Kaji M. Overexpression of CDC20 predicts poor prognosis in primary non-small cell lung cancer patients. J Surg Oncol 2012; 106: 423-30.
[117] Majumder P, Bhunia S, Bhattacharyya J, Chaudhuri A. Inhibiting tumor growth by targeting liposomally encapsulated CDC20siRNA to tumor vasculature: Therapeutic RNA interference. J Control Release. 2014; 180C:100-108.
[118] Kitagawa K, Abdulle R, Bansal PK, Cagney G, Fields S, Hieter P. Requirement of Skp1-Bub1 interaction for kinetochore-mediated activation of the spindle checkpoint. Mol Cell 2003; 11: 1201-13.
[119] Liu D, Zhang N, Du J, *et al.* Interaction of Skp1 with CENP-E at the midbody is essential for cytokinesis. Biochem Biophys Res Commun 2006; 345: 394-402.
[120] Freed E, Lacey KR, Huie P, *et al.* Components of an SCF ubiquitin ligase localize to the centrosome and regulate the centrosome duplication cycle. Genes Dev 1999; 13: 2242-57.
[121] Wang X, Babu JR, Harden JM, *et al.* The mitotic checkpoint protein hBUB3 and the mRNA export factor hRAE1 interact with GLE2p-binding sequence (GLEBS)-containing proteins. J Biol Chem 2001; 276: 26559-67.
[122] Blower MD, Nachury M, Heald R, Weis K. A Rae1-containing ribonucleoprotein complex is required for mitotic spindle assembly. Cell 2005; 121: 223-34.
[123] Sitterlin D. Characterization of the Drosophila Rae1 protein as a G1 phase regulator of the cell cycle. Gene 2004; 326: 107-16.
[124] Pritchard CE, Fornerod M, Kasper LH, van Deursen JM. RAE1 is a shuttling mRNA export factor that binds to a GLEBS-like NUP98 motif at the nuclear pore complex through multiple domains. J Cell Biol 1999; 145: 237-54.

[125] Babu JR, Jeganathan KB, Baker DJ, Wu X, Kang-Decker N, van Deursen JM. Rae1 is an essential mitotic checkpoint regulator that cooperates with Bub3 to prevent chromosome missegregation. J Cell Biol 2003; 160: 341-53.

[126] Williams BC, Karr TL, Montgomery JM, Goldberg ML. The Drosophila l(1)*ZW10* gene product, required for accurate mitotic chromosome segregation, is redistributed at anaphase onset. J Cell Biol 1992; 118: 759-73.

[127] Scaërou F, Aguilera I, Saunders R, Kane N, Blottière L, Karess R. The rough deal protein is a new kinetochore component required for accurate chromosome segregation in Drosophila. J Cell Sci 1999; 112: 3757-68.

[128] Scaërou F, Starr DA, Piano F, Papoulas O, Karess RE, Goldberg ML. The *ZW10* and Rough Deal checkpoint proteins function together in a large, evolutionarily conserved complex targeted to the kinetochore. J Cell Sci 2001; 114: 3103-14.

[129] Karess RE, Glover DM. rough deal: a gene required for proper mitotic segregation in Drosophila. J Cell Biol 1989; 109: 2951-61.

[130] Karess R. Rod-*ZW10-ZWILCH*: a key player in the spindle checkpoint. Trends Cell Biol 2005; 15: 386-92.

[131] Williams BC, Li Z, Liu S, *et al. ZWILCH*, a New Component of the *ZW10* / ROD Complex Required for Kinetochore Functions. Mol Biol Cell 2003;14: 1379-91.

[132] Kops GJPL, Kim Y, Weaver BAA, *et al. ZW10* links mitotic checkpoint signaling to the structural kinetochore. J Cell Biol 2005; 169: 49-60.

[133] Mao Y, Abrieu A, Cleveland DW. Activating and silencing the mitotic checkpoint through CENP-E-dependent activation/inactivation of BubR1. Cell 2003; 114: 87-98.

[134] The PyMOL Molecular Graphics System, Version 1.7 Schrödinger, LLC.

CHAPTER 3

ErbB Receptors as a Therapeutic Target in Metastatic Cancer Disease

Adriano Angelucci*

Department of Biotechnological and Applied Clinical Sciences, University of L'Aquila, L'Aquila, Italy

Abstract: The very early intuition by Paget about the molecular features of metastasis has been observed in the field of therapeutic opportunities only in the last few years with the development of targeted therapy. However, to date, the diagnosis of metastases is associated in the majority of cases with the loss of any therapeutic hope. According to present knowledge, metastatic spread is considered a part of a long process in which tumor cells gain new properties regarding their cellular function, including invasion and adaptive survival. This gain of function is based on the expression of new molecular markers that may be potential therapeutic targets in blocking tumor diffusion. The epidermal growth receptor family (ErbB) comprises four members that are frequently upregulated in advanced tumor stages and have been associated with the metastatic potential of several tumors. Several inhibitors specific for one ErbB receptor have been demonstrated to be effective antitumor agents in primary cancer, but their utilization is restricted to ErbB-overexpressing tumors and limited by toxicity problems, drug resistance and molecular desensitization. However, new studies indicate that ErbB inhibitors may provide a much-needed therapeutic option, mainly for patients with metastases. In order to illustrate the potential of ErbB family members as therapeutic targets in blocking metastases, we summarize the latest molecular evidence and the results of clinical trials.

Keywords: Cancer metastasis, clinical trials, EGF, epidermal growth factor, HER2, targeted therapy, tumor invasion, trastuzumab, tyrosine kinases.

ErbB RECEPTORS IN CANCER PROGRESSION

ErbB Receptors: Structure and Functions

ErbB (avian erythroblastic leukemia viral oncogene homolog) receptors, because their ubiquitous expression in carcinomas and function as master regulators of

***Corresponding Author Adriano Angelucci:** Department of Biotechnological and Applied Clinical Sciences, University of L'Aquila, *via* Vetoio, Coppito 2, 67100 L'Aquila, Italy; Tel: +39-862-433550; Fax: +39-862-433523; E-mail: adriano.angelucci@univaq.it

cancer cell survival and proliferation, have been extensively studied as anti-tumor targets. However, one of the most important lessons derived from these studies was the necessity to have a deep understanding of the mechanisms controlling ErbB receptor activation. For this reason, the first part of this review is dedicated to the molecular features that have a major impact on treatment decisions about the use of ErbB inhibitors in metastatic disease.

The ErbB receptors belong to the family of protein tyrosine kinases (class I receptor protein kinases) and comprise four members: ErbB1 (epidermal growth factor receptor, EGFR; chromosomal location 7p12.3-p12.1); ErbB2 (neuroblastoma or glioblastoma-derived, NEU; human epidermal growth factor receptor 2, HER2; chromosomal location 17q21.1); ErbB3 (human epidermal growth factor receptor 3, HER3; chromosomal location 12q13); ErbB4 (human epidermal growth factor receptor 4, HER4; chromosomal location 2q33.3-q34). The ErbB proteins have four regions: one projects outside the cell, containing the site for binding extracellular ligands, and consists of four domains (I-IV); the second is embedded in the membrane; the third and the fourth project into the cytoplasm and contain the kinase domain and several tyrosine phosphorylation sites, respectively (Fig. **1**). ErbB3 contains the extracellular ligand-binding domain but lacks the intracellular tyrosine kinase moiety due to substitutions in critical residues in its kinase domain [1].

Under physiological conditions, the activation of signaling pathways downstream of ErbB receptors is regulated by their level of expression and the availability of their ligands. The ligands of ErbB receptors are structurally related polypeptides grouped in the EGF family. ErbB1 specifically binds to epidermal growth factor (EGF), transforming growth factor alpha (TGF-α), epigen (EPGN), amphiregulin (AR), epiregulin (EPR), betacellulin (BTC), and heparin binding EGF (HB-EGF). The last three ligands can also bind ErbB4. The EGF family of proteins includes other important ligands, *i.e.* neuregulins (NRGs, also known as NEU differentiation factor, NDF or heregulins, HRGs), that have key roles in the development of the heart and neuronal system, as well as in the formation of neuromuscular synapses. NRGs bind ErbB3 (NRG1 and 2) and ErbB4 (NRG1, 2, 3 and 4) (Fig. **2**). The ErbB2 receptor does not bind directly to any known ligand and functions as a preferential co-receptor for the other members of the ErbB family. Ligand binding to ErbB receptors stimulates the formation of receptor homo or heterodimers and, in turn, the cross-phosphorylation of specific residues in the C-terminal tail of the partnering receptor (Fig. **1**).

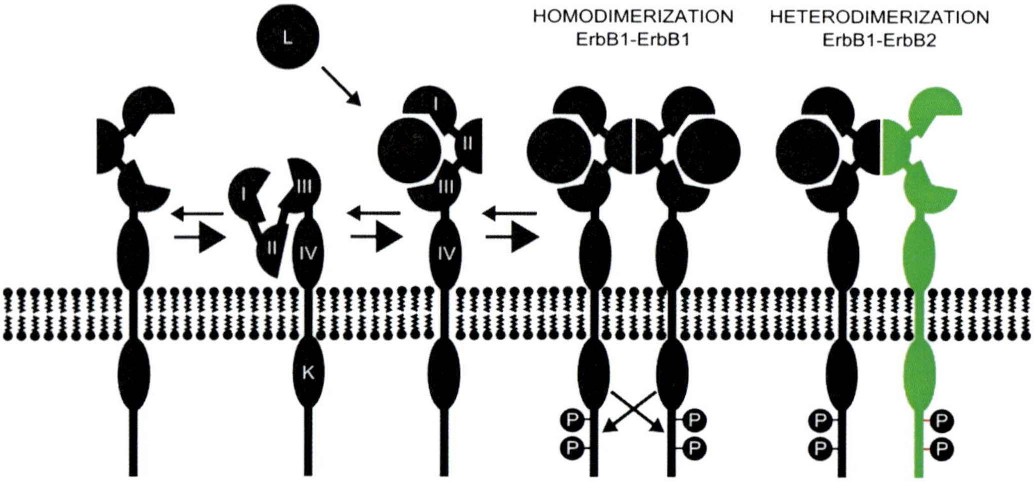

Fig. (1): Structure and activation of ErbB receptors. The unbound receptor is prevalently present on the cell membrane in the closed form. The ligand (L) binding to domain I and III stabilizes the open form of the receptor in which domain II permits homodimerization or heterodimerization. The formation of a dimer stimulates the phosphorylation of the docking region by the kinase domain (K).

The pattern of all the possible combinations of ErbB receptor dimers and ligands produces complex activation profiles. The degree of activation by a particular ligand to a receptor is variable and may justify the functional predominance of certain combinations of dimers over others [2]. Moreover, there are preferred heterodimers that form between ErbB2 and ErbB receptors in response to specific EGF family peptides [3]. For example, several biochemical studies have shown that ErbB2 is the preferred dimerization partner for ErbB3 and ErbB4 upon NRG stimulation [3, 4]. BTC promotes ErbB4 as well as ErbB1 dimers with ErbB2, but not with ErbB3. EGF primarily induces ErbB1/ErbB2 heterodimers [5].

Recent studies have permitted the clarification of the process of ligand-induced receptor dimerization. The crystal structure of ErbB receptors has revealed that extracellular domains I and III are responsible for ligand binding, and that ligands are not directly involved in receptor dimerization [6, 7]. The dimerization function is performed by residues in domain II that are normally masked in the unliganded form of the receptor. Only ErbB2 differs significantly in the native conformation of its extracellular domain. ErbB2 has a unique conformation in which domain II is always available for receptor-receptor binding (Fig. **1**) [8].

Receptor dimerization results in auto- and trans-phosphorylation of intracellular domains. The phosphorylated forms of these receptors then serve as docking sites for several proteins containing Src homology 2 (SH2) or phosphotyrosine binding (PTB) domains that function as second messengers responsible for transducing downstream signaling cascades (Fig. **2**). Different combinations of dimers can drive specific signaling cascades. The differentiation in downstream signaling pathways is mainly mediated by three different mechanisms: the presence of several docking sites within each receptor, a distinct pattern of docking sites among different members (for an accurate description of the phosphotyrosine interactome, see [9]) (Fig. **2**), and new signaling properties acquired by heterodimers [10, 11]. At present, it is unclear if each ErbB family member has a specific signaling role, but several indications suggest that ErbB1 and ErbB4 function as pivotal controllers, while ErbB2 and ErbB3 are modulators. In fact, ErbB1 and ErbB4 are the only two fully functional receptors of the family, and they can activate similar downstream processes in response to their different ligands. Moreover, ErbB1 and ErbB4 are rarely co-expressed in the same cell. On the other hand, ErbB2 and ErbB3 are usually described as the preferred binding partners of ErbB1 of ErbB4, and differences in the interaction partner, especially for ErbB3, indicate a specific role of the heterodimer [9]. Because compensatory activation by heterodimerization could be the reason for resistance phenomena, the use of a broad spectrum inhibitor could result in more effective in blocking downstream signaling. Canertinib is a next generation tyrosine kinase inhibitor able to alkylate and irreversibly inhibit the activation of ErbB1, 2 and 4 [12]. In preclinical models, canertinib was found to be very selective for ErbB receptors, and it exhibited a broad spectrum of antiproliferative activity in several different types of cancer, including colorectal carcinoma, head and neck carcinoma and breast cancer (BrCa) [13, 14]. The use of pan-ErbB inhibitors has opened new therapeutic perspectives, as recently demonstrated by the preclinical and clinical use of neratinib, an oral, small-molecule inhibitor that irreversibly binds to pan-ErbB receptor tyrosine kinases [15, 16].

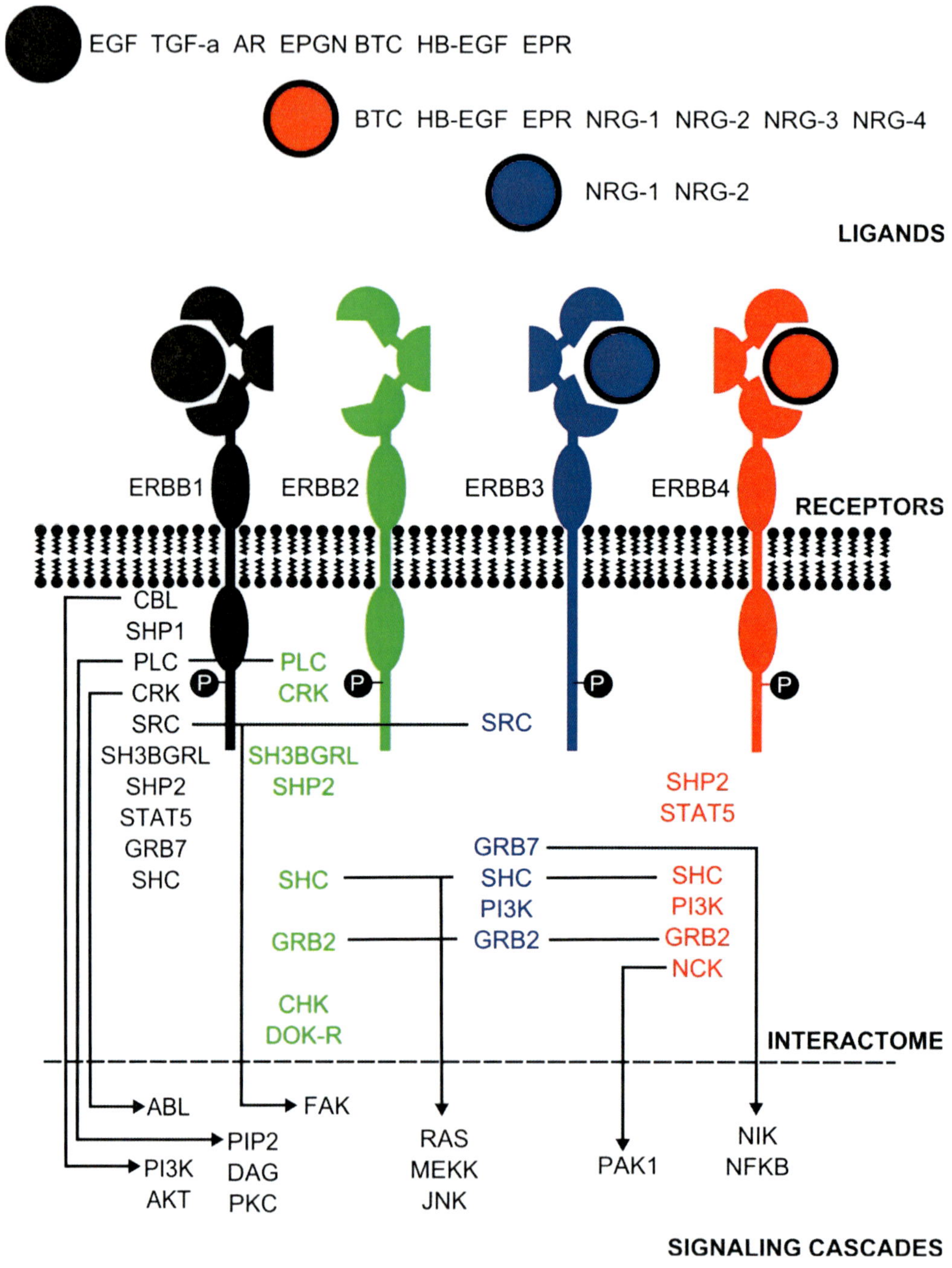

Fig. (2): The signaling flux modulated by ErbB receptors is schematically divided into distinct spatial and temporal layers. The specificity of ligands and adaptor proteins is indicated by the same color of the receptor. In the signaling cascade, only representative factors are shown.

Modulation of ErbB Receptor Signaling

In addition to heterodimerization, other mechanisms of modulation of ErbB receptors signaling have been described. These include the status of signaling molecules in downstream intracellular pathways, receptor endocytosis and the expression of variant forms of receptors. There is a general consensus on the hypothesis that alterations in key downstream molecules involved in ErbB signaling is one of most frequently encountered mechanisms involved in the resistance to ErbB inhibitors [17]. In this regard, it has been hypothesized that the PI3K/AKT axis is the main signaling pathway involved in resistance to anti-ErbB1 agents [18]. In the presence of a constitutively active PI3K/AKT pathway, sensitivity to the ErbB1 inhibitor gefitinib was restored by inhibiting PI3K [19].

The ErbB receptors are downmodulated through receptor-mediated endocytosis. Endocytosis regulates the persistence of signaling after ligand-induced activation. Significantly, ligand/receptor complexes that remain stable within endosomes (such as EGF/ErbB1) are efficiently degraded, while other complexes that are more dynamic (such as those containing TGF-α and NRG) are associated with receptor recycling. This mechanism of control is particularly important for ErbB1 [20] and may be contrasted by overexpression of ErbB2 [21].

Another source of signaling complexity may derive from the existence of variant forms. Alternative protein forms of ErbB receptors are generated by differential splicing or proteolytic processing. Variant forms of ErbB1, ErbB2 and ErbB3 have been frequently described in cancers. A variant form of ErbB2 is thought to have a role in carcinogenesis [22], while an extracellularly truncated form of ErbB2 has been associated with lymph node metastasis [23].

Further complications in the mechanisms controlling ErbB signaling have been described in *D. melanogaster*, but these await confirmation in mammals [24].

Physiological Functions of ErbB Receptors

Data from studies regarding the physiological roles of ErbB receptors may help anti-cancer therapeutic approaches in two important ways: targeted therapies may promote side effects when the target is physiologically relevant and the provision of anti-tumor efficacy through an indirect mechanism targeting tumor-associated normal cells. In fact, it is well-known that neighboring normal cells play an important adjuvant role in the growth of tumor cells both at primary and metastatic sites.

Under physiological conditions, ErbB receptors are expressed at highly variable levels in a variety of tissues and cells of epithelial, mesothelial, endothelial, and neuronal origin where they elicit broad biological functions, including organ development, maintenance of cell proliferation and differentiation, and the regulation of tissue homeostasis [25]. Animal models have demonstrated that ErbB members are fundamental in many phases of development. Studies utilizing null mice have demonstrated that multiple abnormalities, usually lethal at different stages of development, are associated with ErbB receptors. These studies strengthen the hypothesis that ErbBs regulate a wide range of cellular activities. Mice lacking ErbB receptors die mainly due to severely abnormal development of the ventricles, peripheral nervous system and gastrointestinal lining.

ErbB1-/- mice have defects in semilunar valve formation [26], in the central and peripheral nervous system, in bone formation [27, 28] and they also display several abnormalities in epithelial tissues [29-31]. The study of neuronal defects in ErbB1 deficient mice have permitted the association between ErbB1 activation and the proliferation and differentiation of astrocytes and the survival and migration of postmitotic neurons [32, 33]. ErbB2 null mice embryos also have lethal cardiac defects [34]. Other authors have shown that ErbB2, normally expressed in Schwann and muscle cells, is essential for the *in vivo* development of the neuromuscular junction [35]. Most ErbB3-knockout embryos die before birth, without Schwann cell precursors and Schwann cells that normally accompany peripheral axons of sensory and motor neurons [36]. ErbB4 deficient mouse embryos develop a severe abnormal neuronal morphology compatible with a model in which ErbB4 signaling provides patterning information essential for the proper migration of neural crest cells [37]. This abnormal migration of neurons is also associated with other defective phenotypes found in mice lacking neuronal ErbB4 expression [38].

ErbB receptors are also implicated in postnatal somatic growth. One of the first biological activities of ErbB1 activation to be recognized *in vivo* was its ability to accelerate epidermal differentiation, causing premature eyelid opening in newborn mice [39]. In normal skin, ErbB1 is expressed mainly in the basal layer of the epidermis, and it has been shown to stimulate cell cycle progression of normal epidermal keratinocytes through autocrine and paracrine mechanisms. Activation of ErbB receptors plays an important role in the regulation of cell proliferation, as well as differentiation in various tissues, including the mammary gland [40], the gastrointestinal tract [41], and the nervous system [33].

In the mammary gland, all four ErbB receptors are expressed in cell type- and developmental stage-specific patterns [42, 43]. The major function of ErbB1 is in promoting ductal growth, while ErbB2 and ErbB4 have a key role in lobuloalveolar differentiation and lactation. Studies on the development of the mammary gland have highlighted significant data regarding how the specificity of action of ErbB receptors is regulated by their ligands. These data indicate that although functional redundancy in the roles of ErbB ligands is frequent, some ligands make specific contributions to mammary gland development. For example, AR expression is particularly elevated during duct development, and its deficiency, but not that of EGF or TGF-α, is associated with impaired ductal growth [44]. Recent findings have also linked ErbB members to cognitive dysfunctions. Silberberg concluded that NRG1 and ErbB4 are components of a biological pathway involved in schizophrenia, perhaps by affecting neuronal migration and resulting in alterations in cortical connectivity [45].

In the last few years, several studies have demonstrated some important functions of EGF and EGF-like ligands in regulating bone growth and remodeling (see review [46]). ErbB1 seems to be involved in the regulation of the metabolism of all the principal cell types present in bone, allowing the proper development of the long bones. In particular, ErbB1 signaling promotes proliferation but prohibits differentiation or maturation of growth plate chondrocytes and metaphyseal bone osteoblasts, and ErbB1 ligands also promote the formation and function of bone resorptive osteoclasts. In addition, ErbB1 signaling appears to regulate bone homeostasis and regeneration potential by promoting proliferation but suppressing differentiation of bone marrow mesenchymal stem cells.

Oncogenic Functions of ErbB Receptors

The ErbB receptor-activated signaling pathway was first proposed as a potential target for anti-cancer therapy in the early 1980s, after studying ErbB1, the prototypic member of the ErbB family [47]. Aberrant signaling from ErbB receptors has been implicated in the pathogenesis of a number of different tumors, including skin, breast, colorectal, head and neck, glioblastoma, lung, ovarian, and pancreatic cancer [48]. Several observations indicate that abnormalities in the expression of ErbB1 and/or its ligands are common features in the development of skin tumors. In studies on transgenic mice, overexpression of TGF-α targeted to the epidermis led to the development of hyperplasia, hyperkeratosis, papillomas, and squamous cell carcinomas [49]. Whether amplified wild-type ErbB1 in the absence of ligands contributes to oncogenesis remains to be established [50, 51]. A family with germ line mutations in ErbB1 has been identified [52]. In this family of European descent, six family members in three generations had lung cancer, three with the broncholoalveolar carcinoma subtype of adenocarcinoma. The variable oncogenic potential demonstrated by overexpression of a single ErbB receptor suggests the importance of cooperation among different members of the family. Overexpression of ErbB1 in the mouse mammary gland induces infrequent adenocarcinomas, while ErbB2 overexpression induces more frequent mammary tumors with relatively short latency [53, 54]. In addition, the ErbB2 receptor is able to induce with high efficiency the transformation of fibroblasts, and ErbB1 is almost 100-fold weaker than ErbB2 in its transforming ability [55, 56]. Although the data are not always in agreement, the overexpression of ErbB2 in NSCLC may stimulate the activation of ErbB1 and consequently sensitize to ErbB1 inhibitor treatment [57]. ErbB2 overexpression in normal fibroblasts augments the effect of EGF on the transformed phenotype [58], while ErbB4-induced transformation of fibroblasts requires co-expression of either ErbB1 or ErbB2 [59, 60].

Oncogenic Activation: Mutation *vs* Overexpression

The pro-oncogenic role of ErbB receptors depend on abnormal activation caused by gain-of-function somatic mutations, by gene amplification, or by protein overexpression. The contribution of each of these mechanisms is highly variable in distinct tumors and does not permit the formulation of a unique hypothesis. The hunt for somatic mutations has frequently failed in several cancers. However, ErbB1 gene mutations have been reported in many tumors, and in nearly all cases, alterations have been reported in tumors with ErbB1 amplification [61]. It is plausible that, for the ErbB1 receptor, the concomitant presence of amplification and activation mutations offer a net advantage in terms of tumor survival. Although non-small cell lung cancer (NSCLC) expresses ErbB1 at a variable rate of 40%-85%, somatic mutations in the tyrosine kinase domain of ErbB1 have been identified in about 10% of these tumors [62]. Two of the most commonly occurring ErbB1 somatic mutations, ErbB1 L858R and ErbB1 Del(746-750), enhance downstream ErbB1 signaling pathways and influence cell survival [63, 64]. A mutant ErbB1 (ErbB1vIII) that lacks 267 amino acids from its extracellular domain, resulting in the formation of a new, tumor-specific target, is found in 27% of breast carcinomas and 52% of gliomas [65]. ErbB1 kinase domain mutations are almost exclusively found in a small population of NSCLC, and rare mutations are also found in head and neck cancers (SCCHN), cholangiocarcinomas, and cancers of the colon, esophagus and pancreas [66-69]. The frequency and the clinical impact of mutations in ErbB3 and ErbB4 remain to be elucidated.

Other aspects limit the contribution of ErbB1 somatic mutations in tumorigenesis. First, experience from clinical trials suggests that ErbB kinase mutation status is a poor predictor of patient survival [70]. Second, the effect of these mutations seems to be cell type-specific, in terms of both overall activation and heterodimerization with specific ErbB members [71]. Interestingly, mutations in more than one of the genes for ErbB receptors are rarely encountered in a single tumor.

Overexpression is a more frequent event with respect to mutation in different tumors. Hyperexpression associated with ErbB1 gene amplification is seen in more than 50% of glioblastomas [72]. Protein overexpression without gene amplification has been reported in 12-38% of glioblastomas [73, 74] and in 55% of colorectal cancer tumors [75], suggesting that multiple ways of deregulation in ErbB1 expression may exist at the translational and post-translational levels. ErbB1 overexpression is observed in >50% of BrCas and correlates with estrogen receptor-negative status, poor tumor grade, and aneuploidy [76]. Up to 90% of high-grade astrocytic gliomas express ErbB1, which is associated with ErbB1 gene amplification in 40–50% of glioblastoma multiforme [72, 77]. The presence of an increased copy number of wild-type ErbB1 renders some tumors sensitive to treatment with the ErbB1 inhibitor, gefitinib, providing a strong correlation with the outcome, especially survival, with respect to ErbB1 mutation [57].

Early observations indicated that the *erbb2* gene is frequently amplified in tumor cells. On the contrary, an activated mutant form of ErbB2 is rarely found in human cancers [78]. Mutations in the kinase domain of ErbB2 have been identified in a small number of NSCLCs [79]. An activating mutation (Val to Glu 659) in ErbB2 gene was shown to increase metastatic potential in a CRC murine experimental model [80]. Overexpression of the wild-type ErbB2 protein, amplification of the ErbB2 gene, or both, occur in 20-25% of BrCa [81]. By microarray analysis, it was possible to describe a specific subtype of ErbB2-overexpressing BrCa [82]. These studies have reinforced the hypothesis of a strict association between the ErbB2 positive BrCa subtype and a high rate of recurrence and short disease-free intervals after adjuvant chemotherapy. Distant metastases are more frequent in the ErbB2 overexpressing subtype than other BrCa subtypes, and leads to a poorer prognosis in the BrCa subgroup. To date, ErbB2 status, together with ER status, is thought the most important prognostic factor of BrCa [83]. Patients with ErbB2-positive metastatic BrCa are less likely to respond to hormone treatment than ErbB2-negative patients, and their survival expectation is also shorter [84].

ErbB3 is overexpressed or amplified in cell lines [85] and primary tumor tissues from human BrCa [86]. Moreover, high ErbB3 protein expression has been linked with a poor prognosis in NSCLC [87] and oral squamous cell carcinoma [88]. At the same time, the overexpression of ErbB3 or ErbB4 seems to be more important when co-expressed with ErbB1 or ErbB2 rather than as a driving event. ErbB3 expression is frequently seen in association with ErbB2 overexpression in several cancers, including breast, bladder, and melanoma [89-91]. The co-expression of ErbB4 appears to be biologically significant in childhood medulloblastomas [92].

ErbB RECEPTORS AND METASTASIS

Expression of ErbB Receptors During Tumor Progression

Cancer is the second leading cause of death in western countries. The probability of developing an invasive cancer is 50% in men and 33% in women. The mean probability of finding metastases in cancer patients at diagnosis is 20% in all tumors, and is particularly high in cancers of the lung, pancreas, stomach and ovary. The five-year survival rate with the presence of metastasis dramatically decreases to less than 30% with respect to confined tumors [93]. Although their involvement in carcinogenesis is probably limited, data have accumulated in the last few years, mainly regarding ErbB1 and ErbB2, to suggest that ErbB receptors have a pivotal role in tumor progression. ErbB1 is upregulated during the metastatic progression of different tumors. Enhanced activity or overexpression of ErbB1 has been associated with tumor progression and poor survival in head and neck [94], gastrointestinal tract [95], bladder [96], and colon cancers [97]. Moreover, ErbB1 is expressed in 80% of invasive ductal adenocarcinomas of the pancreas [98]. ErbB1 is also a biomarker of lymph node metastasis and extracapsular spread of oral tongue squamous carcinoma [99]. In addition, also when expressed at a high frequency in the primary tumor, such as for SCCHN, microarray analysis has revealed the presence of a more aggressive TGF-α-expressing tumor subpopulation that demonstrated a higher propensity to metastasize [100]. Moreover, as verified by preclinical models, ErbB1 expression is fundamental in resuming a high proliferation rate in dormant metastatic cells [101]. In other tumors, the involvement of ErbB1 in progression is less clear and is probably linked to the expression of specific mutants or variants, such as for NSCLC. Preclinical studies seem to indicate an effective action of ErbB receptor inhibitors in blocking the metastatic spread of various tumor cells. The oral administration of the ErbB1 tyrosine kinase inhibitor, PKI 166, inhibited progressive growth and metastasis of human pancreatic cancer implanted orthotopically in nude mice [102]. In mouse models, gefitinib inhibited the formation of metastases in murine hepatocellular carcinoma tumors [103] and in PCa [104].

A significant correlation between a more aggressive course of cancer disease and ErbB2 overexpression has been frequently described in different cancers. Early studies conducted in BrCa demonstrated that high levels of expression of ErbB2 were positively correlated with lymph node metastasis [81, 105]. This phenomenon is confirmed by the *in vivo* observation that NIH 3T3 fibroblasts transformed with an activating mutant form of ErbB2 gene became high metastatic [106]. More recently, it was demonstrated that the overexpression of wild-type ErbB2 can promote the invasive and metastatic potential of a human BrCa cell line [107].

The expression of ErbB2 protein in colorectal cancer (CRC) tissue correlates closely with liver metastasis, but not with lymphatic or lung metastases [108, 109]. The ErbB2 positivity rate (65%), as determined by immunohistochemistry, was significantly higher in metastatic liver tumors than in primary tumors of the stomach (38%) [110]. ErbB2 protein-positive staining was detected in 7, 16 and 29% of early, advanced and recurrent or inoperable metastatic stomach cancers, respectively [111]. Although data from NSCLC are not always in concordance, a significant, unfavorable prognostic effect of ErbB2 overexpression has been shown in many studies [112]. Interestingly, while the overexpression of ErbB1 alone does not have a prognostic value in NSCLC, synchronous overexpression of ErbB1 and ErbB2 at the protein level predicts increased recurrence risk and may predict decreased survival in patients with stage I NSCLC [113].

Hormone-dependent cancers, prostate cancer (PCa) and BrCa, despite all available therapeutic approaches, evolve frequently toward a hormone refractory, metastatic phase. It has been postulated that this type of progression is supported by the activation of growth factor receptors, including the ErbB receptors. During antihormone challenge in BrCa, the induction of ErbB1 can comprise an important mechanism for promoting residual growth, cell survival signaling activity and metastatic progression [114]. ErbB2-overexpressing cancers are usually associated with a poor prognosis and account for about 30% of metastatic BrCa in women. For this reason, and since the first observation in 1987, ErbB2 amplification is used in breast carcinoma as an independent prognostic indicator of patient survival and is correlated with the occurrence of metastasis and micrometastatic bone marrow disease [81, 115]. However, ErbB2-overexpression in BrCa does not increase the probability of developing bone metastases. Recent studies suggest that the nature of the effect of ErbB2 status on distant recurrence rates vary considerably from site to site and is dependent on ER status. For liver, distant lymph node and bone recurrences, there is a significant effect of ErbB2 overexpression, independent of ER status [116]. Circulating levels of the extracellular domain of ErbB2 are elevated in 35-40% of patients with metastatic BrCa and are associated with a poorer prognosis in these patients [117]. The detection of ErbB2 status in metastatic patients with PCa has been suggested as a marker of an unfavorable prognosis and for predicting the interval to recurrence after endocrine therapy [118]. Whether ErbB2 status is stable during BrCa metastasis is currently debated. Previous studies have indicated that ErbB2 amplification can be evaluated reliably in material from either primary or metastatic tumors in most patients [119], and that paired primary tumors and distant metastatic lesions have highly concordant ErbB2 status when analyzed by immunohistochemistry or fluorescent *in situ* hybridization (FISH) [120]. However, recent data have demonstrated that a true discordant rate exists between the expression of the ErbB2 receptor in relapsed lesions and primary BrCa [121, 122]. This evidence suggests that a percentage of ErbB2-positive primary BrCa, generally <30%, could progress independently from ErbB2 expression.

Several studies have demonstrated ErbB2 protein overexpression and/or gene amplification in a subset of PCa patients, especially in the androgen-independent phase of the disease [123-126]. Interestingly, androgen deprivation therapy appears to exert positive selective pressure on the overexpression of ErbB2 in PCa [127-129]. Different explanations for this phenomenon have been formulated. In a compensatory way, ErbB may activate hormone receptors in the absence of the ligand, as suggested by evidence that ErbB2, when overexpressed, enhances androgen receptor transactivating activity, even in the absence of androgens [130]. On the other hand, estrogen/ER signaling has been associated with the suppression of the growth factor receptor tyrosine kinase ErbB1 at the transcriptional level in various ER+ BrCa models *in vitro* [131, 132]. The absence of the hormone is a permissive event for the overexpression of ErbB receptors. ErbB3 has been found overexpressed in bone metastases in PCa patients, as a secreted variant [133], or translocated into the nucleus [134]. The biological significance of these observations remains to be elucidated.

ErbB Receptors and Tumor Invasion

ErbB receptors promote migration and invasion of tumor cells. It is well-known that EGF is a potent promoter of wound healing, stimulating the migration of intestinal epithelial cells into the wounded area [135]. It is not always possible to associate a given biological response with the activity of a single ErbB receptor or to understand the relative role of homodimers and heterodimers in promoting invasion [5, 136]. However, several studies have suggested that ErbB2 plays a pivotal role in modulating migration and invasion. Overexpression of ErbB2 was sufficient to induce cell migration in NIH 3T3 fibroblast cells [137] and in BrCa cells [138]. Moreover, ErbB2 activation by heterodimerization appears to be a necessary event for BrCa cell migration through the extracellular matrix [138]. The leading role of ErbB2 in the migration of tumor cells is supported by several considerations. For example, cells devoid of functional ErbB2 receptors are not induced to migrate and invade, even in the presence of EGF-related peptides. Therefore, it is thought that migration induced by ErbB1, 3 and 4 is mediated by ErbB2 activation; it is likely that the role of ErbB2 in migration is to diversify receptor transphosphorylation events and to provide unique downstream effector molecules that specifically link ErbB receptors to the migration and invasion machinery of cells. This specificity is achieved only by heterodimers containing ErbB2 but not by homodimers. In this context, it is significant that studies using controlled dimerization systems show that ErbB1-ErbB2 heterodimers qualitatively differ from ErbB2 homodimers by promoting the invasion of breast epithelial cells. However, because instances in which ErbB2-null cells can migrate in response to EGF family peptides have been described, compensatory mechanisms may exist according to the cell type and physiological condition. ErbB1 or ErbB4 overexpressing fibroblasts are stimulated to migrate *via* EGF and HB-EGF, respectively [139]. Moreover, treatment of human squamous cell carcinomas of head and neck cancer with the anti-ErbB1 blocking antibody cetuximab significantly reduced their ability to invade surrounding tissues, including bone [140]. Also, in BrCa cells, the activation of overexpressed ErbB1 was sufficient to induce a moderate level of migration in the absence of ErbB2

[138], and ligand availability could play a central role in the modulation of this phenomenon. NRG1 is a factor likely to promote tumor formation independently of ErbB2 overexpression [141]. Interestingly, NRG1 overexpression promotes BrCa tumorigenicity and metastasis independently of ErbB2 overexpression and may account for cases of poor prognosis in the absence of ErbB2 amplification. Blockage of NRGs expression results in nearly complete inhibition of tumor metastasis *in vivo* [141].

ErbB receptor homodimerization as well as heterodimerization activate multiple signaling pathways regulating cytoskeletal rearrangements and cellular migration (Fig. **2**). Several parallel pathways downstream of ErbB1, including phospholipase C-γ and phosphatidylinositol 3-kinase (PI 3-kinase)/AKT, are required for EGF stimulation of cell migration in intestinal epithelial cells [135]. EGF stimulation induces the phosphorylation of paxillin to create docking sites for the adaptor protein CrkII [142]. In turn, CrkII activates Rac1 and promotes lamellipodium formation, cell motility, and invasion. The invasive process induced by ErbB receptors requires ERK activity and CAS/CRK coupling (coupling of the adaptor proteins p130CAS (Crk-associated substrate) and c-CrkII) [138]. ERK can phosphorylate myosin light chain kinase, leading to increased myosin phosphorylation and motor activity during cell migration [143].

Tumor Growth at Distant Sites

Tumor growth at distant sites is possible only if tumor cells adapt to environmental conditions very different to those present at the primary site. As previously discussed, the oncogenic role of ErbB receptors develops early during tumor progression, and the ErbB phenotype could represent an advantage for metastatic growth, depending on the availability of ligands at the new site. While at the primary site, the constitutive activation of ErbB receptors is the result of a progressive co-evolution of tumor and stromal cells [144], the situation is very different for single or a few tumor cells invading new tissues. However, two aspects suggest a positive role for ErbB receptors in the early phases of metastatic spread: the ubiquitous distribution of ErbB receptors and ligands in human tissues and the adaptation potential of the ErbB receptor (Fig. **3**).

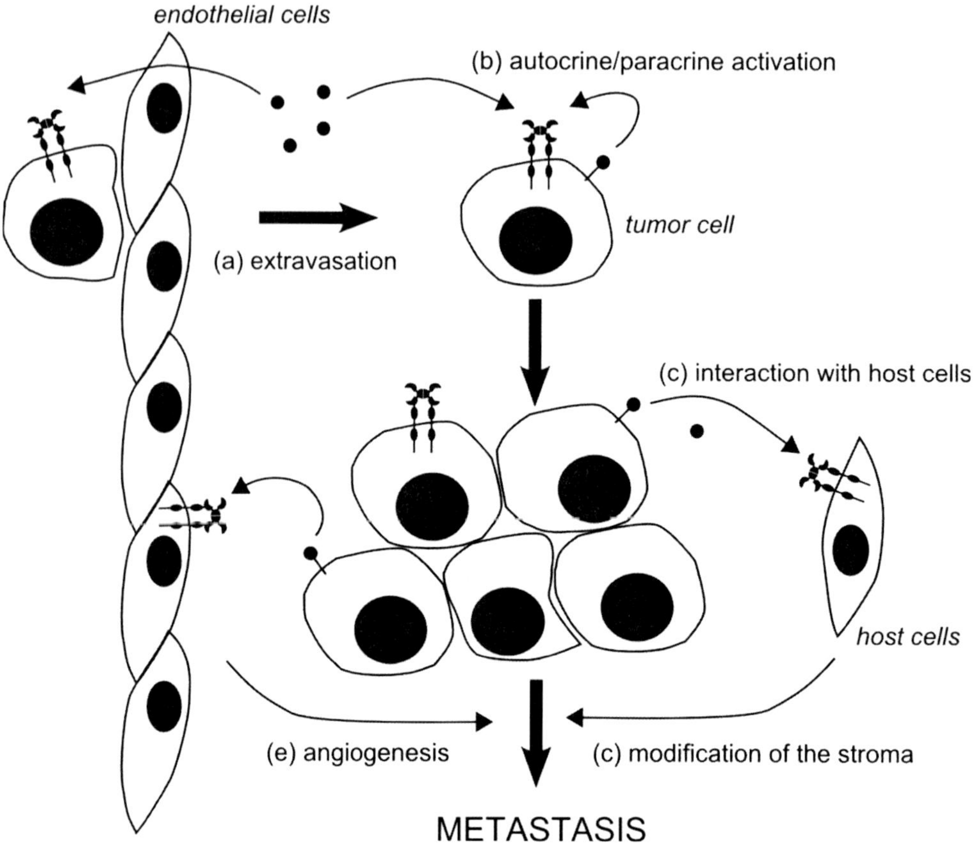

Fig. (3): ErbB receptor-dependent events involved in the formation of a metastasis. (a) Extravasation is directed by ErbB ligands that function as chemotactic factors. (b) The activation of ErbB receptors by an autocrine/paracrine loop sustains the initial phases of tumor growth. (c) Complex paracrine interactions with host cells are dependent on the expression of ErbB receptors and (d) contribute to the formation of a favorable "soil" for tumor cells, *i.e.* "seeds". (e) Tumor-associated endothelial cells are stimulated to change their ErbB receptor expression pattern toward a pro-angiogenic phenotype.

Tissue Distribution of ErbB Receptor Ligands

In the absence of an activating mutation, ErbB receptors remain dependent on the availability of ligands. Some EGF-like proteins, including EGF and TGF-α, have been detected in several tissues, while the expression of other ligands seems to be restricted to a few organs. RT-PCR analysis of human tissues detected strong EGF expression in the kidney, salivary gland, cerebrum, and prostate, moderate expression in the trachea and thyroid, and low expression in the bone marrow, heart, spleen, thymus, uterus, and colon. No expression was detected in the adrenal gland, liver, lung, cerebellum, placenta, and small intestine [145]. TGF-α is expressed in many human tissues, as indicated by northern blot analysis. Expression levels of TGF-α mRNA are particularly elevated in the kidney, brain, and pancreas [146]. On the contrary, EPR is expressed only in the placenta, peripheral blood leukocytes, and macrophages [146], and the physiological function of NRGs appears limited to a few tissues, including the nervous system, heart, breast, and skeletal muscle [147]. Most of these growth factors are synthesized as cell membrane-associated precursors that are biologically active and can interact with receptors on metastatic tumor cells.

The overexpression in an autocrine manner of a specific ligand represents an important mechanism in sustaining tumor growth in the absence of ligands in the host microenvironment [148]. It has been previously demonstrated that co-expression of different EGF-like peptides is a common phenomenon in human carcinogenesis (for a review, see [149]). For example, co-expression of TGFα and AR occurs in most human colon, breast, lung, and ovarian carcinomas [150-154]. A tumor phenotype comprising overexpression of EGF-like peptides and receptors may confer an undoubted advantage to micrometastases in the early phases of growth.

Adaptation Ability of ErbB Receptors

A role of ErbB receptors in tumor growth may be consolidated at the metastatic site because of intrinsic "plasticity" mechanisms (Fig. **4**): amplification of ErbB gene expression, the activation of compensatory downstream signaling due to the formation of different dimers with a broad spectrum of possible ligands, and ErbB transactivation. Data from many studies clearly suggest that co-expression of two or more ErbB receptors frequently occur in human carcinomas. ErbB receptors can cooperate with other members of the family by inducing resistance to a specific ErbB receptor inhibitor or by leading to the activation of additional intracellular pathways. In some situations, this cooperation is particularly important. For example, in some cancer models, the loss of ErbB2 activation could also inhibit ErbB1-dependent proliferation [155].

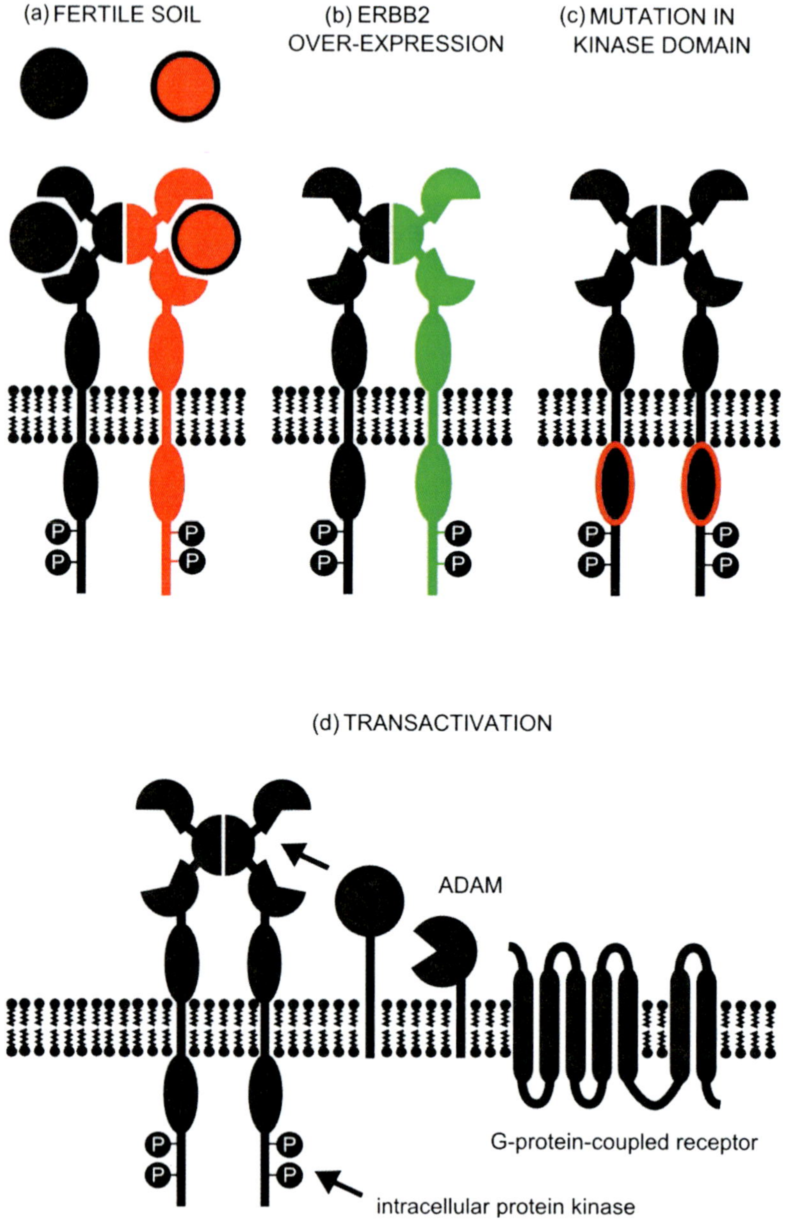

Fig. (4): The ErbB receptor activation mechanisms relevant in metastatic dissemination. (**a**) The formation of ErbB heterodimers allows the extension in the number of possible ligands and renders cancer growth more probable in different "soils". (**b**) ErbB2 overexpression permits the activation of ErbB dimers without ligands. (**c**) Mutations in the kinase domains generate intrinsically activated ErbB1 forms; (**d**) G-protein coupled receptors, but also other membrane proteins, can stimulate the release of ligands through the proteolytic activity of ADAMs, or the direct phosphorylation of the ErbB receptor docking domain.

The term transactivation refers to mechanisms activating the ErbB receptor in dependence of other signaling pathways (Fig. **4**). Transactivation of ErbB receptors can be induced by chemokines, integrins, and G-protein-coupled receptors (GPCRs). There are two main modalities described in the transactivation of ErbB1: in the first, the release of the ligand is controlled in a autocrine manner (reviewed in [156]); in the second, the activation of ErbB1 is a ligand-independent event [157]. EGF-like growth factors are produced as transmembrane precursors, and the shedding of their active forms is controlled by proteases. The best model that fits this phenomenon is the "triple membrane-passing signal" (TMPS), first described by Prenzel for a GPCR [158]. Extracellular ligands, including bombesin, lysophosphatidic acid (LPA), and endothelin 1 (ET1), activate GPCR that in turn release membrane-bound ErbB1 ligands through the proteolytic action of metalloproteases. Significantly, inhibitors of ET1, already in clinical use for their ability to interact with bone marrow stromal cells and block the osteoblastic response during bone metastasis of PCa, have been demonstrated to directly target the survival of PCa cells, suggesting a new function in their antimetastatic potential [159]. The participation of metalloproteinases in ErbB1 transactivation has been well-established; it involves the shedding of membrane-bound ErbB1 ligands by members of the A Disintegrin And Metalloenzyme (ADAM) family of metalloproteases. However, a close relationship between other secreted or membrane-linked proteases and ErbB1 activation has been suggested. In fact, in studies with broad spectrum inhibitors, serine proteases [160] and metalloproteases [161, 162] have been identified as potential mediators of ErbB receptor ligand shedding. Most of these proteases are constitutively overexpressed in invading and metastatic tumor cells. Moreover, the broad-spectrum MMP inhibitor GM6001 prevents ErbB1 phosphorylation at both the Tyr1068 and Tyr845 residues [163]. In the presence of sphingosine 1-phosphate, MT1-MMP stimulates ErbB1 transactivation through a process that is dependent upon GPCR signaling and Src activities and leads to enhanced cellular migration [164]. Recent findings suggest that the cross-talk between proteases and ErbB1 might sustain the ability of tumor cells to form bone metastases. In particular, the urokinase plasminogen activator (uPA/uPAR) axis is able to stimulate the osteotropism of PCa cells in the absence of ErbB1 or ErbB2 overexpression through the transactivation of ErbB1 [165]. Moreover, this mechanism is also associated with the upregulation of metalloprotease 9 (MMP9). The transactivation of ErbB1 by uPAR has been also shown in BrCa, where it appears to mediate cellular invasiveness rather than proliferation [166].

The ligand-independent transactivation of ErbB1 was also attributed to an intracellular mechanism. Intracellular kinases are able to phosphorylate specific residues of ErbB1, stimulating the formation of the active form of the receptor. These kinases includes Src [167], Pkc [168], and Pyk2 [169], intracellular messengers that are frequently associated with a metastatic phenotype. However, the causal role of these kinases as activators of ErbB1 is debated, and this has been described sporadically in specific cell models. The situation is complicated by the concomitant role of the same kinases as downstream signaling targets of ErbB1.

Interaction with Host Cells

It has been proposed that, in the initial steps of metastasis formation, many tumors lie dormant until a tumor-mediated switch in the local equilibrium between negative and positive regulators of growth occurs. This molecular perturbation may involve a paracrine interaction through the ErbB axis between tumor and host cells (Fig. **3**). Targeting ErbB receptors in stromal cells could increase the potential of targeted therapy, but to date this has not been fully considered. We have to consider that ErbB1, for example, shows a ubiquitous expression pattern, because PCR amplification products are obtained in most tissues tested [145]. Although this aspect was previously underestimated, the co-evolution of tumor and tumor-associated stroma is increasingly recognized as a potential therapeutic target.

A well-documented crosstalk based upon the ErbB axis involves the interaction between the tumor and endothelial cells (Fig. **3**). A comparative analysis of the expression profiles of the four ErbB receptors shows that normal endothelial cells express ErbB2, ErbB3, and ErbB4. However, in a significant manner, it has been demonstrated that tumor-associated endothelial cells undergo a phenotypic switch, expressing mainly ErbB1, ErbB2 and ErbB4, but not ErbB3 [170]. This phenomenon, reported to date only by immunohistochemical analysis of tumor xenografts [171], may have important consequences in future therapy. Tumor-associated endothelial cells expressing ErbB1 are sensitive to the paracrine stimulation by tumor cells that sustains endothelial cell proliferation and migration, and in turn angiogenesis. ErbB1 tyrosine kinase inhibitors have been shown to block the proliferation and motility of endothelial cells *in vitro* [172, 173]. Furthermore, these agents were found to produce significant levels of apoptosis only in tumor-associated endothelial cells that express the active form of the ErbB1 receptor [174]. The ErbB1 inhibitor PKI 166 repressed growth in the bone of nude mice in both renal cell carcinomas and androgen-independent PCa [104, 175]. Treatment with PKI 166 produced a significant reduction in the levels of ErbB1 phosphorylation in both tumor cells and tumor-associated endothelial cells. This observation suggests that the ability to block tumor growth in the bone by anti-ErbB1 agents is also due to a direct effect on angiogenesis.

Active interaction with the microenvironment is particularly important in high osteotropic cancers, including BrCa and PCa. The propensity to metastasize to the bone could be explained by a complex interaction between metastatic tumor cells and the host microenvironment. ErbB ligands in the bone microenvironment modulate bone cell proliferation and differentiation. EGF- and TGF-α–dependent stimulation of bone resorption and osteoclastogenesis is accompanied by decreased osteoprotegerin (OPG) expression and sustained production of receptor activator of nuclear factor kappa-B ligand (RANKL) by bone stromal cells [176, 177]. Human bone stromal cells express ErbB1, and its activation by ligands produced by tumor cells leads to the release of the osteoclastogenic factor RANKL, that in turn triggers remodeling of the mineralized bone matrix [165, 177]. At the same time, bone stromal cells can produce TGF-α and AR that modulate tumor growth [177]. In addition, ErbB1 is expressed by osteoblasts, and its activation stimulates osteoblast proliferation and decreases mineralization [178]. ErbB1 ligands may also function by an autocrine loop, stimulating the release of cytokines by BrCa cells that directly influence osteoclastogenesis or indirectly stimulate ErbB1 signaling within bone cells. The key cytokine produced by BrCa cells in this way is parathyroid hormone related protein (PTHrP), which is able to stimulate RANKL expression and inhibit OPG expression in cells of the osteoblast lineage [179]. In addition, PTHrP induces the expression and shedding of AR and TGF-α, thereby increasing the availability of ErbB ligands in the bone microenvironment.

ISSUES FROM CLINICAL TRIALS

The rationale for the use of ErbB receptors as target for antimetastatic therapy was proposed several years ago, on the basis of the promising results obtained with a recombinant humanized monoclonal antibody used in monotherapy in ErbB2-overexpressing metastatic BrCa. Objective responses were seen in about 10% of the patients, and included one complete remission [180]. Since the initial approval of trastuzumab for clinical use in metastatic patients in 1998, data from clinical trials have led to the approval by the FDA and EMA of several other ErbB inhibitors for metastatic disease. This number is estimated to grow in the near future (Table **1**).

The timeline for the development of ErbB receptor inhibitors is characterized by the synthesis of new compounds with higher specificity and potency. These inhibitors include two main categories: antibodies (mAb) directed against the extracellular domain and small tyrosine kinase inhibitors (TKI) that bind the intracellular kinase domain of ErbB receptors. Currently, several potent anti-ErbB agents are available for clinical studies: the ErbB1 receptor tyrosine kinase inhibitors gefitinib (ZD1839, Iressa) and erlotinib (OSI-774, Tarceva), the dual ErbB1 and ErbB2 receptor tyrosine kinase inhibitor lapatinib (GW-572016), the pan-ErbB receptor tyrosine kinase inhibitor canertinib (CI-1033), the human–murine chimeric anti-ErbB1 monoclonal antibody cetuximab, the anti-ErbB1 monoclonal antibody panitumumab, and the humanized anti-ErbB2 monoclonal antibody trastuzumab.

The rationale for the use of ErbB-targeted therapy is based on two different aspects of the metastatic process: in blocking cancer cell spread from the primary site and in ameliorating the prognosis in metastatic patients. The results from clinical trials using ErbB inhibitors have not equated with the expectations of such exciting preclinical data. The reasons for clinical disappointment have not been completely clarified, but two main aspects are currently considered with

Table 1: Drugs Approved by the Food and Drug Administration (FDA) or European Medicine Agency (EMA) for Use in Patients with Metastatic Disease

Drug	Drug Trade Name	Class and Target	Updated Therapeutic Indication	First Approval Date & Institution
Trastuzumab	Herceptin	mAb ErbB2	**Breast cancer**: as a single agent or in combination with cisplatinum in combination with paclitaxel, docetaxel or an aromatase inhibitor in ErbB2-overexpressing metastatic cancer (a)(b) **Gastric and gastroesophageal junction cancer:** for patients with ErbB2-positive metastatic cancer who have not received previous therapy for metastatic disease (e)(f).	(a) 1998 FDA (b) 2000 EMA (c) 2010 FDA (d) 2010 EMA
Cetuximab	Erbitux	mAb ErbB1	**Colorectal carcinoma**: as a single agent after chemotherapy failure or in combination with irinotecan or in combination with FOLFIRI (or FOLFOX)* for first-line treatment in ErbB1-expressing and wild-type KRas metastatic cancer (a) (b) **Squamous cell carcinoma of the head and neck**: use after chemotherapy failure as a single agent or in combination with platinum-based therapy or radiotherapy in locally, regionally advanced or metastatic cancer (c)(d)	(a) 2004 FDA (b) 2004 EMA (c) 2006 FDA (d) 2008 EMA
Erlotinib	Tarceva	TKI ERBB1	**Non-small-cell lung cancer**: as a single agent after chemotherapy failure, or as first-line treatment in cancer with exon 19 deletions or exon 21 substitution mutations in ErbB1, or as maintenance treatment after cisplatinum treatment in ErbB1-positive advanced or metastatic cancer (a)(b) **Pancreatic cancer**: in combination with gemcitabine for the first-line treatment of patients with locally advanced, unresectable or metastatic cancer (c)(d)	(a) 2004 FDA (b) 2005 EMA (c) 2005 FDA (d) 2005 EMA
Panitumumab	Vectibix	mAb ErbB1	**Colorectal carcinoma**: As a single agent for the treatment of patients with ErbB1-expressing and KRas wild-type metastatic cancer of the colon or rectum with disease progression on or following chemotherapy regimens	2006 FDA 2007 EMA
Lapatinib	Tykerb	TKI ErbB1, ErbB2	**Breast cancer**: in combination with capecitabine for treatment of patients with metastatic cancer overexpressing ErbB2 and after prior chemotherapy or trastuzumab (a)(b) or in combination with trastuzumab or chemotherapy or an aromatase inhibitor (c)	(a) 2007 FDA (b) (c) 2008 EMA
Pertuzumab	Perjeta	mAb ErbB2	**Breast cancer**: as neoadjuvant treatment in combination with trastuzumab and docetaxel in locally advanced (a)(b) or metastatic (b) ErbB2-positive cancer	(a) 2012 FDA (b) 2013 EMA

* "FOLFOX" chemotherapy = oxaliplatin, 5-fluorouracil and folinic acid; "FOLFIRI" chemotherapy = irinotecan, 5-fluorouracil and folinic acid.

increasing attention: the presence of mutations and the pattern of expression of ErbB members. To date, the emergence of drug resistance, generally within a year of commencing therapy, is likely to be one of most relevant problems. In fact, specific mutations could be associated with resistance to a particular treatment. For this reason, genetic screening for specific mutations other than gene amplifications could be a fundamental predictive marker. This evidence has been extensively described in NSCLC. Second-site mutations in one of the exons encoding the ErbB1 kinase domain are observed in about half of drug-resistant tumors that resume growth during treatment with ErbB1 inhibitors [181]. In the Iressa Dose Evaluation in Advanced Lung Cancer trials, response to gefitinib was reported in 46% of patients with ErbB1 mutations, in 29% of patients with increased gene copy numbers by FISH, and in only 9% of patients with neither mutations nor amplification [182]. However in other cases, the correlation between genotype and therapeutic response is more ambiguous and gene overexpression or mutation does not represent a suitable predictive marker. For example, although ErbB1 is overexpressed in up to 70% of NSCLC [153, 183], only modest objective responses, between 12 and 18%, were observed with gefitinib in phase II trials [184, 185]. At the same time, it has also been observed that responses to erlotinib in patients with NSCLC did not show any correlation with ErbB1 expression [186]. For the interpretation of such results, it could be useful to consider the mechanisms of adaptability of ErbB receptors (heterodimerization, transactivation) and the interaction between tumor cells and the microenvironment.

ErbB2-Targeting Agents

The efficacy of the ErbB2 inhibitor trastuzumab has been extensively evaluated in both early disease and metastatic settings. In fact, in 1998, it was approved by the FDA for the first-line treatment of ErbB2-positive metastatic BrCa, and in 2005, it was approved for use in combination with chemotherapy for non-metastatic ErbB-positive BrCa. In recent years, several reports from large clinical trials evaluating the impact of adjuvant trastuzumab in disease-free survival and overall survival have been presented [187-189].

In the international multicenter randomized trial HERA, 1 or 2 years of trastuzumab treatment after standard neoadjuvant or adjuvant chemotherapy was compared with the observation group. Although each arm was comprised of 58% node-positive patients, trastuzumab reduced the incidence of distant events with respect to the control arm (9% *vs* 14%) and significantly prolonged overall survival after a median follow-up of two years [189]. In another trial, women with ErbB-positive, node-positive or high-risk node-negative BrCa who were assigned to receive trastuzumab for nine weeks with chemotherapy had better distant event-free survival than those treated with chemotherapy only (17.4% *vs* 25.9%) [190]. Patients with stage I-III ErbB2-positive BrCa treated with adjuvant trastuzumab had an increased metastases-free survival rate with respect to untreated patients [191]. These promising results have vigorously prompted the evaluation of the efficacy and safety of long-term adjuvant trastuzumab treatment in combination with standard chemotherapy by the North Central Cancer Treatment Group (NCCTG) N9831 and the National Surgical Adjuvant Breast and Bowel Project (NSABP) B-31 trials. These trials were designed similarly, and both started in 2000. The 2011 report was indicated that of women in the trastuzumab arm, 85.8% were alive without evidence of recurrence with respect to 75.8% in the control arm. The percentage of patients with local, regional, or distant recurrence was significantly reduced from 20.6% in the control arm to 11.7% in the trastuzumab arm [192].

As a single agent against metastatic BrCa, trastuzumab, in agreement with the initial studies, has been confirmed to produce response rates similar or better than those of many single-agent chemotherapeutic agents, but with more restricted toxicity. Because combining trastuzumab with chemotherapy can result in synergistic antitumor activity, further trials have evaluated the use of trastuzumab in combination with other forms of chemotherapy, including vinorelbine, docetaxel, anthracyclines, and platinum agents. Objective clinical responses were observed in 24% of patients with ErbB2 overexpressing metastatic BrCa treated with trastuzumab and cisplatin. These response rates were higher than those reported for either single agent alone [193]. The addition of trastuzumab to chemotherapy (doxorubicin, epirubicin, cyclophosphamide or paclitaxel) was associated with a longer time to disease progression, a higher rate of objective response, a longer duration of response, and a lower rate of death at one year [194-198]. Although questions regarding the efficacy of various combinations and dosing schedules are in many cases not yet resolved, some recent phase II and III clinical trials have offered important indications. Very significant results were obtained with first-line trastuzumab combined with docetaxel. In the M77001 study group that recruited 186 patients with ErbB2-positive metastatic BrCa, the combination was significantly superior to docetaxel alone in terms of the overall response rate (61% *vs* 34%), with little additional toxicity [199]. The addition of first-line carboplatin to paclitaxel and trastuzumab significantly improved the objective response rate in a randomized, multicenter phase III trial that recruited 196 women [200]. A international phase II trial demonstrated that vinorelbine plus trastuzumab is one of the most active treatment regimens for patients with ErbB2-positive metastatic BrCa and demonstrated a very favorable safety profile allowing prolonged treatment with long-term survival [201]. The effectiveness of the combinations vinorelbine/trastuzumab and taxane/trastuzumab as first-line treatment has been confirmed by other authors who observed response rates greater than 40% [195].

Although trastuzumab provides substantial clinical benefits when used either as monotherapy or in combination with a number of chemotherapeutic agents, we may consider three important adverse features. First, accurate assessment of ErbB2 status is essential to ensure that the patients are likely to benefit from trastuzumab treatment. In fact, only patients with immunohistochemistry 3+ (and in some case 2+) or FISH-positive disease have experienced the greatest clinical advantage [202]. Treatment with trastuzumab has been associated with important adverse events, including serious infusion-related reactions, cardiotoxicity, and severe neutropenia. For this reason, some authors have expressed doubts on the use of trastuzumab, recommending its use only in controlled clinical trials under vigilant cardiac monitoring [203, 204]. A third aspect that renders the use of trastuzumab questionable derives from the evidence that 10% to 34% of patients receiving trastuzumab in combination with chemotherapy developed isolated CNS metastases as the first site of tumor progression [205-207]. This evidence has important consequences in the interpretation of results. In fact, the predilection to metastasize to the brain is observed even in the presence of an objective response of the tumor at other sites. This has been explained by the filtering function of the blood–brain barrier on the antibody trastuzumab [208]. This confirms that trastuzumab treatment is directly effective on cancer cells that have already disseminated to metastatic sites. Trastuzumab was recently approved for the use in metastatic gastric cancer following positive, but modest, results from phase III clinical trials; this represents the first targeted therapy in gastric cancer. In the Trastuzumab for Gastric Cancer (ToGA) trial, standard chemotherapy (5-fluorouracil/capecitabine plus cisplatin) was compared with chemotherapy plus trastuzumab. The median of progression-free survival was increased by trastuzumab from 5.5 months to 6.7 months [209].

ErbB1-Targeting Agents

While the evaluation of ErbB2-targeted drugs is strictly linked to BrCa studies due to the frequent amplification of ErbB2 in this tumor, inhibitors of ErbB1 have been tested as antimetastatic agents in a wider spectrum of tumors, generating very heterogeneous results. Gefitinib has been used in tumors in which progression is frequently associated with ErbB1 expression, such as SCCHN, CRC, NSCLC, pancreatic, and renal carcinoma. Although gefitinib is extensively considered for the clinical treatment of NSCLC, the results have been frequently discouraging (reviewed in [210]). In metastatic disease, the use of gefitinib as a single agent does not appear particularly efficacious, as observed in the treatment of heavily pretreated metastatic BrCa patients [211], with previously treated CRC patients [212], or in SCCHN [213]. Interestingly, in these cases, several investigators were unable to reveal a significant inhibition of ErbB1 activation with gefitinib therapy [212, 214]. At present, the interest in gefitinib has shifted to its use in combination with chemotherapy, and the available data suggest an increased therapeutic efficacy. Patients with metastatic ErbB1-positive CRC received gefitinib combined with simplified FOLFOX6 (oxaliplatin plus folinic acid and 5-fluorouracil) as first-line therapy, and 71% of the patients had complete or partial responses [215]. Complete plus partial responses were observed in 22 out of 41 patients treated with gefitinib in combination with docetaxel as first-line treatment in women with metastatic BrCa [216]. The sequential administration of docetaxel and gefitinib was well-tolerated and moderately active against advanced pre-treated NSCLC [217]. The combination of chemotherapy and erlotinib seems to have similarly promising activity in metastatic patients. Patients with metastatic CRC that progressed and were intolerant to first-line chemotherapy when treated with capecitabine, oxaliplatin, and erlotinib demonstrated a relatively higher response rate and progression-free survival time compared with previous reports of chemotherapy alone [218]. Cetuximab, a human–murine chimeric antibody against ErbB1, binds to the second domain of the receptor, thereby blocking the ligand-receptor interaction and prompting receptor internalization. Cetuximab has been shown to have significant activity as a single agent in tumors resistant to chemotherapy [219]. Treatment with cetuximab was particularly effective in metastatic CRC, in which a significant percentage of complete responses was reported [220]. Other phase II and III studies have shown significant responses to treatment in variable proportions of patients with SCCHN when cetuximab was used as first- or second-line treatment in combination with chemotherapy [221].

As previously discussed, one of the limitations to the use of ErbB inhibitors resides in the formation of heterodimers. ErbB inhibitors have generally restricted specificity toward only one member of the ErbB family, so the signaling generated by heterodimerization or by compensatory activation of other members of the family remain unaffected by inhibition. For this reason, dual inhibitors have been designed and tested in preclinical and clinical trials. The first of such inhibitors to be approved for use in clinical practice in metastatic patients is lapatinib (Table **1**). Lapatinib monotherapy has also been evaluated in ErbB2-positive locally advanced or metastatic BrCa in a trastuzumab-naïve setting. Although effective in providing better progression-free survival, first-line monotherapy with lapatinib does not seem to offer a significant benefit over that of single-agent trastuzumab [222]. Promising preclinical studies have provided the foundation for the evaluation of lapatinib in two clinical settings: in combination with trastuzumab, and for the treatment of trastuzumab-resistant BrCa. Notably, the use of lapatinib for the treatment of trastuzumab resistant-metastatic BrCa in an initial phase I clinical trial indicated a partial response [223]. Phase II clinical trials of confirmed the effectiveness of lapatinib as a single agent in patients with refractory metastatic BrCa resistant to trastuzumab and in heavily pretreated tumors [195, 224]. A randomized phase III clinical trial compared lapatinib alone or in combination with trastuzumab in trastuzumab-refractory ErbB2-positive metastatic BrCa. The trial found a small but statistically significant improvement in progression-free survival, with an increase from 8.1 to 12.0 weeks with the combination [225]. Better results are expected for the treatment of brain metastases with lapatinib due to the ability of this drug to penetrate the blood-brain barrier. Treatment with lapatinib resulted in a significant reduction in CNS metastases in animal models [226], and retrospective analyses of trials evaluating patients with CNS metastases treated with lapatinib plus capecitabine have revealed a statistically significant reduction in CNS metastatic progression [227, 228]. Lapatinib is an orally bioavailable molecule; however, frequent severe gastrointestinal and skin toxicity limits the dose that can be safely used. Other monoclonal antibodies are being investigated in clinical trials as an alternative or in combination with trastuzumab. Pertuzumab, an ErbB2 dimerization inhibitor, is active and well-tolerated in patients with metastatic ErbB2-positive BrCa who had experienced progression during prior trastuzumab therapy [229]. The CLEOPATRA phase III trial compared the efficacy of pertuzumab, trastuzumab, and docetaxel in patients with ErbB2-positive first-line metastatic BrCa. Treatment with pertuzumab resulted in superior progression-free survival (18.5 *vs* 12.4 months) without increasing the risk of cardiac dysfunction associated with trastuzumab [230]. Thus, pertuzumab has been recently approved as a neoadjuvant treatment in combination with trastuzumab and docetaxel in locally advanced or metastatic ErbB2-positive cancer.

COMMENTS AND PERSPECTIVES

The use of ErbB inhibitors has greatly contributed to the use of targeted therapy in metastatic disease. Supported by solid rationale and several favorable preclinical studies, trials using different ErbB receptor inhibitors have documented many cases of complete response in desperate clinical situations. The way is open, but the results are far from expectations. The reasons for the disappointing results are to date largely unknown, but the current knowledge permit us some considerations. The initial design of ErbB inhibitors provided a molecule specific for a single member of the ErbB family. However, targeting heterodimers may represent in some cases a better therapeutic strategy, as demonstrated by promising results obtained with lapatinib, and more recently with canertinib and neratinib. Moreover, the absence of a widely accepted predictive marker, measured by standardized methods, on the outcome of ErbB-targeted therapy needs to be addressed. The individuation of a good predictive marker is not easy as expected; in fact, the response to ErbB inhibitors is affected by many factors, including the presence of mutations in the receptor and the oncogenic expression of important downstream signaling intermediates. For this reason, a more inclusive molecular characterization of tumors appears to be a key prerequisite in selecting responsive patients who are eligible for ErbB-targeted therapy. In addition, this is aspect is particularly important when we consider that metastatic disease is associated with a very abnormal genotype that is not always identical to that of the original primary tumor. In conclusion, the use of pan-ErbB inhibitors in parallel with a wider genetic characterization of single tumors could represent an important advancement in the cure of metastatic disease.

ABBREVIATIONS

ADAM = A disintegrin and metalloenzyme

AR = Amphiregulin

BTC = Betacellulin

BrCa = Breast cancer

CRC = Colon carcinoma

FDA = U.S. Food and Drug Administration

FISH = Fluorescent *in situ* hybridization

EGF = Epidermal growth factor

EMA = European Medicine Agency

EPGN = Epigenin

EPR = Epiregulin

ErbB = Avian erythroblastic leukemia viral oncogene homolog

GPCR = G-protein-coupled receptor

HB-EGF = Heparin binding epidermal growth factor

NRG = Neuregulin

NSCLC = Non-small cell lung cancer

OPG = Osteoprotegerin

PCa = Prostate carcinoma

PI3K = Phosphatidylinositol 3-kinase

PTHrP = Parathyroid hormone related protein

RANKL = Receptor activator of nuclear factor kappa-B ligand

SCCHN = Squamous cell carcinoma of head and neck cancers

TGF-α = Transforming growth factor alpha

ACKNOWLEDGEMENTS

None declared.

CONFLICT OF INTEREST

The author confirms that this chapter contents have no conflict of interest.

DISCLOSURE

The chapter submitted for the eBook Series entitled **"Advances in Cancer Drug Targets, Volume 2"** is an update of our article in **Current Cancer Drug Targets, Volume 9, Issue 1, 2009, pp. 1-18,** with additional text and references.

REFERENCES

[1] Guy PM, Platko JV, Cantley LC, *et al.* Insect cell-expressed p180erbB3 possesses an impaired tyrosine kinase activity. Proc Natl Acad Sci USA 1994 Aug 16; 91(17): 8132-6.

[2] Harari D, Yarden Y. Molecular mechanisms underlying ErbB2/HER2 action in breast cancer. Oncogene 2000 Dec 11; 19(53): 6102-14.

[3] Tzahar E, Waterman H, Chen X, *et al.* A hierarchical network of interreceptor interactions determines signal transduction by Neu differentiation factor/neuregulin and epidermal growth factor. Mol Cell Biol 1996 Oct; 16(10): 5276-87.
[4] Graus-Porta D, Beerli RR, Daly JM, *et al.* ErbB-2, the preferred heterodimerization partner of all ErbB receptors, is a mediator of lateral signaling. Embo J 1997 Apr 1; 16(7): 1647-55.
[5] Riese DJ, 2nd, Stern DF. Specificity within the EGF family/ErbB receptor family signaling network. Bioessays 1998 Jan; 20(1): 41-8.
[6] Garrett TP, McKern NM, Lou M, *et al.* Crystal structure of a truncated epidermal growth factor receptor extracellular domain bound to transforming growth factor alpha. Cell 2002 Sep 20; 110(6): 763-73.
[7] Ogiso H, Ishitani R, Nureki O, *et al.* Crystal structure of the complex of human epidermal growth factor and receptor extracellular domains. Cell 2002 Sep 20; 110(6): 775-87.
[8] Garrett TP, McKern NM, Lou M, *et al.* The crystal structure of a truncated ErbB2 ectodomain reveals an active conformation, poised to interact with other ErbB receptors. Mol Cell 2003 Feb; 11(2): 495-505.
[9] Schulze WX, Deng L, Mann M. Phosphotyrosine interactome of the ErbB-receptor kinase family. Mol Syst Biol 2005; 1: 2005 0008.
[10] Olayioye MA, Graus-Porta D, Beerli RR, *et al.* ErbB-1 and ErbB-2 acquire distinct signaling properties dependent upon their dimerization partner. Mol Cell Biol 1998 Sep; 18(9): 5042-51.
[11] Olayioye MA, Beuvink I, Horsch K, *et al.* ErbB receptor-induced activation of stat transcription factors is mediated by Src tyrosine kinases. J Biol Chem 1999 Jun 11; 274(24): 17209-18.
[12] Smaill JB, Palmer BD, Rewcastle GW, *et al.* Tyrosine kinase inhibitors. 15. 4-(Phenylamino)quinazoline and 4-(phenylamino)pyrido[d]pyrimidine acrylamides as irreversible inhibitors of the ATP binding site of the epidermal growth factor receptor. J Med Chem 1999 May 20; 42(10): 1803-15.
[13] Nyati MK, Maheshwari D, Hanasoge S, *et al.* Radiosensitization by pan ErbB inhibitor CI-1033 *in vitro* and *in vivo*. Clin Cancer Res 2004 Jan 15; 10(2): 691-700.
[14] Allen LF, Lenehan PF, Eiseman IA, *et al.* Potential benefits of the irreversible pan-erbB inhibitor, CI-1033, in the treatment of breast cancer. Semin Oncol 2002 Jun; 29(3 Suppl 11): 11-21.
[15] Jankowitz RC, Abraham J, Tan AR, *et al.* Safety and efficacy of neratinib in combination with weekly paclitaxel and trastuzumab in women with metastatic HER2positive breast cancer: an NSABP Foundation Research Program phase I study. Cancer Chemother Pharmacol 2013 Dec; 72(6): 1205-12.
[16] Awada A, Dirix L, Manso Sanchez L, *et al.* Safety and efficacy of neratinib (HKI-272) plus vinorelbine in the treatment of patients with ErbB2-positive metastatic breast cancer pretreated with anti-HER2 therapy. Ann Oncol 2013 Jan; 24(1): 109-16.
[17] Park BH, Davidson NE. PI3 kinase activation and response to Trastuzumab Therapy: what's neu with herceptin resistance? Cancer Cell 2007 Oct; 12(4): 297-9.
[18] Moasser MM, Basso A, Averbuch SD, *et al.* The tyrosine kinase inhibitor ZD1839 ("Iressa") inhibits HER2-driven signaling and suppresses the growth of HER2-overexpressing tumor cells. Cancer Res 2001 Oct 1; 61(19): 7184-8.

[19] Bianco R, Shin I, Ritter CA, *et al.* Loss of PTEN/MMAC1/TEP in EGF receptor-expressing tumor cells counteracts the antitumor action of EGFR tyrosine kinase inhibitors. Oncogene 2003 May 8; 22(18): 2812-22.

[20] Baulida J, Kraus MH, Alimandi M, *et al.* All ErbB receptors other than the epidermal growth factor receptor are endocytosis impaired. J Biol Chem 1996 Mar 1; 271(9): 5251-7.

[21] Huang G, Chantry A, Epstein RJ. Overexpression of ErbB2 impairs ligand-dependent downregulation of epidermal growth factor receptors *via* a post-transcriptional mechanism. J Cell Biochem 1999 Jul 1; 74(1): 23-30.

[22] Kwong KY, Hung MC. A novel splice variant of HER2 with increased transformation activity. Mol Carcinog 1998 Oct; 23(2): 62-8.

[23] Christianson TA, Doherty JK, Lin YJ, *et al.* NH2-terminally truncated HER-2/neu protein: relationship with shedding of the extracellular domain and with prognostic factors in breast cancer. Cancer Res 1998 Nov 15; 58(22): 5123-9.

[24] Freeman M. Complexity of EGF receptor signalling revealed in Drosophila. Curr Opin Genet Dev 1998 Aug; 8(4): 407-11.

[25] Olayioye MA, Neve RM, Lane HA, *et al.* The ErbB signaling network: receptor heterodimerization in development and cancer. Embo J 2000 Jul 3; 19(13): 3159-67.

[26] Chen B, Bronson RT, Klaman LD, *et al.* Mice mutant for Egfr and Shp2 have defective cardiac semilunar valvulogenesis. Nat Genet 2000 Mar; 24(3): 296-9.

[27] Sibilia M, Wagner B, Hoebertz A, *et al.* Mice humanised for the EGF receptor display hypomorphic phenotypes in skin, bone and heart. Development 2003 Oct; 130(19): 4515-25.

[28] Wang K, Yamamoto H, Chin JR, *et al.* Epidermal growth factor receptor-deficient mice have delayed primary endochondral ossification because of defective osteoclast recruitment. J Biol Chem 2004 Dec 17; 279(51): 53848-56.

[29] Miettinen PJ, Berger JE, Meneses J, *et al.* Epithelial immaturity and multiorgan failure in mice lacking epidermal growth factor receptor. Nature 1995 Jul 27; 376(6538): 337-41.

[30] Sibilia M, Wagner EF. Strain-dependent epithelial defects in mice lacking the EGF receptor. Science 1995 Jul 14; 269(5221): 234-8.

[31] Threadgill DW, Dlugosz AA, Hansen LA, *et al.* Targeted disruption of mouse EGF receptor: effect of genetic background on mutant phenotype. Science 1995 Jul 14; 269(5221): 230-4.

[32] Kornblum HI, Hussain R, Wiesen J, *et al.* Abnormal astrocyte development and neuronal death in mice lacking the epidermal growth factor receptor. J Neurosci Res 1998 Sep 15; 53(6): 697-717.

[33] Sibilia M, Steinbach JP, Stingl L, *et al.* A strain-independent postnatal neurodegeneration in mice lacking the EGF receptor. Embo J 1998 Feb 2; 17(3): 719-31.

[34] Morris JK, Lin W, Hauser C, *et al.* Rescue of the cardiac defect in ErbB2 mutant mice reveals essential roles of ErbB2 in peripheral nervous system development. Neuron 1999 Jun; 23(2): 273-83.

[35] Lin W, Sanchez HB, Deerinck T, *et al.* Aberrant development of motor axons and neuromuscular synapses in erbB2-deficient mice. Proc Natl Acad Sci USA 2000 Feb 1; 97(3): 1299-304.

[36] Schmucker J, Ader M, Brockschnieder D, *et al.* erbB3 is dispensable for oligodendrocyte development *in vitro* and *in vivo*. Glia 2003 Oct; 44(1): 67-75.

[37] Golding JP, Trainor P, Krumlauf R, *et al.* Defects in pathfinding by cranial neural crest cells in mice lacking the neuregulin receptor ErbB4. Nat Cell Biol 2000 Feb; 2(2): 103-9.
[38] Flames N, Long JE, Garratt AN, *et al.* Short- and long-range attraction of cortical GABAergic interneurons by neuregulin-1. Neuron 2004 Oct 14; 44(2): 251-61.
[39] Cohen S. Isolation of a mouse submaxillary gland protein accelerating incisor eruption and eyelid opening in the new-born animal. J Biol Chem 1962 May; 237: 1555-62.
[40] Xie W, Paterson AJ, Chin E, *et al.* Targeted expression of a dominant negative epidermal growth factor receptor in the mammary gland of transgenic mice inhibits pubertal mammary duct development. Mol Endocrinol 1997 Nov; 11(12): 1766-81.
[41] Barnard JA, Beauchamp RD, Russell WE, *et al.* Epidermal growth factor-related peptides and their relevance to gastrointestinal pathophysiology. Gastroenterology 1995 Feb; 108(2): 564-80.
[42] Schroeder JA, Lee DC. Dynamic expression and activation of ERBB receptors in the developing mouse mammary gland. Cell Growth Differ 1998 Jun; 9(6): 451-64.
[43] Darcy KM, Zangani D, Wohlhueter AL, *et al.* Changes in ErbB2 (her-2/neu), ErbB3, and ErbB4 during growth, differentiation, and apoptosis of normal rat mammary epithelial cells. J Histochem Cytochem 2000 Jan; 48(1): 63-80.
[44] Luetteke NC, Qiu TH, Fenton SE, *et al.* Targeted inactivation of the EGF and amphiregulin genes reveals distinct roles for EGF receptor ligands in mouse mammary gland development. Development 1999 Jun; 126(12): 2739-50.
[45] Silberberg G, Darvasi A, Pinkas-Kramarski R, *et al.* The involvement of ErbB4 with schizophrenia: association and expression studies. Am J Med Genet B Neuropsychiatr Genet 2006 Mar 5; 141(2): 142-8.
[46] Xian CJ. Roles of epidermal growth factor family in the regulation of postnatal somatic growth. Endocr Rev 2007 May; 28(3): 284-96.
[47] Shimizu N, Kondo I, Gamou S, *et al.* Genetic analysis of hyperproduction of epidermal growth factor receptors in human epidermoid carcinoma A431 cells. Somat Cell Mol Genet 1984 Jan; 10(1): 45-53.
[48] Mendelsohn J, Baselga J. The EGF receptor family as targets for cancer therapy. Oncogene 2000 Dec 27; 19(56): 6550-65.
[49] Amundadottir LT, Nass SJ, Berchem GJ, *et al.* Cooperation of TGF alpha and c-Myc in mouse mammary tumorigenesis: coordinated stimulation of growth and suppression of apoptosis. Oncogene 1996 Aug 15; 13(4): 757-65.
[50] Greulich H, Chen TH, Feng W, *et al.* Oncogenic transformation by inhibitor-sensitive and -resistant EGFR mutants. PLoS Med 2005 Nov; 2(11): e313.
[51] Velu TJ, Beguinot L, Vass WC, *et al.* Epidermal-growth-factor-dependent transformation by a human EGF receptor proto-oncogene. Science 1987 Dec 4; 238(4832): 1408-10.
[52] Bell DW, Gore I, Okimoto RA, *et al.* Inherited susceptibility to lung cancer may be associated with the T790M drug resistance mutation in EGFR. Nat Genet 2005 Dec; 37(12): 1315-6.
[53] Guy CT, Webster MA, Schaller M, *et al.* Expression of the neu protooncogene in the mammary epithelium of transgenic mice induces metastatic disease. Proc Natl Acad Sci USA 1992 Nov 15; 89(22): 10578-82.
[54] Brandt R, Eisenbrandt R, Leenders F, *et al.* Mammary gland specific hEGF receptor transgene expression induces neoplasia and inhibits differentiation. Oncogene 2000 Apr 20; 19(17): 2129-37.

[55] Schechter AL, Stern DF, Vaidyanathan L, *et al.* The neu oncogene: an erb-B-related gene encoding a 185,000-Mr tumour antigen. Nature 1984 Dec 6-12; 312(5994): 513-6.

[56] Di Fiore PP, Segatto O, Taylor WG, *et al.* EGF receptor and erbB-2 tyrosine kinase domains confer cell specificity for mitogenic signaling. Science 1990 Apr 6; 248(4951): 79-83.

[57] Cappuzzo F, Varella-Garcia M, Shigematsu H, *et al.* Increased HER2 gene copy number is associated with response to gefitinib therapy in epidermal growth factor receptor-positive non-small-cell lung cancer patients. J Clin Oncol 2005 Aug 1; 23(22): 5007-18.

[58] Kokai Y, Myers JN, Wada T, *et al.* Synergistic interaction of p185c-neu and the EGF receptor leads to transformation of rodent fibroblasts. Cell 1989 Jul 28; 58(2): 287-92.

[59] Alimandi M, Romano A, Curia MC, *et al.* Cooperative signaling of ErbB3 and ErbB2 in neoplastic transformation and human mammary carcinomas. Oncogene 1995 May 4; 10(9): 1813-21.

[60] Zhang K, Sun J, Liu N, *et al.* Transformation of NIH 3T3 cells by HER3 or HER4 receptors requires the presence of HER1 or HER2. J Biol Chem 1996 Feb 16; 271(7): 3884-90.

[61] Frederick L, Wang XY, Eley G, *et al.* Diversity and frequency of epidermal growth factor receptor mutations in human glioblastomas. Cancer Res 2000 Mar 1; 60(5): 1383-7.

[62] Johnson BE, Janne PA. Epidermal growth factor receptor mutations in patients with non-small cell lung cancer. Cancer Res 2005 Sep 1; 65(17): 7525-9.

[63] Sordella R, Bell DW, Haber DA, *et al.* Gefitinib-sensitizing EGFR mutations in lung cancer activate anti-apoptotic pathways. Science 2004 Aug 20; 305(5687): 1163-7.

[64] Jiang J, Greulich H, Janne PA, *et al.* Epidermal growth factor-independent transformation of Ba/F3 cells with cancer-derived epidermal growth factor receptor mutants induces gefitinib-sensitive cell cycle progression. Cancer Res 2005 Oct 1; 65(19): 8968-74.

[65] Wikstrand CJ, Hale LP, Batra SK, *et al.* Monoclonal antibodies against EGFRvIII are tumor specific and react with breast and lung carcinomas and malignant gliomas. Cancer Res 1995 Jul 15; 55(14): 3140-8.

[66] Gwak GY, Yoon JH, Shin CM, *et al.* Detection of response-predicting mutations in the kinase domain of the epidermal growth factor receptor gene in cholangiocarcinomas. J Cancer Res Clin Oncol 2005 Oct; 131(10): 649-52.

[67] Lee JW, Soung YH, Kim SY, *et al.* Somatic mutations of EGFR gene in squamous cell carcinoma of the head and neck. Clin Cancer Res 2005 Apr 15; 11(8): 2879-82.

[68] Nagahara H, Mimori K, Ohta M, *et al.* Somatic mutations of epidermal growth factor receptor in colorectal carcinoma. Clin Cancer Res 2005 Feb 15; 11(4): 1368-71.

[69] Kwak EL, Kim S, Zhang J, *et al.* Mammary tumorigenesis following transgenic expression of a dominant negative CHK2 mutant. Cancer Res 2006 Feb 15; 66(4): 1923-8.

[70] Tsao MS, Sakurada A, Cutz JC, *et al.* Erlotinib in lung cancer - molecular and clinical predictors of outcome. N Engl J Med 2005 Jul 14; 353(2): 133-44.

[71] Amann J, Kalyankrishna S, Massion PP, *et al.* Aberrant epidermal growth factor receptor signaling and enhanced sensitivity to EGFR inhibitors in lung cancer. Cancer Res 2005 Jan 1; 65(1): 226-35.

[72] McLendon RE, Wikstrand CJ, Matthews MR, *et al.* Glioma-associated antigen expression in oligodendroglial neoplasms. Tenascin and epidermal growth factor receptor. J Histochem Cytochem 2000 Aug; 48(8): 1103-10.

[73] Chaffanet M, Chauvin C, Laine M, *et al.* EGF receptor amplification and expression in human brain tumours. Eur J Cancer 1992; 28(1): 11-7.

[74] Tsugu A, Kijima H, Yamazaki H, *et al.* Localization of aberrant messenger RNA of epidermal growth factor receptor (EGFR) in malignant glioma. Anticancer Res 1997 May-Jun; 17(3C): 2225-32.

[75] Alvarez G, Perry A, Tan BR, *et al.* Expression of epidermal growth factor receptor in squamous cell carcinomas of the anal canal is independent of gene amplification. Mod Pathol 2006 Jul; 19(7): 942-9.

[76] Klijn JG, Berns PM, Schmitz PI, *et al.* The clinical significance of epidermal growth factor receptor (EGF-R) in human breast cancer: a review on 5232 patients. Endocr Rev 1992 Feb; 13(1): 3-17.

[77] Libermann TA, Nusbaum HR, Razon N, *et al.* Amplification and overexpression of the EGF receptor gene in primary human glioblastomas. J Cell Sci Suppl 1985; 3: 161-72.

[78] Semba K, Kamata N, Toyoshima K, *et al.* A v-erbB-related protooncogene, c-erbB-2, is distinct from the c-erbB-1/epidermal growth factor-receptor gene and is amplified in a human salivary gland adenocarcinoma. Proc Natl Acad Sci USA 1985 Oct; 82(19): 6497-501.

[79] Stephens P, Hunter C, Bignell G, *et al.* Lung cancer: intragenic ERBB2 kinase mutations in tumours. Nature 2004 Sep 30; 431(7008): 525-6.

[80] Yusa K, Sugimoto Y, Yamori T, *et al.* Low metastatic potential of clone from murine colon adenocarcinoma 26 increased by transfection of activated c-erbB-2 gene. J Natl Cancer Inst 1990 Oct 17; 82(20): 1633-6.

[81] Slamon DJ, Clark GM, Wong SG, *et al.* Human breast cancer: correlation of relapse and survival with amplification of the HER-2/neu oncogene. Science 1987 Jan 9; 235(4785): 177-82.

[82] Sorlie T, Perou CM, Tibshirani R, *et al.* Gene expression patterns of breast carcinomas distinguish tumor subclasses with clinical implications. Proc Natl Acad Sci USA 2001 Sep 11; 98(19): 10869-74.

[83] Kim MJ, Ro JY, Ahn SH, *et al.* Clinicopathologic significance of the basal-like subtype of breast cancer: a comparison with hormone receptor and Her2/neu-overexpressing phenotypes. Hum Pathol 2006 Sep; 37(9): 1217-26.

[84] Leitzel K, Teramoto Y, Konrad K, *et al.* Elevated serum c-erbB-2 antigen levels and decreased response to hormone therapy of breast cancer. J Clin Oncol 1995 May; 13(5): 1129-35.

[85] Kraus MH, Issing W, Miki T, *et al.* Isolation and characterization of ERBB3, a third member of the ERBB/epidermal growth factor receptor family: evidence for overexpression in a subset of human mammary tumors. Proc Natl Acad Sci USA 1989 Dec; 86(23): 9193-7.

[86] Naidu R, Yadav M, Nair S, *et al.* Expression of c-erbB3 protein in primary breast carcinomas. Br J Cancer 1998 Nov; 78(10): 1385-90.

[87] Yi ES, Harclerode D, Gondo M, *et al.* High c-erbB-3 protein expression is associated with shorter survival in advanced non-small cell lung carcinomas. Mod Pathol 1997 Feb; 10(2): 142-8.

[88] Shintani S, Funayama T, Yoshihama Y, *et al.* Prognostic significance of ERBB3 overexpression in oral squamous cell carcinoma. Cancer Lett 1995 Aug 16; 95(1-2): 79-83.

[89] Lemoine NR, Barnes DM, Hollywood DP, *et al.* Expression of the ERBB3 gene product in breast cancer. Br J Cancer 1992 Dec; 66(6): 1116-21.

[90] Rajkumar T, Stamp GW, Hughes CM, *et al.* c-erbB3 protein expression in ovarian cancer. Clin Mol Pathol 1996 Aug; 49(4): M199-M202.

[91] Bodey B, Bodey B, Jr., Groger AM, *et al.* Clinical and prognostic significance of the expression of the c-erbB-2 and c-erbB-3 oncoproteins in primary and metastatic malignant melanomas and breast carcinomas. Anticancer Res 1997 Mar-Apr; 17(2B): 1319-30.

[92] Gilbertson RJ, Perry RH, Kelly PJ, *et al.* Prognostic significance of HER2 and HER4 coexpression in childhood medulloblastoma. Cancer Res 1997 Aug 1; 57(15): 3272-80.

[93] Jemal A, Murray T, Ward E, *et al.* Cancer statistics, 2005. CA Cancer J Clin 2005 Jan-Feb; 55(1): 10-30.

[94] Chua DT, Nicholls JM, Sham JS, *et al.* Prognostic value of epidermal growth factor receptor expression in patients with advanced stage nasopharyngeal carcinoma treated with induction chemotherapy and radiotherapy. Int J Radiat Oncol Biol Phys 2004 May 1; 59(1): 11-20.

[95] Jonjic N, Kovac K, Krasevic M, *et al.* Epidermal growth factor-receptor expression correlates with tumor cell proliferation and prognosis in gastric cancer. Anticancer Res 1997 Sep-Oct; 17(5B): 3883-8.

[96] Neal DE, Sharples L, Smith K, *et al.* The epidermal growth factor receptor and the prognosis of bladder cancer. Cancer 1990 Apr 1; 65(7): 1619-25.

[97] Radinsky R, Risin S, Fan D, *et al.* Level and function of epidermal growth factor receptor predict the metastatic potential of human colon carcinoma cells. Clin Cancer Res 1995 Jan; 1(1): 19-31.

[98] Tobita K, Kijima H, Dowaki S, *et al.* Epidermal growth factor receptor expression in human pancreatic cancer: Significance for liver metastasis. Int J Mol Med 2003 Mar; 11(3): 305-9.

[99] Zhou X, Temam S, Oh M, *et al.* Global expression-based classification of lymph node metastasis and extracapsular spread of oral tongue squamous cell carcinoma. Neoplasia 2006 Nov; 8(11): 925-32.

[100] Chung CH, Parker JS, Karaca G, *et al.* Molecular classification of head and neck squamous cell carcinomas using patterns of gene expression. Cancer Cell 2004 May; 5(5): 489-500.

[101] Aguirre Ghiso JA, Kovalski K, Ossowski L. Tumor dormancy induced by downregulation of urokinase receptor in human carcinoma involves integrin and MAPK signaling. J Cell Biol 1999 Oct 4; 147(1): 89-104.

[102] Solorzano CC, Baker CH, Tsan R, *et al.* Optimization for the blockade of epidermal growth factor receptor signaling for therapy of human pancreatic carcinoma. Clin Cancer Res 2001 Aug; 7(8): 2563-72.

[103] Matsuo M, Sakurai H, Saiki I. ZD1839, a selective epidermal growth factor receptor tyrosine kinase inhibitor, shows antimetastatic activity using a hepatocellular carcinoma model. Mol Cancer Ther 2003 Jun; 2(6): 557-61.

[104] Kim SJ, Uehara H, Karashima T, *et al.* Blockade of epidermal growth factor receptor signaling in tumor cells and tumor-associated endothelial cells for therapy of androgen-independent human prostate cancer growing in the bone of nude mice. Clin Cancer Res 2003 Mar; 9(3): 1200-10.

[105] Lacroix H, Iglehart JD, Skinner MA, *et al.* Overexpression of erbB-2 or EGF receptor proteins present in early stage mammary carcinoma is detected simultaneously in matched primary tumors and regional metastases. Oncogene 1989 Feb; 4(2): 145-51.

[106] Yu DH, Hung MC. Expression of activated rat neu oncogene is sufficient to induce experimental metastasis in 3T3 cells. Oncogene 1991 Nov; 6(11): 1991-6.

[107] Tan M, Yao J, Yu D. Overexpression of the c-erbB-2 gene enhanced intrinsic metastasis potential in human breast cancer cells without increasing their transformation abilities. Cancer Res 1997 Mar 15; 57(6): 1199-205.

[108] Ishida H, Sadahiro S, Suzuki T, *et al.* c-erbB-2 protein expression and clinicopathologic features in colorectal cancer. Oncol Rep 2000 Nov-Dec; 7(6): 1229-33.

[109] Ougolkov A, Yamashita K, Bilim V, *et al.* Abnormal expression of E-cadherin, beta-catenin, and c-erbB-2 in advanced gastric cancer: its association with liver metastasis. Int J Colorectal Dis 2003 Mar; 18(2): 160-6.

[110] Yokoyama H, Ikehara Y, Kodera Y, *et al.* Molecular basis for sensitivity and acquired resistance to gefitinib in HER2-overexpressing human gastric cancer cell lines derived from liver metastasis. Br J Cancer 2006 Dec 4; 95(11): 1504-13.

[111] Chariyalertsak S, Sugano K, Ohkura H, *et al.* Comparison of c-erbB-2 oncoprotein expression in tissue and serum of patients with stomach cancer. Tumour Biol 1994; 15(5): 294-303.

[112] Nakamura H, Kawasaki N, Taguchi M, *et al.* Association of HER-2 overexpression with prognosis in nonsmall cell lung carcinoma: a metaanalysis. Cancer 2005 May 1; 103(9): 1865-73.

[113] Onn A, Correa AM, Gilcrease M, *et al.* Synchronous overexpression of epidermal growth factor receptor and HER2-neu protein is a predictor of poor outcome in patients with stage I non-small cell lung cancer. Clin Cancer Res 2004 Jan 1; 10(1 Pt 1): 136-43.

[114] Gee JM, Harper ME, Hutcheson IR, *et al.* The antiepidermal growth factor receptor agent gefitinib (ZD1839/Iressa) improves antihormone response and prevents development of resistance in breast cancer *in vitro*. Endocrinology 2003 Nov; 144(11): 5105-17.

[115] Pantel K, Izbicki JR, Angstwurm M, *et al.* Immunocytological detection of bone marrow micrometastasis in operable non-small cell lung cancer. Cancer Res 1993 Mar 1; 53(5): 1027-31.

[116] Hess KR, Esteva FJ. Effect of HER2 status on distant recurrence in early stage breast cancer. Breast Cancer Res Treat 2013 Jan; 137(2): 449-55.

[117] Hayes DF, Yamauchi H, Broadwater G, *et al.* Circulating HER-2/erbB-2/c-neu (HER-2) extracellular domain as a prognostic factor in patients with metastatic breast cancer: Cancer and Leukemia Group B Study 8662. Clin Cancer Res 2001 Sep; 7(9): 2703-11.

[118] Nishio Y, Yamada Y, Kokubo H, *et al.* Prognostic significance of immunohistochemical expression of the HER-2/neu oncoprotein in bone metastatic prostate cancer. Urology 2006 Jul; 68(1): 110-5.

[119] Gong Y, Booser DJ, Sneige N. Comparison of HER-2 status determined by fluorescence *in situ* hybridization in primary and metastatic breast carcinoma. Cancer 2005 May 1; 103(9): 1763-9.

[120] Gancberg D, Di Leo A, Cardoso F, *et al.* Comparison of HER-2 status between primary breast cancer and corresponding distant metastatic sites. Ann Oncol 2002 Jul; 13(7): 1036-43.

[121] Amir E, Miller N, Geddie W, *et al.* Prospective study evaluating the impact of tissue confirmation of metastatic disease in patients with breast cancer. J Clin Oncol 2012 Feb 20; 30(6): 587-92.

[122] Niikura N, Liu J, Hayashi N, *et al.* Loss of human epidermal growth factor receptor 2 (HER2) expression in metastatic sites of HER2-overexpressing primary breast tumors. J Clin Oncol 2012 Feb 20; 30(6): 593-9.

[123] Oxley JD, Winkler MH, Gillatt DA, *et al.* Her-2/neu oncogene amplification in clinically localised prostate cancer. J Clin Pathol 2002 Feb; 55(2): 118-20.

[124] Reese DM, Small EJ, Magrane G, *et al.* HER2 protein expression and gene amplification in androgen-independent prostate cancer. Am J Clin Pathol 2001 Aug; 116(2): 234-9.

[125] Ross JS, Sheehan CE, Hayner-Buchan AM, *et al.* Prognostic significance of HER-2/neu gene amplification status by fluorescence *in situ* hybridization of prostate carcinoma. Cancer 1997 Jun 1; 79(11): 2162-70.

[126] Morote J, de Torres I, Caceres C, *et al.* Prognostic value of immunohistochemical expression of the c-erbB-2 oncoprotein in metastasic prostate cancer. Int J Cancer 1999 Aug 20; 84(4): 421-5.

[127] Shi Y, Brands FH, Chatterjee S, *et al.* Her-2/neu expression in prostate cancer: high level of expression associated with exposure to hormone therapy and androgen independent disease. J Urol 2001 Oct; 166(4): 1514-9.

[128] Gravina GL, Festuccia C, Angelucci A, *et al.* Long-term presence of androgens and anti-androgens modulate EGF-receptor expression and MAP-kinase phosphorylation in androgen receptor-prostate positive cancer cells. Int J Oncol 2004 Jul; 25(1): 97-104.

[129] Signoretti S, Montironi R, Manola J, *et al.* Her-2-neu expression and progression toward androgen independence in human prostate cancer. J Natl Cancer Inst 2000 Dec 6; 92(23): 1918-25.

[130] Yeh S, Lin HK, Kang HY, *et al.* From HER2/Neu signal cascade to androgen receptor and its coactivators: a novel pathway by induction of androgen target genes through MAP kinase in prostate cancer cells. Proc Natl Acad Sci USA 1999 May 11; 96(10): 5458-63.

[131] Yarden RI, Wilson MA, Chrysogelos SA. Estrogen suppression of EGFR expression in breast cancer cells: a possible mechanism to modulate growth. J Cell Biochem Suppl 2001; Suppl 36: 232-46.

[132] Wilson MA, Chrysogelos SA. Identification and characterization of a negative regulatory element within the epidermal growth factor receptor gene first intron in hormone-dependent breast cancer cells. J Cell Biochem 2002; 85(3): 601-14.

[133] Chen N, Ye XC, Chu K, *et al.* A secreted isoform of ErbB3 promotes osteonectin expression in bone and enhances the invasiveness of prostate cancer cells. Cancer Res 2007 Jul 15; 67(14): 6544-8.

[134] Cheng CJ, Ye XC, Vakar-Lopez F, *et al.* Bone microenvironment and androgen status modulate subcellular localization of ErbB3 in prostate cancer cells. Mol Cancer Res 2007 Jul; 5(7): 675-84.

[135] Polk DB. Epidermal growth factor receptor-stimulated intestinal epithelial cell migration requires phospholipase C activity. Gastroenterology 1998 Mar; 114(3): 493-502.

[136] Hynes NE, Stern DF. The biology of erbB-2/neu/HER-2 and its role in cancer. Biochim Biophys Acta 1994 Dec 30; 1198(2-3): 165-84.

[137] Verbeek BS, Adriaansen-Slot SS, Vroom TM, *et al.* Overexpression of EGFR and c-erbB2 causes enhanced cell migration in human breast cancer cells and NIH3T3 fibroblasts. FEBS Lett 1998 Mar 20; 425(1): 145-50.

[138] Spencer KS, Graus-Porta D, Leng J, *et al.* ErbB2 is necessary for induction of carcinoma cell invasion by ErbB family receptor tyrosine kinases. J Cell Biol 2000 Jan 24; 148(2): 385-97.

[139] Elenius K, Paul S, Allison G, *et al.* Activation of HER4 by heparin-binding EGF-like growth factor stimulates chemotaxis but not proliferation. Embo J 1997 Mar 17; 16(6): 1268-78.

[140] Huang SM, Li J, Harari PM. Molecular inhibition of angiogenesis and metastatic potential in human squamous cell carcinomas after epidermal growth factor receptor blockade. Mol Cancer Ther 2002 May; 1(7): 507-14.

[141] Tsai MS, Shamon-Taylor LA, Mehmi I, *et al.* Blockage of heregulin expression inhibits tumorigenicity and metastasis of breast cancer. Oncogene 2003 Feb 6; 22(5): 761-8.

[142] Nakashima N, Rose DW, Xiao S, *et al.* The functional role of CrkII in actin cytoskeleton organization and mitogenesis. J Biol Chem 1999 Jan 29; 274(5): 3001-8.

[143] Klemke RL, Cai S, Giannini AL, *et al.* Regulation of cell motility by mitogen-activated protein kinase. J Cell Biol 1997 Apr 21; 137(2): 481-92.

[144] Salomon DS, Normanno N, Ciardiello F, *et al.* The role of amphiregulin in breast cancer. Breast Cancer Res Treat 1995; 33(2): 103-14.

[145] Groenestege WM, Thebault S, van der Wijst J, *et al.* Impaired basolateral sorting of pro-EGF causes isolated recessive renal hypomagnesemia. J Clin Invest 2007 Aug; 117(8): 2260-7.

[146] Toyoda H, Komurasaki T, Uchida D, *et al.* Distribution of mRNA for human epiregulin, a differentially expressed member of the epidermal growth factor family. Biochem J 1997 Aug 15; 326 (Pt 1): 69-75.

[147] Falls DL. Neuregulins: functions, forms, and signaling strategies. Exp Cell Res 2003 Mar 10; 284(1): 14-30.

[148] DeWitt AE, Dong JY, Wiley HS, *et al.* Quantitative analysis of the EGF receptor autocrine system reveals cryptic regulation of cell response by ligand capture. J Cell Sci 2001 Jun; 114(Pt 12): 2301-13.

[149] Normanno N, Bianco C, De Luca A, *et al.* The role of EGF-related peptides in tumor growth. Front Biosci 2001 May 1; 6: D685-707.

[150] Saeki T, Stromberg K, Qi CF, *et al.* Differential immunohistochemical detection of amphiregulin and cripto in human normal colon and colorectal tumors. Cancer Res 1992 Jun 15; 52(12): 3467-73.

[151] Normanno N, Kim N, Wen D, *et al.* Expression of messenger RNA for amphiregulin, heregulin, and cripto-1, three new members of the epidermal growth factor family, in human breast carcinomas. Breast Cancer Res Treat 1995 Sep; 35(3): 293-7.

[152] Panico L, D'Antonio A, Salvatore G, *et al.* Differential immunohistochemical detection of transforming growth factor alpha, amphiregulin and CRIPTO in human normal and malignant breast tissues. Int J Cancer 1996 Jan 3; 65(1): 51-6.

[153] Fontanini G, De Laurentiis M, Vignati S, *et al.* Evaluation of epidermal growth factor-related growth factors and receptors and of neoangiogenesis in completely resected stage I-IIIA non-small-cell lung cancer: amphiregulin and microvessel count are independent prognostic indicators of survival. Clin Cancer Res 1998 Jan; 4(1): 241-9.

[154] D'Antonio A, Losito S, Pignata S, *et al.* Transforming growth factor alpha, amphiregulin and cripto-1 are frequently expressed in advanced human ovarian carcinomas. Int J Oncol 2002 Nov; 21(5): 941-8.

[155] Jannot CB, Beerli RR, Mason S, *et al.* Intracellular expression of a single-chain antibody directed to the EGFR leads to growth inhibition of tumor cells. Oncogene 1996 Jul 18; 13(2): 275-82.

[156] Harris RC, Chung E, Coffey RJ. EGF receptor ligands. Exp Cell Res 2003 Mar 10; 284(1): 2-13.

[157] Zwick E, Hackel PO, Prenzel N, *et al.* The EGF receptor as central transducer of heterologous signalling systems. Trends Pharmacol Sci 1999 Oct; 20(10): 408-12.

[158] Prenzel N, Zwick E, Daub H, *et al.* EGF receptor transactivation by G-protein-coupled receptors requires metalloproteinase cleavage of proHB-EGF. Nature 1999 Dec 23-30; 402(6764): 884-8.

[159] Banerjee S, Hussain M, Wang Z, *et al. In vitro* and *in vivo* molecular evidence for better therapeutic efficacy of ABT-627 and taxotere combination in prostate cancer. Cancer Res 2007 Apr 15; 67(8): 3818-26.

[160] Pandiella A, Bosenberg MW, Huang EJ, *et al.* Cleavage of membrane-anchored growth factors involves distinct protease activities regulated through common mechanisms. J Biol Chem 1992 Nov 25; 267(33): 24028-33.

[161] Arribas J, Coodly L, Vollmer P, *et al.* Diverse cell surface protein ectodomains are shed by a system sensitive to metalloprotease inhibitors. J Biol Chem 1996 May 10; 271(19): 11376-82.

[162] Dempsey PJ, Meise KS, Yoshitake Y, *et al.* Apical enrichment of human EGF precursor in Madin-Darby canine kidney cells involves preferential basolateral ectodomain cleavage sensitive to a metalloprotease inhibitor. J Cell Biol 1997 Aug 25; 138(4): 747-58.

[163] Santiskulvong C, Rozengurt E. Galardin (GM 6001), a broad-spectrum matrix metalloproteinase inhibitor, blocks bombesin- and LPA-induced EGF receptor transactivation and DNA synthesis in rat-1 cells. Exp Cell Res 2003 Nov 1; 290(2): 437-46.

[164] Langlois S, Nyalendo C, Di Tomasso G, *et al.* Membrane-type 1 matrix metalloproteinase stimulates cell migration through epidermal growth factor receptor transactivation. Mol Cancer Res 2007 Jun; 5(6): 569-83.

[165] Angelucci A, Gravina GL, Rucci N, *et al.* Suppression of EGF-R signaling reduces the incidence of prostate cancer metastasis in nude mice. Endocr Relat Cancer 2006 Mar; 13(1): 197-210.

[166] Guerrero J, Santibanez JF, Gonzalez A, *et al.* EGF receptor transactivation by urokinase receptor stimulus through a mechanism involving Src and matrix metalloproteinases. Exp Cell Res 2004 Jan 1; 292(1): 201-8.

[167] Monaghan-Benson E, McKeown-Longo PJ. Urokinase-type plasminogen activator receptor regulates a novel pathway of fibronectin matrix assembly requiring Src-dependent transactivation of epidermal growth factor receptor. J Biol Chem 2006 Apr 7; 281(14): 9450-9.

[168] Stewart JR, O'Brian CA. Protein kinase C-{alpha} mediates epidermal growth factor receptor transactivation in human prostate cancer cells. Mol Cancer Ther 2005 May; 4(5): 726-32.

[169] Keely SJ, Calandrella SO, Barrett KE. Carbachol-stimulated transactivation of epidermal growth factor receptor and mitogen-activated protein kinase in T(84) cells is mediated by intracellular ca(2+), PYK-2, and p60(src). J Biol Chem 2000 Apr 28; 275(17): 12619-25.
[170] Amin DN, Hida K, Bielenberg DR, *et al.* Tumor endothelial cells express epidermal growth factor receptor (EGFR) but not ErbB3 and are responsive to EGF and to EGFR kinase inhibitors. Cancer Res 2006 Feb 15; 66(4): 2173-80.
[171] Baker CH, Kedar D, McCarty MF, *et al.* Blockade of epidermal growth factor receptor signaling on tumor cells and tumor-associated endothelial cells for therapy of human carcinomas. Am J Pathol 2002 Sep; 161(3): 929-38.
[172] Sini P, Wyder L, Schnell C, *et al.* The antitumor and antiangiogenic activity of vascular endothelial growth factor receptor inhibition is potentiated by ErbB1 blockade. Clin Cancer Res 2005 Jun 15; 11(12): 4521-32.
[173] Hirata A, Ogawa S, Kometani T, *et al.* ZD1839 (Iressa) induces antiangiogenic effects through inhibition of epidermal growth factor receptor tyrosine kinase. Cancer Res 2002 May 1; 62(9): 2554-60.
[174] Baker CH, Pino MS, Fidler IJ. Phosphorylated epidermal growth factor receptor on tumor-associated endothelial cells in human renal cell carcinoma is a primary target for therapy by tyrosine kinase inhibitors. Neoplasia 2006 Jun; 8(6): 470-6.
[175] Weber KL, Doucet M, Price JE, *et al.* Blockade of epidermal growth factor receptor signaling leads to inhibition of renal cell carcinoma growth in the bone of nude mice. Cancer Res 2003 Jun 1; 63(11): 2940-7.
[176] Zhu J, Jia X, Xiao G, *et al.* EGF-like ligands stimulate osteoclastogenesis by regulating expression of osteoclast regulatory factors by osteoblasts: implications for osteolytic bone metastases. J Biol Chem 2007 Sep 14; 282(37): 26656-64.
[177] Normanno N, De Luca A, Aldinucci D, *et al.* Gefitinib inhibits the ability of human bone marrow stromal cells to induce osteoclast differentiation: implications for the pathogenesis and treatment of bone metastasis. Endocr Relat Cancer 2005 Jun; 12(2): 471-82.
[178] Qin L, Tamasi J, Raggatt L, *et al.* Amphiregulin is a novel growth factor involved in normal bone development and in the cellular response to parathyroid hormone stimulation. J Biol Chem 2005 Feb 4; 280(5): 3974-81.
[179] Gilmore JL, Scott JA, Bouizar Z, *et al.* Amphiregulin-EGFR signaling regulates PTHrP gene expression in breast cancer cells. Breast Cancer Res Treat 2008 Aug; 110(3): 493-505.
[180] Baselga J, Tripathy D, Mendelsohn J, *et al.* Phase II study of weekly intravenous recombinant humanized anti-p185HER2 monoclonal antibody in patients with HER2/neu-overexpressing metastatic breast cancer. J Clin Oncol 1996 Mar; 14(3): 737-44.
[181] Kobayashi S, Ji H, Yuza Y, *et al.* An alternative inhibitor overcomes resistance caused by a mutation of the epidermal growth factor receptor. Cancer Res 2005 Aug 15; 65(16): 7096-101.
[182] Bell DW, Lynch TJ, Haserlat SM, *et al.* Epidermal growth factor receptor mutations and gene amplification in non-small-cell lung cancer: molecular analysis of the IDEAL/INTACT gefitinib trials. J Clin Oncol 2005 Nov 1; 23(31): 8081-92.
[183] Rusch V, Klimstra D, Venkatraman E, *et al.* Overexpression of the epidermal growth factor receptor and its ligand transforming growth factor alpha is frequent in resectable non-small cell lung cancer but does not predict tumor progression. Clin Cancer Res 1997 Apr; 3(4): 515-22.

[184] Fukuoka M, Yano S, Giaccone G, *et al.* Multi-institutional randomized phase II trial of gefitinib for previously treated patients with advanced non-small-cell lung cancer (The IDEAL 1 Trial) [corrected]. J Clin Oncol 2003 Jun 15; 21(12): 2237-46.

[185] Kris MG, Natale RB, Herbst RS, *et al.* Efficacy of gefitinib, an inhibitor of the epidermal growth factor receptor tyrosine kinase, in symptomatic patients with non-small cell lung cancer: a randomized trial. Jama 2003 Oct 22; 290(16): 2149-58.

[186] Perez-Soler R. The role of erlotinib (Tarceva, OSI 774) in the treatment of non-small cell lung cancer. Clin Cancer Res 2004 Jun 15; 10(12 Pt 2): 4238s-40s.

[187] Romond EH, Perez EA, Bryant J, *et al.* Trastuzumab plus adjuvant chemotherapy for operable HER2-positive breast cancer. N Engl J Med 2005 Oct 20; 353(16): 1673-84.

[188] Piccart-Gebhart MJ, Procter M, Leyland-Jones B, *et al.* Trastuzumab after adjuvant chemotherapy in HER2-positive breast cancer. N Engl J Med 2005 Oct 20; 353(16): 1659-72.

[189] Smith I, Procter M, Gelber RD, *et al.* 2-year follow-up of trastuzumab after adjuvant chemotherapy in HER2-positive breast cancer: a randomised controlled trial. Lancet 2007 Jan 6; 369(9555): 29-36.

[190] Joensuu H, Bono P, Kataja V, *et al.* Fluorouracil, epirubicin, and cyclophosphamide with either docetaxel or vinorelbine, with or without trastuzumab, as adjuvant treatments of breast cancer: final results of the FinHer Trial. J Clin Oncol 2009 Dec 1; 27(34): 5685-92.

[191] Musolino A, Ciccolallo L, Panebianco M, *et al.* Multifactorial central nervous system recurrence susceptibility in patients with HER2-positive breast cancer: epidemiological and clinical data from a population-based cancer registry study. Cancer 2011 May 1; 117(9): 1837-46.

[192] Perez EA, Romond EH, Suman VJ, *et al.* Four-year follow-up of trastuzumab plus adjuvant chemotherapy for operable human epidermal growth factor receptor 2-positive breast cancer: joint analysis of data from NCCTG N9831 and NSABP B-31. J Clin Oncol 2011 Sep 1; 29(25): 3366-73.

[193] Pegram MD, Slamon DJ. Combination therapy with trastuzumab (Herceptin) and cisplatin for chemoresistant metastatic breast cancer: evidence for receptor-enhanced chemosensitivity. Semin Oncol 1999 Aug; 26(4 Suppl 12): 89-95.

[194] Slamon DJ, Leyland-Jones B, Shak S, *et al.* Use of chemotherapy plus a monoclonal antibody against HER2 for metastatic breast cancer that overexpresses HER2. N Engl J Med 2001 Mar 15; 344(11): 783-92.

[195] Burnstein H, Storniolo AM, Franco S, *et al.* A phase II, open-label, multicenter study of lapatinib in two cohorts of patients with advanced or metastatic breast cancer who have progressed while receiving trastuzumabcontaining regimens. Ann Oncol 2004; 15 (Suppl 3): iii27.

[196] O'Shaughnessy J, Vukelja SJ, Marsland T, *et al.* Phase II trial of gemcitabine plus trastuzumab in metastatic breast cancer patients previously treated with chemotherapy: preliminary results. Clin Breast Cancer 2002 May; 3 Suppl 1: 17-20.

[197] Gori S, Colozza M, Mosconi AM, *et al.* Phase II study of weekly paclitaxel and trastuzumab in anthracycline- and taxane-pretreated patients with HER2-overexpressing metastatic breast cancer. Br J Cancer 2004 Jan 12; 90(1): 36-40.

[198] Burris H, 3rd, Yardley D, Jones S, *et al.* Phase II trial of trastuzumab followed by weekly paclitaxel/carboplatin as first-line treatment for patients with metastatic breast cancer. J Clin Oncol 2004 May 1; 22(9): 1621-9.

[199] Marty M, Cognetti F, Maraninchi D, *et al.* Randomized phase II trial of the efficacy and safety of trastuzumab combined with docetaxel in patients with human epidermal growth factor receptor 2-positive metastatic breast cancer administered as first-line treatment: the M77001 study group. J Clin Oncol 2005 Jul 1; 23(19): 4265-74.

[200] Robert N, Leyland-Jones B, Asmar L, *et al.* Randomized phase III study of trastuzumab, paclitaxel, and carboplatin compared with trastuzumab and paclitaxel in women with HER-2-overexpressing metastatic breast cancer. J Clin Oncol 2006 Jun 20; 24(18): 2786-92.

[201] Chan A, Martin M, Untch M, *et al.* Vinorelbine plus trastuzumab combination as first-line therapy for HER 2-positive metastatic breast cancer patients: an international phase II trial. Br J Cancer 2006 Oct 9; 95(7): 788-93.

[202] Mass RD, Press MF, Anderson S, *et al.* Evaluation of clinical outcomes according to HER2 detection by fluorescence *in situ* hybridization in women with metastatic breast cancer treated with trastuzumab. Clin Breast Cancer 2005 Aug; 6(3): 240-6.

[203] Venturini M, Bighin C, Monfardini S, *et al.* Multicenter phase II study of trastuzumab in combination with epirubicin and docetaxel as first-line treatment for HER2-overexpressing metastatic breast cancer. Breast Cancer Res Treat 2006 Jan; 95(1): 45-53.

[204] Tan-Chiu E, Yothers G, Romond E, *et al.* Assessment of cardiac dysfunction in a randomized trial comparing doxorubicin and cyclophosphamide followed by paclitaxel, with or without trastuzumab as adjuvant therapy in node-positive, human epidermal growth factor receptor 2-overexpressing breast cancer: NSABP B-31. J Clin Oncol 2005 Nov 1; 23(31): 7811-9.

[205] Burstein HJ, Lieberman G, Slamon DJ, *et al.* Isolated central nervous system metastases in patients with HER2-overexpressing advanced breast cancer treated with first-line trastuzumab-based therapy. Ann Oncol 2005 Nov; 16(11): 1772-7.

[206] Bendell JC, Domchek SM, Burstein HJ, *et al.* Central nervous system metastases in women who receive trastuzumab-based therapy for metastatic breast carcinoma. Cancer 2003 Jun 15; 97(12): 2972-7.

[207] Bria E, Cuppone F, Fornier M, *et al.* Cardiotoxicity and incidence of brain metastases after adjuvant trastuzumab for early breast cancer: the dark side of the moon? A meta-analysis of the randomized trials. Breast Cancer Res Treat 2008 May; 109(2): 231-9.

[208] Stemmler HJ, Schmitt M, Harbeck N, *et al.* Application of intrathecal trastuzumab (Herceptintrade mark) for treatment of meningeal carcinomatosis in HER2-overexpressing metastatic breast cancer. Oncol Rep 2006 May; 15(5): 1373-7.

[209] Bang YJ, Van Cutsem E, Feyereislova A, *et al.* Trastuzumab in combination with chemotherapy *versus* chemotherapy alone for treatment of HER2-positive advanced gastric or gastro-oesophageal junction cancer (ToGA): a phase 3, open-label, randomised controlled trial. Lancet 2010 Aug 28; 376(9742): 687-97.

[210] Barlesi F, Tchouhadjian C, Doddoli C, *et al.* Gefitinib (ZD1839, Iressa) in non-small-cell lung cancer: a review of clinical trials from a daily practice perspective. Fundam Clin Pharmacol 2005 Jun; 19(3): 385-93.

[211] von Minckwitz G, Jonat W, Fasching P, *et al.* A multicentre phase II study on gefitinib in taxane- and anthracycline-pretreated metastatic breast cancer. Breast Cancer Res Treat 2005 Jan; 89(2): 165-72.

[212] Rothenberg ML, LaFleur B, Levy DE, *et al.* Randomized phase II trial of the clinical and biological effects of two dose levels of gefitinib in patients with recurrent colorectal adenocarcinoma. J Clin Oncol 2005 Dec 20; 23(36): 9265-74.

[213] Kirby AM, A'Hern RP, D'Ambrosio C, *et al.* Gefitinib (ZD1839, Iressa) as palliative treatment in recurrent or metastatic head and neck cancer. Br J Cancer 2006 Mar 13; 94(5): 631-6.

[214] Cohen EE, Rosen F, Stadler WM, *et al.* Phase II trial of ZD1839 in recurrent or metastatic squamous cell carcinoma of the head and neck. J Clin Oncol 2003 May 15; 21(10): 1980-7.

[215] Zampino MG, Magni E, Massacesi C, *et al.* First clinical experience of orally active epidermal growth factor receptor inhibitor combined with simplified FOLFOX6 as first-line treatment for metastatic colorectal cancer. Cancer 2007 Aug 15; 110(4): 752-8.

[216] Ciardiello F, Troiani T, Caputo F, *et al.* Phase II study of gefitinib in combination with docetaxel as first-line therapy in metastatic breast cancer. Br J Cancer 2006 Jun 5; 94(11): 1604-9.

[217] Pallis AG, Christofillakis C, Tselepatiotis E, *et al.* Sequential administration of docetaxel followed by maintenance gefitinib, as salvage treatment in patients with advanced NSCLC: a multicenter phase II trial. Lung Cancer 2007 Jan; 55(1): 101-7.

[218] Meyerhardt JA, Zhu AX, Enzinger PC, *et al.* Phase II study of capecitabine, oxaliplatin, and erlotinib in previously treated patients with metastastic colorectal cancer. J Clin Oncol 2006 Apr 20; 24(12): 1892-7.

[219] Cunningham D, Humblet Y, Siena S, *et al.* Cetuximab monotherapy and cetuximab plus irinotecan in irinotecan-refractory metastatic colorectal cancer. N Engl J Med 2004 Jul 22; 351(4): 337-45.

[220] Reynolds NA, Wagstaff AJ. Cetuximab: in the treatment of metastatic colorectal cancer. Drugs 2004; 64(1): 109-18; discussion 19-21.

[221] Burtness B. Cetuximab and cisplatin for chemotherapy-refractory squamous cell cancer of the head and neck. J Clin Oncol 2005 Aug 20; 23(24): 5440-2.

[222] Vogel CL, Cobleigh MA, Tripathy D, *et al.* Efficacy and safety of trastuzumab as a single agent in first-line treatment of HER2-overexpressing metastatic breast cancer. J Clin Oncol 2002 Feb 1; 20(3): 719-26.

[223] Burris HA, 3rd, Hurwitz HI, Dees EC, *et al.* Phase I safety, pharmacokinetics, and clinical activity study of lapatinib (GW572016), a reversible dual inhibitor of epidermal growth factor receptor tyrosine kinases, in heavily pretreated patients with metastatic carcinomas. J Clin Oncol 2005 Aug 10; 23(23): 5305-13.

[224] Blackwell KL, Kaplan EH, Franco SX, *et al.* A phase II, open-label, multicenter study of GW572016 in patients with trastuzumab-refractory metastatic breast cancer. J Clin Oncol 2004; 22 (14S): 3006.

[225] Blackwell KL, Burstein HJ, Storniolo AM, *et al.* Randomized study of Lapatinib alone or in combination with trastuzumab in women with ErbB2-positive, trastuzumab-refractory metastatic breast cancer. J Clin Oncol 2010 Mar 1; 28(7): 1124-30.

[226] Gril B, Palmieri D, Bronder JL, *et al.* Effect of lapatinib on the outgrowth of metastatic breast cancer cells to the brain. J Natl Cancer Inst 2008 Aug 6; 100(15): 1092-103.

[227] Cameron D, Casey M, Press M, *et al.* A phase III randomized comparison of lapatinib plus capecitabine *versus* capecitabine alone in women with advanced breast cancer that has progressed on trastuzumab: updated efficacy and biomarker analyses. Breast Cancer Res Treat 2008 Dec; 112(3): 533-43.

[228] Metro G, Foglietta J, Russillo M, *et al.* Clinical outcome of patients with brain metastases from HER2-positive breast cancer treated with lapatinib and capecitabine. Ann Oncol 2011 Mar; 22(3): 625-30.

[229] Baselga J, Gelmon KA, Verma S, *et al.* Phase II trial of pertuzumab and trastuzumab in patients with human epidermal growth factor receptor 2-positive metastatic breast cancer that progressed during prior trastuzumab therapy. J Clin Oncol 2010 Mar 1; 28(7): 1138-44.

[230] Miles D, Baselga J, Amadori D, *et al.* Treatment of older patients with HER2-positive metastatic breast cancer with pertuzumab, trastuzumab, and docetaxel: subgroup analyses from a randomized, double-blind, placebo-controlled phase III trial (CLEOPATRA). Breast Cancer Res Treat 2013 Nov; 142(1): 89-99.

Advances in Cancer Drug Targets, Vol. 2, 2014, 127-174

CHAPTER 4

Anti-Tumour Effects of Bisphosphonates - What have we Learned from *In Vivo* Models?

Hannah K. Brown and Ingunn Holen*

Academic Unit of Clinical Oncology, University of Sheffield, Sheffield, UK

Abstract: Bisphosphonates are extensively used to treat cancer-induced bone disease in a range of solid and bone derived tumours, where they reduce the incidence of skeletal related events and improve patients' quality of life. Recent reports indicate that bisphosphonates may also prevent recurrence of breast cancer at peripheral sites, suggesting that these drugs may have anti-cancer activity outside the skeleton and effects on a range of tumour cell types have been reported *in vitro*. These positive results have subsequently been supported by investigations of effects of bisphosphonates on tumour growth *in vivo,* both in bone and at peripheral sites. A reduction of tumour burden and in cancer-induced bone disease following bisphosphonate treatment is demonstrated in several model systems, including breast and prostate cancer, osteosarcoma and multiple myeloma. In addition, bisphosphonates have been shown to significantly reduce growth of human tumour cells implanted subcutaneously in immunocompromised mice. However, the majority of *in vivo* studies reporting anti-tumour effects have used high doses and frequent administration of bisphosphonates, and the clinical relevance of these data have therefore been the subject of considerable debate. Bisphosphonates may hold greater promise as anti-tumour agents when used in combination with cytotoxic drugs, and several *in vivo* studies have reported substantial increased inhibition of tumour growth and improved survival when bisphosphonates have been added to standard chemotherapy regimens. This review will summarise the published data on anti-tumour effects of bisphosphonates reported from *in vivo* models, alone and in combination with other anti-cancer agents, and highlight the main lessons learned and future challenges in this field.

Keywords: Bone metastases, breast cancer, cancer-induced bone disease, prostate cancer.

INTRODUCTION

Different types of solid tumours and haematological malignancies show a predilection of metastases to bone, with breast, prostate and lung cancer being the

***Corresponding Author Ingunn Holen:** Academic Unit of Clinical Oncology, Medical School, University of Sheffield, Beech Hill Road, Sheffield S10 2RX, UK; Tel: + 44 (0) 114 271 3854;
E-mail: I.Holen@Sheffield.ac.uk

Atta-ur-Rahman (Ed)

most common types. 65-70% of breast cancer patients with advanced disease develop bone metastases and death is often due to the development of metastatic lesions and not because of the primary tumour [1]. Cancer spread to bone results in development of osteolytic, osteoblastic or mixed lesions, depending on the type of primary cancer. The associated skeletal morbidity is high, with a pathophysiology of bone fractures, hypercalcemia of malignancy and spinal cord compression. Cancer-induced bone disease is generally treated with an anti-neoplastic and a palliative regimen, the latter including radiotherapy, administration of analgesia and occasionally orthopaedic surgery to improve quality of life. In addition, bisphosphonates are effective inhibitors of bone resorption, resulting in pain relief and reduced incidence of skeletal skeletal-related events [2, 3]. Zoledronic acid, ibandronate and pamidronate belong to the group of nitrogen-containing bisphosphonates (NBPs) with increased potency compared to the non-nitrogen containing counterparts like clodronate. Inhibition of bone resorption is mediated through inhibition of osteoclast activity at micromolar concentrations [4-6], which NBPs cause by inhibition of key enzymes of the mevalonate pathway [7-9], and non-NBPs by inducing intracellular accumulation of cytotoxic ATP analogues [10].

Apart from the effects on bone resorption, there is increasing interest in the potential anti-tumour effects of bisphosphonates, and evidence is emerging from *in vitro* and *in vivo* studies suggesting an anti-cancer effect on a range of different tumour cells. However, the exact cellular and molecular mechanisms involved in the proposed anti-tumour effects of bisphosphonates remain to be elucidated. One major difficulty in pinpointing these is the separation between direct effects on cancer cells and those mediated through alterations of the bone microenvironment. Although the majority of the published studies conclude that the bone-mediated, indirect effects on tumour cells are predominantly *via* inhibition of bone resorption, data are currently emerging that osteoblasts (and potentially other cells) as well as the vasculature are also affected by NBPs and may thus affect tumour cell homing, progression and growth in bone. In addition, the putative metastatic niche in bone may be altered by bisphosphonate treatment potentially leading to anti-tumour effects, however, this remains to be thoroughly investigated. When using *in vivo* models, a separation of indirect and direct activity is possible by *e.g.* subcutaneous implantation of tumour cells, which allows the investigation of the effects on cancer cells without bone involvement. As it will be illustrated by a number of studies described in this review, it is likely that a combination of both direct and indirect factors co-operate to generate the reduction in tumour growth caused by bisphosphonates. New clinical applications of these drugs are currently emerging. For example, treatment-induced bone loss caused by aromatase inhibitors in treatment of estrogen receptor-positive breast cancer may be counteracted by bisphosphonates, either at the point when increased bone loss is detected or as a preventive therapy [11, 12].

The *in vivo* pharmacokinetics of bisphosphonates have been an important issue for investigations of the potential anti-tumour effects. Because of their high affinity to bone, bisphosphonates are readily cleared from the circulation. In clinical practice, zoledronic acid administration, 4 mg *i.v.* every 3-4 weeks [13], results in peak plasma levels of 1-2 μM for a few hours and declines to only ~1% after 24 hours. In bone, however, zoledronic acid concentrations are thought to reach levels of up to 1000 μM in the resorption pits of actively resorbing osteoclasts [14], a level that may induce cytotoxic effects. It has therefore been proposed that tumour cells within bone could be exposed to a potentially cytotoxic concentration of bisphosphonates, compared to peripheral tumours, although this remains to be proven. The difference in drug distribution between tissues leads to the question whether bisphosphonate concentrations outside bone ever reach cytotoxic levels. Preclinical studies reporting anti-tumour effects of bisphosphonates have frequently used high and/or repeated dosing regimens, resulting in accumulated concentrations well beyond those used in clinic. More recently, attention has turned to the use of combination therapy, where drugs specifically targeting the tumour cells (chemotherapy, endocrine, biological agents) are given together with anti-resorptive agents targeting the bone microenvironment. *In vivo* studies have shown increased inhibition of tumour growth following combined treatment compared to that seen by the use of single therapies, and clinical trials are needed to verify the relevance for human cancer. In addition to affecting established bone metastases, a number of *in vivo* studies have shown that a preventive bisphosphonate schedule (treatment initiated prior to tumour cell implantation) leads to reduced levels of subsequent bone metastases.

The recently reported AZURE trial showed that adjuvant zoledronic acid therapy reduced bone metastasis in post-meonpausal breast cancer patients, supporting that bisphosphonates may have a preventive effect [15]. This article reviews the data from the main *in vivo* studies investigating the anti-tumour effects of bisphosphonate mono- and combination-therapy, summarising their conclusions and pointing out remaining challenges.

BISPHOSPHONATES ALONE – EFFECTS ON TUMOURS IN BONE

Bisphosphonates are commonly used to treat patients with confirmed metastatic bone disease, and a growing number of publications report a potential anti-tumour activity of these compounds, reviewed in [16-19]. Initial studies focused on the effects of bisphosphonates used as single agents in the treatment of cancer-induced bone disease, whereas more recently the effects on tumours in other sites are increasingly investigated. As described in the following sections, there is a considerable body of evidence of anti-tumour effects of bisphosphonates in bone, reducing the extent of bone lesions and bone tumour burden. In contrast, reports of the ability of bisphosphonates to affect tumours that have progressed to colonise bone-associated soft tissue and peripheral tumours are less consistent. A number of different tumour types that grow in bone have been subject to investigation of the effects of bisphosphonate treatment *in vivo*. Both NBPs (zoledronic acid, pamidronate, alendronate, risedronate) as well as non-nitrogen BPs (*e.g.* clodronate) have been used. The effects of bisphosphonates on the early stages of bone metastases development have been investigated using preventive treatment regimens (started either before or at the same time as tumour cell implantation), allowing assessment of tumour cell migration, invasion and adhesion to bone. In addition, therapeutic protocols have been applied to assess the effects on established bone metastases. The range of effects caused by bisphosphonates in these studies is shown in Fig. (**1**). The following sections summarise the data from a number of published studies using single, preventive and/or therapeutic protocols.

Inhibition of Osteolysis but No Effect on Skeletal Tumour Burden

Using zoledronic acid in a mouse model of canine prostate cancer, Thudi *et al.* found no effect of bisphosphonates on skeletal tumour burden despite a reduction in osteolysis [20]. Male nude mice were injected with Ace-1 cells into the left ventricle of the heart and treated with zoledronic acid (100 µg/kg, 2x/week). Neither the preventive (week 1 to 4) nor delayed treatment with zoledronic acid (week 2 to 4) caused a significant change in bone tumour burden when compared to control animals, despite causing significantly decreased osteolytic areas. The inhibition of osteolytic lesions was less pronounced in the delayed treatment group compared to preventive treatment, potentially due to differences in treatment time. Interestingly, these results suggest that a bisphosphonate-induced change of the bone microenvironment by inhibition of osteolysis is not necessarily associated with a reduction in tumour growth and development.

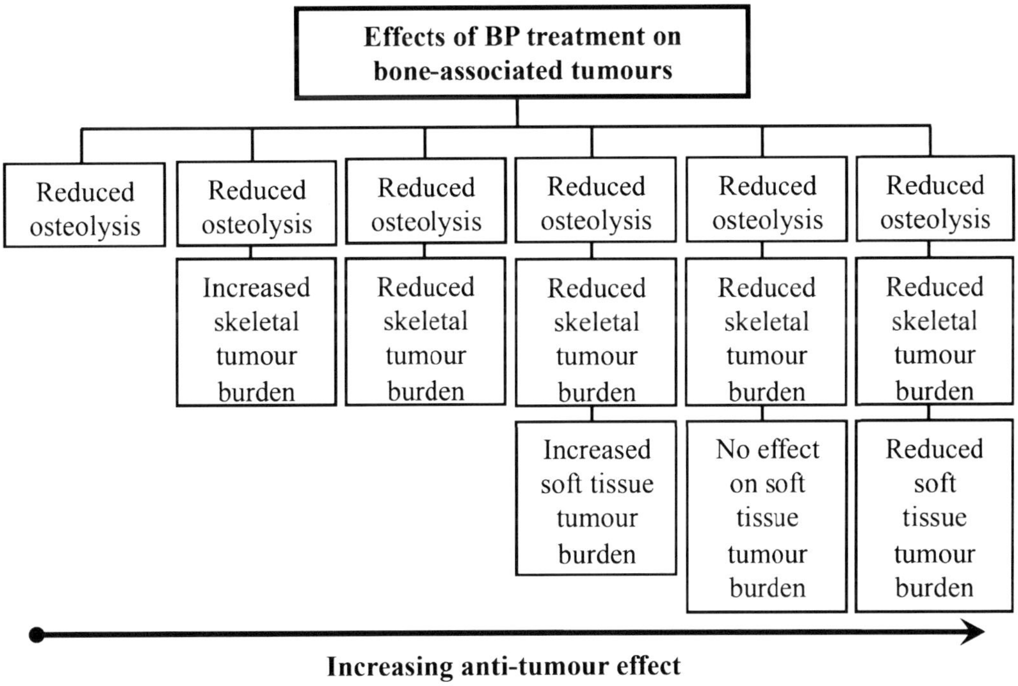

Fig. (1): Anti-tumour effects of bisphosphonates reported from *in vivo* model systems.

A more recent study utilising a mixed osteoblastic and osteolytic prostate cancer model confirmed these results [21]. C57Bl/6 mice were intracardiac injected with RM1 (BM) cells and treated with 20 or 100 µg/kg zoledronic acid every 4 days until day 12. Neither of the two doses significantly reduced total tumour number although bone-sparing effects were detected compared to control. The highest dose lead to an increase in survival in treated compared to control animals ($p=0.031$).

Two studies in models of multiple myeloma also showed that inhibition of bone resorption does not necessarily affect tumour growth in bone. Female C57BL/KaLwRij mice bearing 5TGM1 or 5T33 myeloma cells treated with ibandronate (4 μg/mouse/day), starting on the day of cancer cell implantation had significantly reduced number and size of osteolytic lesions [22]. However, although the ibandronate dose used was 100x higher than the concentration known to inhibit osteolysis, there was no decrease in the tumour area in bone, liver or spleen, or increase in survival, compared to control.

The data are in agreement with a study investigating the effects of ibandronate on 5T2MM myeloma bearing mice [23]. Animals were injected with a single dose of 100 μg ibandronate, or for 4 days, and sacrificed 3 days after the last injection. Single or repeated drug treatment had no effect on tumour cell number and apoptosis in bone when compared to control. These data reflect the results obtained from clinical studies on bisphosphonates, reporting a reduction in bone disease accompanied by improved quality of life, but without significant increases in survival [24, 25]. None of studies described above showed anti-tumour effects in bone [20-23] and only one reported increased survival after BP treatment [21]. Collectively, the data suggest that a reduction in bone resorption does not necessarily result in reduced skeletal tumour burden.

Inhibition of Osteolysis, Increased Tumour Burden in Bone, No Effect on Associated Soft Tissue Tumours

In contrast to the studies described in the previous section, increased bone tumour burden accompanied by reduced osteolysis after bisphosphonate treatment has been reported [26]. The effects of pamidronate on osteolytic lesions caused by Walker 256 carcinosarcoma cells in male Fischer rats was investigated and animals received pamidronate (0.5 mg/kg/day) for 7 days before intramuscular injection of cancer cells into the thigh. Preventive treatment with pamidronate induced a significant increase in trabecular bone thickness showing the expected drug-induced inhibition of osteolysis. A significant increase in tumour area and increased growth rate of cancer cells located in the femur of animals in the preventive group was observed when compared to control. Tumour burden was not increased either in liver, lungs or kidneys, indicating that the effect in bone was somehow associated with the inhibition of bone resorption. This report remains the only one to show increased tumour burden in bone following bisphosphonate treatment, and the exact mechanisms involved were not identified, suggesting that the increased bone-associated tumour burden is a feature of the particular model used in this study.

Inhibition of Osteolysis, Reduced Skeletal Tumour Burden and No Effect on Soft Tissue Tumours

Anti-tumour activity of bisphosphonates on prostate tumour growth in bone has been investigated using nude mice inoculated intratibially with the human prostate cancer cells PC3-GFP, comparing the effects of etidronic acid, pamidronate, 1,1'-diphosphonopropane-2,3'-dicar-bonic acid monohydrate and olpadronate on skeletal tumour burden *in vivo* [27]. Bisphosphonates were administered at 2.6 mmol/L (250 μl/mouse) four weeks prior to, on the day of, and thirty days after tumour cell implantation. A reduction in the severity of osteolytic bone lesions and a decrease in osseous tumour growth were only observed in animals treated with olpadronate. Pamidronate did cause a reduction in tumour burden, but was less effective than olpadronate. The other bisphosphonates tested in this study had no effect on either bone disease or tumour burden, showing that there is great variety in the efficacy of different bisphosphonates, reflecting the differences in potency of the compounds. Using the same prostate cancer model, Burton *et al.* [28] found a reduction in the number of osteolytic lesions and tumour size in bone after administration of pamidronate at high (14.4 mg/kg) but not at low concentrations (2.2 mg/kg). Animals bearing intratibial PC3-GFP tumours were treated with pamidronate 1 month before, on the day of and monthly after tumour cell inoculation. The data suggest a dose-dependent anti-tumour effect of pamidronate, and that a monthly high dose strategy may be beneficial in clinical treatment of prostate cancer.

Nude mice bearing PC3 cells (causing osteolytic lesions) or LuCap 23.1 xenografts (causing osteoblastic lesions) were used by Corey *et al.* to investigate the anti-tumour activity of zoledronic acid [29]. Prostate cancer cells or tissues were engrafted either subcutaneously, to study the drugs effects on soft tissue tumour, or injected intratibially to study effects on bone. Mice bearing established subcutaneous tumours were treated with zoledronic acid (5 μg/mouse, 2x/week) while animals bearing intratibial tumours were treated using a preventive protocol (commencing with cancer cell injection) or a therapeutic protocol (33 or 7 days after tumour cell injection for LuCaP 23.1 or PC-3, respectively). There was no inhibition of subcutaneous tumour growth after zoledronic acid administration, but a significant reduction in osseous tumour cell proliferation and osteolysis. However, zoledronic acid did not cause complete inhibition of tumour cell growth and preventive treatment did not affect tumour take rate when compared to control animals, suggesting no prevention of *de-novo* metastases formation in this model. In conclusion, the data indicate that zoledronic acid can reduce prostate cancer-induced tumour growth in bone but does not affect extra-osseous tumours.

Tumour cells are exposed to a variety of stimulating factors in bone and it has been shown that tumour cells expressing calcium-sensing receptors show increased proliferation when exposed to high calcium levels, as may be the case in an active resorbing bone environment. The effects of reduced calcium levels in bone after anti-resorptive treatment of ACE-1^{Luc} prostate cancer cells seeded onto mineralised matrices (neonatal mouse vertebrae = vossicles) or a non-mineralised collagen matrix followed by subcutaneous implantation into athymic mice were assessed [30]. Treatment with zoledronic acid (200 μg/kg, twice/week) or OPG-Fc (10 mg/kg, 3x/week) both showed bone protective activity compared to control in vossicles, which was associated with a reduction in tumour growth. Treated animals bearing tumour-inoculated collagen matrices did not have reduced tumour burden compared to PBS control. The authors concluded that the inhibitory effect of anti-resorptive agents is mediated through an indirect effect of inhibition of bone resorption and thus decreased calcium release from bone.

Effects of bisphosphonates on tumours in and outside of bone have also been extensively investigated in breast cancer models. Neudert *et al.* injected MDA-MB-231 human breast tumour cells directly into the femoral artery of male athymic rats, resulting in site-specific osteolytic lesions in the tibia and femora [31]. Therapeutic ibandronate (10 μg/kg/day, day 18-30) inhibited progression of established osteolytic lesions and metastases. Complete elimination of tumour growth was not achieved, and it was shown that the therapeutic effect was size-dependent as only small lesions (<6 mm) and the corresponding tumour area shrank significantly, whereas the bigger lesions (>6 mm) were unaffected. When treatment was initiated 3 days prior to cancer cell injection, formation of new osteolytic lesions was decreased, bone structure appeared healthy and animals had reduced incidence of metastases. Small metastatic foci may consist of cells that are bone microenvironment-dependent and therefore more sensitive towards the bisphosphonate-induced changes, whereas with increased size tumours may achieve autocrine (microenvironment-independent) growth. Similarly, Thudi *et al.* reported that the preventive protocol was more effective in the inhibition of osteolysis than the therapeutic protocol, suggesting that bisphosphonates are most effective at the early stages of cancer-induced bone disease when tumour growth and expansion is still dependent on the microenvironment [20].

Early studies by Mundy *et al.* used the 4T1 mouse mammary tumour model to assess the effects of zoledronic acid (day 7: single 0.3 μg/mouse and 0.5 or 5 μg/day) on established tumours following inoculation of 4T1/luc breast cancer cells in the mammary fat pad [32]. A single dose of 0.3 μg zoledronic acid reduced osteolytic areas, and both protocols of the repeated schedule (0.5 or 5 μg/day) were shown to significantly increase 4T1 tumour cell and osteoclast apoptosis in bone metastases. This bone associated anti-tumour effect was also reported by Hiraga *et al.* who determined the effects of ibandronate in a xenograft model of human breast cancer [33]. MDA-MB-231 cells were intracardiac injected and animals were treated with ibandronate (4 μg/mouse/day) from day 21 to 28 when bone metastases were established. The treatment profoundly reduced expansion of the osteolytic lesions and reduced tumour burden in bone, which was associated with increased cancer cell apoptosis but no change in proliferation. The number of osteoclasts was dramatically reduced in treated mice and an increase in apoptotic osteoclasts was observed suggesting that the effects on bone tumour burden were due to drug-induced apoptosis and inhibition of bone resorption. Treatment with ibandronate (4 μg/mouse/day, day 7-28) did not reduce tumour burden, affect tumour cell apoptosis or proliferation when MDA-MB-231 cells were implanted in the mammary fat pad. The data suggest that the anti-cancer activities exhibited by ibandronate are restricted to the bone microenvironment, but it is unclear whether effects seen in bone are due to direct or indirect anti-cancer activity and both mechanisms may contribute to the inhibition of osteolytic bone metastases.

Fournier and colleagues performed two elegant studies aiming to decipher if NBPs exert their anti-tumour effects *via* indirect or direct effects [34, 35]. The group compared risedronate with analogues exhibiting either 70-fold lower bone mineral binding affinity and poor anti-resorptive activities [34] or normal bone binding properties but with a lower ability to inhibit osteoclasts [35]. The first study assessed whether the high affinity of NBPs to bone mineral lowers the anti-tumour effects in bone in a B02 bone metastases model by reducing free drug concentrations [34]. Treatment with NE-10790 (150 μg/kg/day) showed a 70% reduction in bone tumour burden while risedronate induced a 40% inhibition compared to control when measured by non-invasive imaging. It was shown that this anti-tumour effect was not induced by bone sparing activities because 150 μg/kg of NE-10790 did not inhibit osteolysis and risedronate did. When the two drugs were given in combination no additional anti-tumour effects were detected *vs* single treatment. The low bone binding affinity of NE-10790 may cause the BP analogue to be more readily available to tumours growing outside of bone, however, neither risedronate nor NE-10790 exerted anti-neoplastic activity either in a subcutaneous breast tumour model or in a lung metastases model using intravenously injected B16-F10 melanoma cells when compared to vehicle control. In a follow up study [35] the group inverted the strategy and made use of a risedronate analogue (NE-58051) that binds to bone at a similar rate than risedronate but with a 3000-fold lower anti-resorptive activity. NE-58051 or risedronate were given daily at 150 μg/kg from day 0-35 in a B02 bone metastases model. Only risedronate protected bone structure and reduced tumour growth in bone in comparison to NE-58051 or PBS treated mice suggesting that inhibition of osteoclast activity is required to induce anti-neoplastic effects in bone. When the compounds were injected into animals bearing established subcutaneous B02 tumours or in a model of B16-F10 melanoma lung cancer neither of the drugs induced anti-tumour effects. The overall conclusion from these studies was that NBP-induced anti-cancer effects are predominantly mediated through their anti-resorptive activity. However, once the compounds are released from bone they may also be able to target tumour cells directly depending on their proximity.

To date, the strongest evidence of osteoclast independent anti-tumour effects of zoledronic acid is generated in animals with defective osteoclasts [36]. Mice lacking functional osteoclasts ($src^{-/-}$) and wild type (WT) radiation chimeras were treated with zoledronic acid (0.75 µg/mouse) 10 and 3 days before injection of B16-FL melanoma cells. Pre-treatment with zoledronic acid significantly reduced tumour burden in bone by 88% in $src^{-/-}$ radiation chimeras compared to PBS control. WT radiation chimeras treated with zoledronic acid showed a 68% reduction in tumour burden compared to PBS control. The study provides convincing evidence that zoledronic acid can modify tumour growth by mechanisms that do not involve osteoclast inhibition.

The effects of non-nitrogen compared to nitrogen-containing BPs on tumours derived from the human breast cancer cells B02/GFP.2 were assessed in a preventive (from day -1) or therapeutic (day 18 onwards) setting [37]. Zoledronic acid was given daily (3 µg/kg preventive and 7 µg/kg therapeutic), weekly (20 µg/kg preventive and 50 µg/kg therapeutic) or on a single dose schedule (100 µg/kg preventive or therapeutic). The accumulated concentration of 98-100 µg/kg/mouse is estimated to be equivalent to the standard clinical dose (4 mg *i.v.* every 3 to 4 weeks). Clodronate was administered daily at 530 µg/kg, a dose analogous to the oral 1600 mg/day clinical regimen. Zoledronic acid significantly reduced osteolytic bone disease in all settings apart from a single preventive dose. A single therapeutic dose of zoledronic acid reduced skeletal tumour burden but the preventive administration did not. In contrast, preventive or therapeutic administration of clodronate (daily) and zoledronic acid (daily or weekly) significantly reduced tumour burden, with zoledronic acid treatment being superior to clodronate. Taken together, the data suggests that frequent administration of bisphosphonates is necessary to inhibit tumour cell growth in bone, indicating that drug-induced inhibition of osteolysis is associated with the anti-tumour effects. Bisphosphonate administration in adjuvant breast cancer therapy could therefore reduce cancer-induced bone disease but may not be sufficient to affect tumour growth in the soft tissue surrounding affected bones.

In some cases tumours growing in the bone marrow may expand into the adjacent soft tissues, allowing studies of the effects of bisphosphonate treatment on both intra- and/or extra-osseous tumour growth. Van der Pluijm *et al.* used the MDA-231-B/luc+ breast cancer model to investigate the effect of olpadronate on cancer-induced bone metastases [38]. When olpadronate was given in a preventive way (1.6 μmol/kg/day starting 2 days before intracardiac tumour cell injection) the formation of new bone metastases was significantly reduced. Olpadronate also inhibited osteolysis when administered in a therapeutic protocol (1.6 μmol/kg/day, from day 28 to day 46), but the inhibition of bone resorption did not have significant impact on osseous tumour progression when metastases were already established at the time of bisphosphonate administration. It is noteworthy that the observed inhibitory effect on bone metastases was only transient following either of the treatment regimens. In an intra-osseous model, daily injections of pamidronate (16 μmol/kg/day) or olpadronate (1.6 μmol/kg/day) were given from day 3 to 43 after cancer cell implantation. Intra-osseous tumour burden was significantly reduced with either bisphosphonate, but total tumour burden including in the soft tissues surrounding bone, was not. It was suggested that this was due to the drug-induced increase in trabecular bone volume resulting in a limited availability of space within bone, thus boosting cancer cell growth in the adjacent soft tissue. The authors concluded that bisphosphonate treatment did not exert direct anti-tumour effects, and that cancer cell growth was merely redirected from intra- to extra-osseous sites due to space limitations caused by inhibition of bone resorption.

In addition to the investigations on breast and prostate cancer the effects of zoledronic acid on multiple myeloma has been assessed using the 5T2MM model [39]. Mice received zoledronic acid (120 μg/kg, 2x/week) in a long-term protocol (commencing on the day of tumour inoculation, 12 weeks), in a short-term protocol commencing after tumour establishment (4 weeks) or as a single dose after tumours had developed. The short- and long-term protocols inhibited the development of bone lesions accompanied by a reduction of osteoclast numbers, significantly decreased angiogenesis and intra-osseous tumour burden. There was no increase in tumour burden in adjacent soft tissues. Short-term administration of the drug was not able to abolish cancer cell invasion of bone, suggesting that inhibition of resorption on its own and short-term dosing is not sufficient to impede bone associated myeloma cell growth. Importantly, zoledronic acid treatment (120 μg/kg, 2x/week until first signs of morbidity) could prolong disease-free survival significantly (47 *vs* 35 days in control animals) but a single dose did not, despite bone resorption being suppressed. The data show that zoledronic acid treatment of experimental myeloma exhibits significant anti-tumour effects and most importantly prolonged disease-free survival suggesting a beneficial role of bisphosphonate treatment in clinical treatment of human myeloma.

The effects of minodronate (YM529) on osteolytic bone disease, tumour burden and survival in SCID mice intravenously inoculated with the human small-cell lung cancer cells (SCLC) SBC-5 has been reported by Zhang *et al.* [40]. Single injections of YM529 (0.2, 2 or 20 μg/mouse) on day 1 effectively decreased the number of new bone metastases in a dose-dependent manner, whereas lung, liver, lymph nodes and kidney metastases were unaffected. In a separate experiment 2 μg minodronate/mouse were administered as single injections on day 0, 7, 14 or 21 to investigate the effect on different stages of tumour development. Single injections (day 7, 14 or 21) were found to inhibit the formation of new metastases to bone, suggesting that the drug inhibits *de-novo* cancer cell growth and established disease in bone. Surprisingly, a repeated dosing regimen did not augment the effects caused by the single treatments, suggesting a single dose is sufficient to inhibit bone metastases. Although the drug was effective in inhibiting tumour-induced osteolysis, no significant increase in survival rates could be shown after a single administration of YM529 (day 7, 2 μg/mouse). The authors concluded that a combined treatment regimen between cytotoxic agents and bisphosphonates would be required to inhibited both intra- and extra-osseous metastases, as well as prolong survival.

A more intense treatment regimen was chosen to assess the effects of Dichloromethylene bisphosphonate (Cl_2MBP) on Walker carcinoma 256 carcinosarcoma [41]. Cl_2MBP was administered in a short-term dosing regimen (30 mg/kg for 5 days) 7, 3 or 1 week before, on the day of, or 5 days after tumour cell implantation (intratibially or intraarterially) or in a long term protocol (2.5 or 5 mg/kg/day for 3 weeks) where tumour cells were implanted either *s.c.,* intraarterially or intratibially on day 22. Cl_2MBP treatment did not affect tumour growth despite exerting bone-sparing activities. The data indicate that Cl_2MBP has protective effects on bone destruction but is unable to reduce the incidence of tumour cell dissemination to bone or tumour progression, ruling out direct anti-tumour effects.

Inhibition of Osteolysis, Reduced Skeletal - But Increased Soft Tissue Tumour Burden

As described above, bisphosphonates are commonly found to reduce skeletal tumour burden and inhibit osteolysis, but without affecting soft tissue tumour burden, suggesting a microenvironment-dependent anti-tumour effect. In contrast, a few studies have reported a slight increase of tumour mass in thc soft tissuc adjacent to affected bone in bisphosphonate treated animals. Sasaki and colleagues found that risedronate treatment increased soft tissue tumour burden in mice, although there was a reduction in skeletal tumour colonisation [42]. MDA-MB-231 human breast cancer cells were implanted by intracardiac injection. The effects of risedronate in a short-term treatment on established bone metastases (4 μg/mouse/day, day 17-28), the effect of continuous treatment on the development of skeletal metastases (0.4, 4, 40 μg/mouse/day for 28 days, commencing with cancer cell inoculation) and effects of preventive treatment (4 μg/day for 7 days before tumour cell inoculation) were determined. Short-term and preventive administration of 4 μg risedronate significantly reduced the number of osteolytic metastases to bone decreased skeletal tumour volume and osteoclast numbers and increased survival. The same effects were seen in the continuous treatment group, with 4 and 40 μg risedronate being the most effective concentrations. Risedronate treated mice had significantly decreased bone metastases, and a trend towards increased tumour area in surrounding soft tissue was noticed when compared to control, although this was not statistically significant. A similar effect on tumours in soft tissue was seen in the preventive group. No metastases were found in any visceral organs, such as lung and liver. The data suggest that, while treatment with bisphosphonates does reduce skeletal tumour burden and osteolysis, it may cause an increased risk of tumour growth outside bone. These data are in agreement with the conclusion of van der Pluijm *et al.* [38] who proposed that the bisphosphonate-induced limitation of space within bone causes tumours to spread to surrounding soft tissues. Later the same group investigated the effect of the new third generation bisphosphonate YH529 [43]. YH529 was administered at 0.2, 2, 20 μg/mouse/day in the same protocols as described above. In the continuous treatment group (daily for 28 days commencing with cancer cell injection), the number and area of osteolytic lesions was significantly reduced and osseous tumour volume decreased in a dose-dependent manner. Osteoclast numbers were reduced by all doses of YH529. The other treatment protocols (short-term from day 17-28 and preventive from 7 days before tumour cell inoculation) caused similar effects. However, a complete inhibition of cancer cell invasion and establishment of new metastases was not observed following the preventive protocol. Because of the trend towards increased soft tissue tumour burden in their 1995 study, the group investigated the effect of YH529 on cancer cell colonisation of tissue adjacent to affected bones [42]. They found that administration of 0.2 and 2 μg YH529/mouse per day showed a trend towards increased tumour volume in soft tissues surrounding bone, whereas the higher dose of 20 μg/mouse/day reduced it compared to control. These results indicate that, in a clinical setting, prophylactic treatment with a low dose and continuous administration could benefit cancer patients with high risk of skeletal metastases by reducing the incidence of bone metastases. However, the potential increase of tumour growth in soft tissue adjacent to affected bones found following administration of higher concentrations of bisphosphonates requires further preclinical investigation.

A recent study directly aimed to investigate the question whether repeated treatment with zoledronic acid (metronomic administration of 0.0125 mg/kg 2x/week) compared to conventional dosing (single dose of 0.1 mg/kg) could potentiate the anti-tumour effects on MDA-MB-231-TXSA-TGL cell proliferation and bone disease, or in lung and liver metastases, after orthotopic implantation into the mammary fat pad [44]. Tumour cells implanted intratibially or orthotopically progressed more slowly in animals receiving the metronomic treatment compared to a single dose, but tumour growth was not eradicated despite significant bone sparing activities. Assessment of lungs and liver showed that a single dose of zoledronic acid significantly increased tumour burden at the visceral sites compared to animals receiving repeated NBP treatment or PBS.

Importantly, soft tissue tumour burden did not differ between the metronomic Zoledronic acid treatment and PBS control. The study confirms that breast tumour growth can be affected by zoledronic acid in and outside bone albeit only when given frequently. Importantly and in light of the recent AZURE trial showing slightly increased visceral tumour growth in pre-menopausal women receiving zoledronic acid in addition to standard adjuvant treatment [15], the increase in metastases in lungs and liver after bisphosphonate treatment warrants further investigation.

Similar results to the ones observed by Sasaki *et al.* [42, 43] were reported in a study of myeloma-induced bone disease using the SCID human host system [45]. Cells from a cohort of myeloma patients were injected into SCID-hu mice, and animals received either zoledronic acid (0.1 mg/kg/week from week 3), or pamidronate (1.3 mg/kg every 2 weeks from week 4). Both bisphosphonates inhibited bone loss in animals with established osteolysis and caused a strong reduction of tumour growth rate and tumour burden. Interestingly, three animals bearing cells from patients diagnosed with extramedullary disease did not show any anti-myeloma effects but exhibited cancer cell growth in bone as well as in the adjacent tissues despite inhibition of osteolysis. A preventive protocol (zoledronic acid 0.1 mg/kg/week or pamidronate 1.3 mg/kg every 2 weeks, for 3 cycles prior to tumour cell injection) resulted in complete prevention of myeloma cell growth by zoledronic acid, while pamidronate treated mice showed a reduction in tumour burden. However, 3 out of the 5 implanted patient samples resulted in tumour cell growth in the bone surrounding soft tissues. The data suggests indirect anti-tumour activities *via* bisphosphonate-induced changes to the bone microenvironment as only animals bearing the human bone marrow-dependent multiple myeloma cells were affected. These results underline the importance of early intervention in order to prevent tumours from reaching a stage where they are capable of autocrine growth.

Inhibition of Osteolysis, Reduced Skeletal and Soft Tissue Tumour Burden

Most studies investigating effects of bisphosphonates on both skeletal and soft tissue tumour burden did not detect a reduction in the latter, suggesting that the drugs do not exert their major anti-tumour activity outside of the bone microenvironment. As described above, some studies even reported a trend towards enhanced tumour growth adjacent to bone or in soft tissues in animals receiving bisphosphonates [42-45]. In contrast, a reduction in both skeletal and soft tissue tumour burden has been reported by Gao *et al.* [46] in a T-cell leukemia model. The effects of zoledronic acid on osseous and visceral tumours induced by adult T-cell leukaemia *via* over-expression of the HTLV-1–encoded Tax oncoprotein was investigated. Four-week-old Tax+ mice were administered zoledronic acid (0.75 μg/mouse/week) before signs of cancer-induced osteolysis were present and until the end of the experiment at 9 months. Only 17% of zoledronic acid treated Tax+ mice developed bone metastasis, compared to 83% of saline treated animals. In addition, zoledronic acid treated animals showed increased bone density, reduced osteolysis and most interestingly had a significant reduction in tumour formation at peripheral sites ($p<0.01$), accompanied by a significant survival increase ($p<0.01$), compared to control. The data show that frequent, long term, administration of zoledronic acid may exert direct effects on visceral tumours and reduce cancer-induced bone disease, consequently leading to prolonged survival in this experimental leukaemia model. It is noticeable that most studies assessing the effects of bisphosphonates used solid tumour models such as breast, prostate and lung cancer. A direct comparison between these results and those found in haematopoietic malignancies may be difficult, due to the differences in tumour cell type and growth characteristics.

Taken together, the majority of published data support that bisphosphonates exert their anti-tumour effects through inhibition of bone resorption, and that the drugs do not exhibit direct anti-tumour effects at peripheral sites unless high/repeated dosing is used. However, most of these studies were not primarily designed to investigate the effects on soft tissue tumours, or in many cases the occurrence of extra skeletal disease was not evaluated. It is still unclear whether the effects of bisphosphonates on cancer cells seen in bone are due to direct or indirect anti-tumour effects, and it is likely that both mechanisms are involved in the inhibition of bone metastases. Together with the data reported by Gao *et al.* [46], who showed reduced tumour burden at osseous and visceral sites after bisphosphonate treatment, and the fact that most studies have not shown an increase in soft tissue tumour burden, the possibility is raised that bisphosphonates do exert some direct effects on cancer cells, albeit not necessarily independent of the bone microenvironment. Also, the frequent administration of bisphosphonates in a preventive schedule has been shown to be the most effective at protecting bone from metastatic lung [40], breast [31, 37, 38, 42, 43] and prostate cancer [29] as well as multiple myeloma [39, 45] and leukaemia [46]. Currently, clinical treatment with bisphosphonates will only be initiated once bone metastases are confirmed, although pre-clinical studies suggest that the best results would be obtained with an earlier treatment schedule. Despite the beneficial effects of a preventive treatment regimen, it is important to note that none of the studies reported a complete elimination of tumours, suggesting that additional therapy with other anticancer agents is required. An overview of the different effects reported from *in vivo* studies of the anti-tumour effects of bisphosphonates is given in Table **1**.

BISPHOSPHONATES ALONE – EFFECTS ON VISCERAL TUMOURS

The bisphosphonate-induced anti-tumour effects in bone are often attributed to changes of the bone microenvironment, making this a less favorable site for cancer cell growth. The large number of studies investigating the anti-tumour effects in bone possibly reflects the interest in this field with the earliest studies cited in this review being from around 1993. In contrast, the serum concentration following clinical dosing of bisphosphonates may not be sufficient to induce anti-tumour effects outside the skeleton and thus has not attracted as much interest. However, the focus of recent research appears to be shifting towards investigations of extra-skeletal anti-tumour effects. Cells of the tumour microenvironment, such as tumour-associated macrophages (TAMs), are frequently investigated due to increased understanding of their relevance to tumour progression [47]. For example, it has been shown that a single dose of zoledronic acid is sufficient to increase levels of unprenylated Rap1a, a surrogate marker for bisphosphonate uptake, in TAMs located in subcutaneous breast xenografts [48]. Bisphosphonates may thus not only target cells located in bone but may also affect other highly phagocytotic cell types of the tumour microenvironment warranting investigation at non-osseous sites.

Table 1: Effects of Bisphosphonates on Tumours in Bone

Tumour Type	Cells	Bisphosphonate	Effect on Intra-Osseous Tumour	Effect on Associated Soft Tissue Tumour	Effect on Osteolysis	Refs.
Reduced Osteolysis But No Effect on Skeletal Tumour Burden						
Prostate cancer	Ace-1	Zol: 100 µg/kg 2x/w	P & T: no effect	—	P>T: reduced	[20]
Prostate cancer	RM1(BM)	Zol: 20 µg/kg, 100 µg/kg every 4 d	No effect	—	Reduced	[21]
Multiple myeloma	5TGM1 5T33	Iban: 4 µg/m/d	No effect	No effect	Reduced	[22]
Multiple myeloma	5T2MM	Iban: 100 µg/d or single	No effect	No effect	Reduced	[23]
Reduced Osteolysis, Increased Tumour Burden, No Effect on Associated Soft Tissue Tumours						
Carcino-sarcoma	Walker 256	Pam: 0.5 mg/kg/d	Increased	No effect	Reduced	[26]
Reduced Osteolysis and Skeletal Tumour Burden						
Prostate cancer	PC3-GFP	Etidronate, pam, olpa, BPb 2.6 mmol/L, 250 ul/m	Olpa: reduced Pam: reduced Etidronate, BPb: no effect	—	Olpa: reduced Pam, etidronate, BPb: no effect	[27]
Prostate cancer	PC3-GFP	Pam: 2.2 or 14.4 mg/kg	14.4 mg/kg: reduced	—	Reduced	[28]
Prostate cancer	PC-3, LuCap 23.I *s.c.* Intra-osseous	 Zol: 5 µg/m, 2x/w Zol: 5 µg/m, 2x/w	 — P&T: reduced	 No effect —	 — T>P: reduced	[29]
Prostate cancer	Ace-1^{Luc}	Zol: 200 µg/kg, 2x/w	Reduced	—	Reduced	[30]
Breast cancer	MDA-MB-231	Iban: 10 µg/kg/d	T>P: reduced	—	T and P: reduced	[31]
Breast cancer	4T1/luc	Zol: Single: 0.3 µg/m 0.5 µg/d, 5 µg/d	Daily: reduced	—	Single and daily: reduced	[32]
Breast cancer	MDA-MB-231	Iban (T): 4 µg/m/d Iban (P): 4 µg/m/d	Reduced —	— No effect	Reduced —	[33]

(Table 1) contd…..

Tumour Type	Cells	Bisphosphonate	Effect on Intra-Osseous Tumour	Effect on Associated Soft Tissue Tumour	Effect on Osteolysis	Refs.
Breast cancer Melanoma	B02, *i.v.*, *s.c.* B16-F10	Ris, or NE-10790: 150 μg/kg/d	Reduced —	No effect No effect	Reduced	[34]
Breast cancer Melanoma	B02, *i.v.*, *s.c.* B16-F10 (liver, lung)	Ris, or NE-58051: 150 μg/kg/d	Ris; reduced —	No effect No effect	Ris; reduced,	[35]
Melanoma	B16-FL	Zol: 0.75 μg/ mouse, day -10 and -3	Reduced in src$^{-/-}$ and WT radiation chimeras	—	—	[36]
Breast cancer	B02/GFP.2	Zol: 3 μg/kg/d, 7 μg/kg/d, 20 μg/kg/w, 50 μg/kg/w, single 100 μg/kg Clod: 530 μg/kg/d	Zol single: 'T' reduced, P no effect Zol (weekly, daily) > Clod: reduced	No effect	Zol: reduced Clod: no effect	[37]
Breast cancer	MDA-231-B/luc+ Intracardiac Intra-osseous	Olpa: 1.6 μmol/kg/d Olpa 1.6 μmol/kg/d Pam: 16 μmol/kg/d	P: reduced Olpa & Pam: reduced	— Olpa & Pam: no effect	P&T: reduced —	[38]
Multiple myeloma	5T2MM	Zol: 120 μg/kg, 2x/w or single	Reduced	No effect	Reduced	[39]
SCLC	SBC-5	Minodronate: 0.2, 2, 20 μg/m	Single & repeated: reduced	Single: no effect	Single & repeated: reduced	[40]
Carcino-sarcoma	Walker 256 Intra-osseous, i.a. Intra-osseous, i.a., *s.c.*	Cl_2MBP 30 mg/kg 2.5, 5 mg/kg/d	No effect No effect	— No effect	Reduced Reduced	[41]
Inhibition of Osteolysis, Reduced Skeletal But Potential Increase in Associated Soft Tissue Tumour Burden						
Breast cancer	MDA-MB-231	Ris: P: 4 μg/m/d; 0.4, 4, 40 μg/m/d; T: 4 μg/m/d	Reduced	Increased	Reduced	[42]
Breast cancer	MDA-MB-231	YH529: 0.2, 2, 20 μg/m/d	Reduced	0.2, 2 μg/m/d: increased 20 μg/m/d: reduced	Reduced	[43]

(Table 1) contd.....

Tumour Type	Cells	Bisphosphonate	Effect on Intra-Osseous Tumour	Effect on Associated Soft Tissue Tumour	Effect on Osteolysis	Refs.
Breast cancer	MDA-MB-231-TXSA-TGL Intra-osseous, mammary fat pad (lung, liver)	Zol: 0.0125 mg/kg 2x/week, single 0.1 mg/kg	Repeated: reduced, single: no effect	Single: increased at liver/lung, Repeated: no effect	Reduced	[44]
Mutiple myeloma	Patient derived cells	Zol: 0.1 mg/kg/w Pam: 1.3 mg/kg	Zol & Pam: reduced 3: no effect	3: increased	Zol & Pam: reduced	[45]
Reduced osteolysis, skeletal tumour burden and reduced soft tissue tumour burden						
Leukemia	Tax+ mice	Zol: 0.75 µg/m/w	Reduced	Reduced	Reduced	46

Zol: zoledronic acid, Ris: risedronate, Iban: ibandronate, Clod: clodronate, Pam: pamidronate, P= preventive, T=therapeutic, w= week, d= day, m=mouse.

There are several reports of inhibitory effects on visceral tumours in lung cancer models. Matsumoto and colleagues [49] investigated the activity of zoledronic acid on human SCLC SBC-3 cells subcutaneously injected into the flank of male BALB/cA Jcl-nu mice. After reaching a tumour size of 30-50 mm^3, mice received either PBS or zoledronic acid (80 µg/kg) on three consecutive days/week for a total of two weeks. Eight weeks after xenograft implantation, zoledronic acid treated animals had significantly reduced tumour volumes when compared to untreated mice ($p<0.05$), suggesting direct anti-tumour effects. However, administration of zoledronic acid did not abolish tumour growth completely, indicating that combining zoledronic acid with a cytotoxic drug may be required. *In vitro* experiments performed as part of the same study showed an increased anti-tumour effect of zoledronic acid when used in combination with paclitaxel, etoposide, cisplatinum or irinotecan. Further evidence from animal models is required to support the observation that bisphosphonates may be effective against SCLC, but the data suggest that zoledronic acid does exhibit direct anti-tumour effects independent of the bone microenvironment.

A more recent study reported direct anti-tumour effects of zoledronic acid on subcutaneous non-small-cell lung cancer (NSCLC) tumours [50]. The group investigated the effects of a very low dose of zoledronic acid (1 µg/kg/week on day 7, 14 and 21) after line-1 and line-1/lacZ cells were subcutaneously engrafted into the thighs of BALB/cByJ mice. The drug significantly reduced line-1 tumour size ($p<0.05$) and induced significantly prolonged median survival when compared to control animals ($p<0.05$). Examination of line-1/lacZ cells isolated from zoledronic acid treated mice showed inhibition of the cell cycle in S/G2 and M phase and treatment with 100 μM zol for 72 hours *in vitro* did not induce apoptosis. The authors concluded that the drug does exhibit anti-tumour effects on soft tissue NSCLC tumours but not *via* anti-apoptotic effects although this was not tested *in vivo*. It should be noted that the line-1 cells used is a murine lung adenocarcinoma cell line, and further studies are needed to determine whether these results can be reproduced in a human NSCLC model. These data suggest that some tumour types, such as the NSCLC, may be highly sensitive to the effects of zoledronic acid, indicating a promising anti-cancer effect on specific tumours outside bone.

Adenocarcinomas of various organs are known to be associated with malignant pleural effusions, leading to the development of neo-angiogenesis and leaky vasculature. Stathopoulos *et al.* investigated whether the zoledronic acid inhibited the formation and growth of cancer-induced pleural effusions with emphasis on anti-angiogenic effects [51]. Syngeneic C57BL/6 mice were engrafted with murine adenocarcinoma cells of the lungs *via* direct injection into the pleural cavity. Zoledronic acid (100 μg/kg/day) was given either as a preventive (day 3-13) or therapeutic protocol (day 9-13) and caused a significant reduction of tumour spread and intrapleural fluid agglomeration, which was accompanied by reduced recruitment of mononuclear F4/80-positive cells, increased cancer cell apoptosis, reduced neo-angiogenesis and vessel hyperpermeability, leading to a significant increase in survival (therapeutic schedule only). The data indicate that this bisphosphonate may be a promising therapeutic for treatment of malignant pleural effusions of various cancers.

A second study investigating the potential anti-angiogenic effects of zoledronic acid used the HPV/E2 murine model of cervical intraepithelial neoplasia (CIN) and cervical carcinoma [52]. The development of CIN lesions to cervical carcinomas involves neo-angiogenesis, accompanied by up-regulation of MMP-9 and VEGF. Animals with defined CIN-3 (high grade) lesions were injected with zoledronic acid (100 μg/kg/day for 6 weeks) in a preventive protocol, or in a therapeutic trial for 1 month commencing after tumour establishment. Tumour incidence in the preventive schedule and was reduced to 30% (zol) compared to 85% (control) and tumour volume was significantly decreased following either treatment schedule. Further experiments indicated that zoledronic acid exhibited its anti-tumour effects by inducing cancer and epithelial cell apoptosis, but not by inhibiting proliferation. Treatment also reduced MMP-9 activity in CIN lesion and tumour encasing stroma, and decreased MMP-9 expression of cervical tissue-penetrating macrophages. The authors suggest that zoledronic acid might be a promising agent for treatment of cervical cancers *via* reduction of active MMP-9, followed by decreased VEGF levels and subsequently reduced angiogenesis. The anti-angiogenic effect identified in this study suggests that zoledronic acid may have the ability to reduce the growth of a range of tumours, but that a very high cumulative dose of the drug is required to initiate this effect.

Wakchoure and colleagues investigated the effect of risedronate and zoledronic acid on subcutaneously engrafted AB12 mesothelioma cells in BALB/c mice [53]. Animals with established tumours were treated with 15 mg/kg risedronate or 0.5 mg/kg zoledronic acid every six days for four cycles. Both agents significantly inhibited subcutaneous tumour growth when compared to control ($p<0.02$ and $p<0.003$, respectively). However, the effect was transient as after an initial suppression tumours continued growing at a rate comparable to that of untreated animals. For survival experiments animals were injected intraperitoneally with AB12 cells and treatment with PBS, risedronate (15 mg/kg,) or zoledronic acid (0.5 mg/kg, 3x/week for 2 weeks) commenced 6 days later. Zoledronic acid caused a significant increase in median survival when compared to control (43 *vs* 26 days, $p<0.001$), while risedronate treatment had no effect. The same experiment was repeated with mice bearing AC29 mesothelioma cells, and no significantly prolonged survival was observed with either drug. Although the authors concluded that the bisphosphonates tested in this study do exhibit anti-tumour effects against visceral mesothelioma tumours, high doses were required, suggesting that a certain bisphosphonate concentration is required in order to reduce tumour burden in areas outside the bone microenvironment.

The anti-tumour activity of nitrogen-containing bisphosphonates on mesothelioma growth was further supported in a study carried out by Okamoto *et al.* [54]. The human cell lines MSTO-211H or EHMES-10 cells were injected into the pleural cavity of balb/c nude mice before intrapleural administration of a single dose of PBS or zol (40 μg/mouse) on day 3 (preventive) or day 10 (therapeutic). Assessment of MSTO-211H tumour weight at day 25 showed a significant reduction compared to PBS in both protocols although the preventive treatment strategy was more effective. Anti-tumour activity was also seen in EHMES-10 at day 35. The novel intra-pleural administration of zoledronic acid may be avoiding the direct binding of the NBP to bone leading to low drug levels outside of osseous structures.

A study aiming to elucidate the effects of bisphosphonates on visceral metastases of a bone derived tumour was performed by Ory *et al.*, using C3H7He mice inoculated intravenously with the osteosarcoma cell line POS-1, which is known to metastasise readily to lungs without the involvement of a primary bone tumour [55]. Treatment with zoledronic acid (100 μg/kg, 2x/week, 5x/week or 1 mg/kg, 2x/week) commenced 2 days after tumour cell injection. All treatment regimens completely abolished lung tumours in mice surviving 21 days or longer, resulting in significantly increased disease free survival, with the frequent administration of the drug resulting in the most pronounced results. Although the dose of zoledronic acid used in this study is equivalent to the 4 mg clinical dose, the drug was administrated at increased frequency resulting in a high total accumulated dose. The data show that zoledronic acid does exhibit direct anti-tumour effects on osteosarcoma cells without the involvement of bone.

The majority of studies on breast cancer have been performed to investigate the effects of bisphosphonates on cancer-induced bone disease, but there are also recent reports of effects on visceral breast cancer growth. One example is the study by Hiraga *et al.* [56], where mice bearing 4T1/luc tumours were treated either with a single dose of zoledronic acid (0.5 μg or 5 μg/mouse) or intermittently with a total of four doses (days 7, 11, 15 and 19). While a single 5 ug dose did not affect tumour burden in visceral organs, repeated administration significantly reduced bone, lung and liver tumour burden ($p<0.05$) as well as tumour area ($p<0.05$) and number of metastatic foci ($p<0.05$), but without inducing 4T1/luc cell death in the lungs. When comparing the effects of zoledronic acid (32 μg/mouse), clodronate (6 mg/mouse) and pamidronate (360 μg/mouse) injected twice (days 7 and 14), only zoledronic acid caused a significant reduction of metastatic tumour burden in the lungs ($p<0.05$) accompanied by a significant increase in overall survival ($p<0.05$). The authors concluded that the anti-tumour effects induced by zoledronic acid in soft tissues are probably due to inhibition of tumour cell invasion and migration, rather than induction of apoptosis. The data support the hypothesis that bisphosphonates have direct anti-tumour activity, affecting both bone and visceral tumours. The same group previously reported that ibandronate (4 mg/mouse/day, day 21 to 28) had no effect on growth of MDA-MB-231 breast cancer cells in the mammary fat pad or in bone [33], suggesting that only the more potent agents (like zoledronic acid) have anti-tumour effects.

An indirect anti-tumour effect attributed to NBPs is the activation of cytotoxic Vγ9Vδ2 T-cells and it has been shown that these cells can be activated by zoledronic acid-induced IPP and ApppI accumulation in tumour cells [57, 58]. Effects of *in vivo* activation of a cytotoxic T-cell response induced from human peripheral blood monocytes (PBMCs) after zoledronic acid treatment of animals bearing subcutaneous B02 or T47D tumours was assessed [59]. Animals bearing palpable tumours were injected 2x/week for two weeks with zoledronic acid (30 μg/kg), human PBMCs plus IL-2 (10.000U) or human PBMCs plus IL-2 plus zol. A significant growth inhibition in T47D but not B02 tumour growth was reported in the zol+PBMC+IL-2 group compared to single treatments or control animals. Importantly, the anti-tumour effect correlated with γδ-Tcell expansion and IPP/ApppI production in the T47D tumour bearing animals, but not in those with B02 tumours, suggesting direct but selective uptake of zol into the subcutaneous tumour cells. The data showing activation of cytotoxic T-cells post zol treatment may thus explain at least in part some of the reported anti-tumour effects reported in clinical trials. A follow up study [60] showed that T47D tumour cells express significantly more IPP/ApppI than B02 cells after *in vitro* risedronate treatment, thus potentially explaining the differential effects seen *in vivo* between the two tumour cell lines in the previous study. To test if the effect is exclusive to zoledronic acid, the same experimental set up was used as described above using risedronate (150 μg/kg). The previous data was confirmed, with a reduction in T47D but not B02 tumour growth after risedronate+PBMC+ IL-2 treatment. The effects on B02 tumours could transiently be potentiated when

2 mg/kg doxorubicin (2 injections) was added to the treatment regimen. Importantly the data show that NBPs can be internalised into tumours growing outside of bone, however, this does not appear to be sufficient to induce an anti-tumour effect on its own.

The anti-tumour effects of NBPs have also been attributed to anti-angiogenic effects, which were confirmed by treatment of subcutaneous CG5 breast cancer xenografts with zoledronic acid (20 μg/mouse 3x/week, 3 weeks) or the RANKL antibody denosumab (10 mg/kg 2x/week, 4 weeks) [61]. Only the animals treated with the NBP showed reduced tumour angiogenesis as well as a delay in tumour progression when compared to denosumab or vehicle control, supporting the suggested anti-angiogenic and anti-cancer effects of zoledronic acid *in vivo*.

While some studies report anti-tumour effects on visceral tumours, others showed increased tumour burden after bisphosphonate administration. One example is the study by Michigami *et al.*, who investigated the effects of ibandronate on peripheral tumours of breast cancer in two animal models, the 4T1 mouse mammary tumour model and the MDA-231AD/Luc human breast cancer model (intracardiac injection of a clone of MDA-MB-231 cells which selectively develops adrenal and bone metastases) [62]. In both models animals were treated with ibandronate (4 μg/mouse/day) using a therapeutic (days 18-28) or a preventive protocol (days 0-28). In the 4T1 model neither treatment schedule had any effects on the number of lung metastases. Results from the MDA-231AD/Luc model were somewhat different: while the therapeutic treatment did not show any effect on adrenal metastases, the preventive treatment regimen significantly increased both size and number of adrenal metastases. Interestingly, the increase was not seen after preventive administration of ibandronate in combination with doxorubicin (150 μg/mouse, on day 1, 7 and 14), but no significant reduction in tumour burden was observed. Doxorubicin alone, however, did cause a significant suppression of tumour burden in adrenal glands. Because of the conflicting data reported within this study the authors suggest that the increase in adrenal gland tumour burden following preventive bisphosphonate administration is an effect specific for this particular xenograft model. Furthermore, the two animal models used here are fundamentally different which could also influence the response to the drug (*e.g.* host immune response in the 4T1 model). In agreement with this study, Sasaki *et al.* [42, 43] (risedronate or YH529 on breast cancer) and Yaccoby *et al.* [45] (zoledronic acid on multiple myeloma) also reported a trend towards increased soft tissue tumour burden after treatment with bisphosphonates.

In most of the studies described above, the dosing regimens exceed the commonly used clinical dose of bisphosphonates (*e.g.* zoledronic acid *i.v.* 4 mg at 3-4 week intervals; ~100 μg/kg in a mouse) and/or frequent drug administration regimens were used. Even though most studies have shown that bisphosphonates may exhibit direct anti-tumour effects in soft tissues, this remains to be confirmed in a clinical setting. All studies reporting an anti-cancer effect on visceral cancer cells have used zoledronic acid apart from Benzaid *et al.* who used risedronate to induce a cytotoxic T-cell response against subcutaneous breast tumours [60]. In addition pre-treatment of tumour cells prior to introduction into the host with YM529/ONO-5920 appeared to have significant effects on tumour establishment on visceral sites. The data therefore suggests that zoledronic acid exhibits superior anti-tumour activity, which is possibly not associated with its potent anti-resorptive effects. Taken together the effects of bisphosphonates on a range of tumour types indicate effective inhibition of cancer-induced bone disease, but the effects on visceral tumours are more complex, with high doses and frequent dosing often being required to induce inhibition of tumour growth. The data furthermore suggests a potential role for bisphosphonates to modify tumour growth outside the skeleton by affecting cells of the tumour microenvironment including macrophages and cells of the immune system. The cellular target(s) of bisphosphonates in extra-skeletal tumours *in vivo* remain to be firmly established but BPs may affect highly phagocytic cells such as TAMs. A summary of the results discussed in this section is shown in Table **2**.

BISPHOSPHONATES IN COMBINATION WITH ANTI-CANCER AGENTS

Preclinical studies of the effects of bisphosphonates on tumour burden in bone-associated soft tissues and visceral sites have reported somewhat conflicting results, and clinical studies have not generally shown improved survival after bisphos-phonate administration [63-65]. The development of new treatment regimens

Table 2: Effects of Bisphosphonates on Visceral Tumours

Tumour Type	Cells	BP Alone	Estimated Accumulated BP Dose	Effect on Visceral Tumour	Effect on Survival	Refs.
SCLC	SBC-3	Zol: 80 µg/kg 3x/w, 2 weeks	480 µg/kg	Reduced	—	[49]
NSCLC	Line-1	Zol: 1 µg/kg 1x/w, 3 weeks	3 µg/kg	Reduced	Increased	[50]
Pleural effusions	Murine adeno-carcinoma of the lung	Zol: 100 µg/kg/d P: day 3-13 T: day 9-13	P: 1 mg/kg T: 400 µg/kg	P &T: reduced	T: increased	[51]
Cervical cancer	HPV/E2 murine model	Zol: 100 µg/kg/d P: 6 weeks T: 4 weeks	P: 4.2 mg/kg T: 2.8 mg/kg	P&T: reduced	—	[52]
Meso-thelioma	AB12	Ris: 15 mg/kg Zol: 0.5 mg/kg every 6 days/4x	Ris: 60 mg/kg Zol: 2 mg/kg	Ris, Zol: reduced	—	[53]
	AB12	Ris: 15 mg/kg Zol: 0.5 mg/kg 3x/w, 2 weeks	Ris: 90 mg/kg Zol: 3 mg/kg	—	Zol: increased	
	AC29	Ris: 15 mg/kg Zol: 0.5 mg/kg 3x/w, 2 weeks	Ris: 90 mg/kg Zol: 3 mg/kg	—	No effect	
Meso-thelioma	MSTO-211H, EHMES-10	Zol: single dose 40 µg/mouse P: day 3 T: day 10	40 µg/mouse	P>T: reduced	—	[54]
Osteo-sarcoma	POS-1	Zol: 100 µg/kg 2x/w, 5x/w 1 mg/kg 2x/w	200 µg/kg/w 500 µg/kg/w 2 mg/kg/w	Reduced	Increased	[55]
Breast cancer	4T1/luc	Zol: 0.5, 5 µg/m, 1x or 4x	0.5 µg/m 5 µg/m 2 µg/m 20 µg/m	4x 5 µg/mouse: reduced	—	[56]
		Zol: 32 µg/m Clod: 6 mg/m Pam: 360 µg/m, 2x	Zol: 64 µg/m Clod: 12 mg/m Pam: 720 µg/m	Zol: reduced Clod, Pam: no effect	Increased	
Breast cancer	B02, T47D	Zol: 30 µg/kg, hPBMC+IL-2, Zol+hPBMC+IL-2 2x/w, 2 weeks	Zol: 120 µg/kg	Zol+hPBMC+IL-2: T47D: reduced B02: no effect Zol only: no effect	—	[59]

(Table 2) contd…..

Tumour Type	Cells	BP Alone	Estimated Accumulated BP Dose	Effect on Visceral Tumour	Effect on Survival	Refs.
Breast cancer	B02, T47D	Ris: 150 μg/kg, hPBMC+IL-2, Ris+hPBMC+IL-2 2x/w, 2 weeks	Ris: 600 μg/kg	Ris+hPBMC+IL-2: T47D: reduced B02: no effect	—	[60]
Breast cancer	CG5	Zol: 20 μg/m, 3x/w, 3 weeks	180 μg/mouse	Reduced	—	[61]
Breast cancer	4T1/luc, MDA-231AD/Luc	Iban: 4 μg/m/d, P: 4 weeks, T: 10 days	P: 112 μg/m T: 40 μg/m	4T1: No effect MDA-MB-231: P, increased	—	[62]

Zol: zoledronic acid, Ris: risedronate, Iban: ibandronate, Clod: clodronate, Pam: pamidronate, P= preventive, T=therapeutic, w= week, d= day, m=mouse.

is therefore essential to improve therapy for patients with cancer spreading to bone. In clinical practice, treatment of cancer-induced bone disease commonly comprises the administration of cytotoxic drugs in combination with the palliative treatment offered by bisphosphonates. *In vitro* studies have shown that the combination of potent bisphosphonates, such as zoledronic acid, with other cytotoxic agents results in enhanced anti-tumour effects [66]. These have been followed by *in vivo* studies investigating the effects of combination of a range of anti-cancer agents and bisphosphonates, showing increased anti-tumour effects compared to single agent therapy and the main data of these studies will be summarised in the following section.

A number of studies using breast cancer models have reported reduced tumour growth following combination of zoledronic acid with cytotoxic drugs. The murine 4T1 breast cancer model was used to examine the anti-metastatic effect of the chemotherapeutic UFT (tegafur-uracil) in combination with zoledronic acid or either drug alone [67]. Syngeneic female BALB/c mice were injected orthotopically (mammary fat pad) with 4T1 cells resulting in dissemination of the tumour cells to bone. A single injection of zoledronic acid (250 μg/kg, day 7) or administration of UFT (20 mg/kg/day, days 14-21) significantly reduced the area of bone metastases and combination treatment was able to augment this effect. The increased anti-tumour effect supports that combined therapy might be more effective in clinical practice compared to single treatments. However, very high doses of zoledronic acid were used in this study, equivalent to a daily 15 mg *i.v.* injection compared to the standard clinical administration of 4 mg every 3-4 weeks.

The combination of the antibiotic doxycycline and zoledronic acid was tested on Balb/c nu/nu mice injected intracardiac with MDA-MB-231 human breast cancer cells [68]. Doxycycline releasing pellets (~15 mg/kg/day) were transplanted *s.c.* into mice, 3 days prior to tumour cell inoculation and/or zoledronic acid treatment (0.2 µg/mouse every 2 days) commenced on the same day and until the end of the experiment on day 28. Both single treatments and the combination resulted in decreased tumour burden in bone and/or surrounding soft tissues and reduced osteolysis. Interestingly it was reported that zoledronic acid alone resulted in a 93% reduction of tumour area in soft tissue adjacent to the affected bones but only in 73% in total tumour burden, suggesting a direct effect of the drug on tumour cells outside the bone microenvironment. The data are in agreement with the work of Corey *et al.* [29] (zoledronic acid in prostate cancer), and Hiraga *et al.* (zoledronic acid in breast cancer), also reporting inhibition of soft tissue tumour burden following bisphosphonate treatment [56]. The combination of zoledronic acid and doxycycline may therefore be a possible therapeutic strategy for patients with advanced breast cancer.

In a study using the same breast cancer cell line, female BALB/c nu/nu mice were inoculated intratibially with MDA-231-B/luc+ cells and treatment commenced 2 days later with zoledronic acid (37.5, 75 or 150 µg/kg, 5x/week) or risedronate (150 µg/kg, 5x/week), docetaxel (2, 4, or 8 mg/kg, 2x/week) or a combination of both (docetaxel at 4 mg/kg, 2x/week and risedronate at 150 µg/kg, 5x/week) for a period of 5 weeks [69]. All concentrations of both bisphosphonates and the combination schedule prevented osteolytic bone destruction, but docetaxel alone had no effect when compared to control. After combination treatment, no tumour growth in bone was detected in 6 out of 7 mice, while treatment with docetaxel alone prevented tumour growth in only 2 out of 7 mice whereas risedronate alone had no effect. The data show an enhanced anti-tumour effect in bone when bisphosphonates are used in combination with docetaxel, even at concentrations that were shown to be ineffective when given alone.

Recently, the combination of the c-Met inhibitor tivantinib in combination with zoledronic acid was assessed in a preventive (treatment start 3 days after tumour cell injection) and therapeutic setting (treatment start 13 days after tumour cell injection) in a model of breast cancer [70]. The bone metastases of the MDA-MB-231 derived bone-seeking clone 1833/TGL were treated with tivantinib alone (300 mg/kg/day), zoledronic acid (100 mg/kg, every 72 hours), combination of both or vehicle control (PEG 400:20% vitamin E in TPGS [60:40]). Both treatment schedules showed highest efficacy when combination treatment was administered resulting in significant reduction in tumour growth and improved survival compared to control. Overall, preventive treatment was more effective than the therapeutic schedule. Interestingly the same treatments did not significantly reduce growth of established subcutaneous tumours suggesting the synergistic anti-tumour effects of the combination treatment are partly mediated through zol-induced effects on bone (osteoclasts), which was further confirmed in *in vitro* studies showing that the combination treatment did not reduce tumour cell proliferation or migration to a higher extend than tivantinib alone.

The majority of published studies have investigated the effects of combination treatments on tumours growing in bone, and it is therefore not possible to determine whether the reported anti-tumour effects are induced directly, indirectly or as a combination of both mechanisms. Ottewell *et al.* [71] assessed the effects of doxorubicin and zoledronic acid on subcutaneous tumours derived from MDA-G8 human breast cancer cells (subclone of the human breast cancer cell line MDA-MB-436), to determine whether sequential and combined treatment can significantly inhibit extra-osseous tumour growth. MDA-G8 cells were injected *s.c.* in the flank of female MF1 nu/nu mice, and once tumours were palpable animals were treated 1x/week for 6 weeks with saline, doxorubicin (2 mg/kg), zoledronic acid (100 μg/kg), zoledronic acid and doxorubicin together, doxorubicin followed 24 hours later by zoledronic acid, and vice versa. While treatment with either drug alone did not have any significant effect on tumour size compared to saline control, combined administration resulted in approximately 50% reduction in tumour size when compared to tumours treated with doxorubicin alone. Sequential treatment with doxorubicin followed by zoledronic acid caused almost complete abolition of tumour growth, whereas administration of the reverse drug sequence had no effect. Sequential (doxorubicin followed by zoledronic acid) and combined treatment increased cancer cell apoptosis and reduced proliferation while single treatments and zoledronic acid followed by doxorubicin did not. Pathway-specific gene array analysis performed to elucidate changes in gene expression induced by sequential treatment showed that 30 genes involved in cell cycle regulation and apoptosis had been specifically changed. The reduction of tumour growth may also be partly mediated by inhibition of angiogenesis, as both combined and sequential treatment (doxorubicin followed by zoledronic acid) caused a reduction in tumour vascularisation. The cumulative concentrations used in this study, although clinically achievable, still exceed doses used in clinic. The data showed that a sequential administration of doxorubicin 24 hours before zoledronic acid significantly reduces tumour growth outside bone. Zoledronic acid (100 µg/kg weekly for 6 weeks) alone had no effect on extra-skeletal tumours, therefore not supporting the proposed direct anti-tumour activity of zoledronic acid. The authors concluded that sequence-specific combination treatment (doxorubicin followed by zoledronic acid) may be beneficial to patients with early-stage breast cancer, thus even in the absence of bone metastases.

Ottewell and colleagues [72] furthermore showed that the anti-tumour effect of the sequential treatment with dox then zol is not limited to xenograft models with an impaired immune system. The same treatment schedule as previously described (2 mg/kg doxorubicin, 100 µg/kg zoledronic acid, doxorubicin followed 24 hours later by zoledronic acid or PBS as vehicle control), was used 1x/week for 6 weeks in 6-week old immunocompetent PyMT mice, which develop spontaneous mammary gland tumours from the age of 6 weeks. Confirming their previous results, only the sequential treatment inhibited development of palpable mammary tumours in comparison to monotherapy or control which all developed extensive mammary gland tumours. This anti-tumour effect was accompanied by a reduction in Ki67 and increased active-caspase-3 positive cells, as well as a reduction in circulating tumour cells in the dox then zol group compared to control or single treatments. This study further underlines the potential anti-tumour effects of addition of zoledronic acid to cytotoxic treatment of breast cancer growth outside of bone. The authors therefore further underlined the relevance of this treatment schedule and the importance to test sequential administration settings of frequently administered compounds in clinic.

Furthermore, the effects of clinically relevant doses of zoledronic acid and doxorubicin on extra- and intra-osseous tumours were investigated using female BALB/c nude mice bearing MDA-MB-231/B02 human breast tumours in bone [73]. After tumour establishment, mice received saline, doxorubicin (2 mg/kg), zoledronic acid (100 μg/kg), zoledronic acid and doxorubicin simultaneously or doxorubicin followed 24 hours later by zoledronic acid. Animals receiving doxorubicin were administered a second injection of the drug on day 25. Zoledronic acid significantly reduced the area of osteolytic lesions and increased bone volume in all treatment schedules, compared to control or doxorubicin treatment. Sequential treatment with doxorubicin followed by zoledronic acid resulted in significant reduction in intra-osseous tumour volume compared to that seen in all other treatment groups. Extra-osseous tumour volume, defined as the tumour mass growing out of the bone marrow into the surrounding soft tissue, was not affected by any of the treatment schedules. Sequential and simultaneous treatment also significantly reduced the number of proliferating cells in intra-osseous tumours, but not in the parts of the tumours growing outside bone. Tumour cell apoptosis was significantly increased in both intra- and extra-osseous parts of the tumours when animals were treated with the sequential protocol, whereas single administration of either drug had no effect on apoptotic cell death. Sequential treatment was shown to be the most effective in prolonging median survival ($p<0.0001$). In addition, administration of zoledronic acid, alone or in combination, increased mean survival when compared to control or doxorubicin alone. The data indicate that intra-osseous anti-tumour effects can be significantly enhanced when doxorubicin is given 24 hours prior to zoledronic acid, but in contrast extra-osseous parts of the tumours are not affected. The surrounding microenvironment and the local drug concentration in different parts of the tumour may therefore influence the response to treatment. The authors suggest that sequential administration of doxorubicin followed by zoledronic acid may be used in the treatment of advanced breast cancer patients, particularly for those with smaller bone metastases confined to the marrow space.

In a follow-up study the successful treatment regimen was altered to assess whether a preventive treatment regimen using a more clinically relevant single administration of the compounds would inhibit breast tumour establishment in bone [74]. It was shown that the bone microenvironment was extensively modified by a single dose of zoledronic acid +/- doxorubicin (increased trabecular bone volume, reduced osteoclast and osteoblast numbers on trabecular bone surfaces on day 23), which was accompanied by a transient inhibition of tumour development in bone compared to single treatments and PBS control. The data suggest that although a single dose of zoledronic acid +/- doxorubicin is sufficient to protect bone when given as preventive treatment, repeated treatment is necessary to inhibit tumour progression.

The effects of combination treatments have also been explored in prostate cancer models. Kim *et al.* [75] investigated the effects of zoledronic acid, paclitaxel and STI571 (Imatinib mesylate, Gleevec) using PC-3MM2 prostate cancer cells implanted into the tibia of nude mice, leading to tumour growth in bone and the development of lymph node metastases. Animals were treated for a total of 5 weeks with paclitaxel (8 mg/kg, 1x/week), STI571 (50 mg/kg/day), zoledronic acid (25 μg/kg, 2x/day), or with a combination of two or three of the drugs. Treatment with zoledronic acid and/or paclitaxel did not decrease bone tumour burden or lymph node metastases but STI571 administration reduced bone and lymph node tumour incidence and weight. The latter was also observed after single treatment with zoledronic acid. The combination of all three agents was found to be the most effective at reducing bone tumour burden ($p<0.001$ *vs* control), tumour weight ($p<0.001$ *vs* control), inhibition of bone loss and most importantly induced a significant decrease in lymph node metastases. The anti-metastatic effects were shown to be associated with reduced osteoclast activity, increased tumour cell apoptosis and a decrease in proliferation, suggesting that both direct and indirect mechanisms were involved. It is important to note that the observed anti-tumour effects of zoledronic acid may be due to the extremely high dosing regimen chosen for this study. The data indicate that a treatment regimen designed to target different stages of the heterogenic tumour growth and dissemination might be a possible new therapeutic approach for prostate cancer patients.

Brubaker and colleagues used male SCID mice bearing intratibial LuCap prostate cancer xenografts to determine the effects of a 7-week treatment with zoledronic acid (0.1 mg/kg, 2x/week), docetaxel (20 mg/kg every 2 weeks) and a combination of both [76]. Zoledronic acid alone induced a decrease in tumour volume compared to control, and a decrease in tumour volume and an increase in bone volume was seen in the combination group. Combination and bisphosphonate only schedules were also shown to significantly reduce the numbers of osteoclasts, but no treatment regimen affected osteoblast numbers. When tumour burden was assessed *via* measurement of prostate specific antigen (PSA) serum levels, only the combined schedule significantly reduced PSA levels indicating reduced tumour growth. However, when intra-osseous tumour volume was assessed by histomorphometry, zoledronic acid given alone and in combination induced a reduction in tumour volume. Note that low concentrations of zoledronic acid (0.1 mg/kg) alone are effective in inhibiting prostate cancer cell growth in bone, which is further enhanced in the combination treatment, but repeated administration results in a cumulative drug concentration exceeding those used in clinic. The data suggests that zoledronic acid sensitizes prostate cancer cells to docetaxel treatment, resulting in an additive anti-tumour effect of the two drugs.

Synergistic effects between the histone deacetylase inhibitor panobinostat and zoledronic acid through increasing ROS levels and inhibition of the MVA pathway were recently reported in an *in vivo* model of prostate cancer without involvement of bone [77]. Subcutaneously injected DU145 cells were left to establish tumours for approximately 1 week before treatment for 5 days/week for 3 weeks with panobinostat (15 mg/kg/day), zoledronic acid (0.1 mg/kg, 3 days/week), the combination of both or vehicle control. The combination treatment induced a significant reduction in tumour volume compared to vehicle treated mice with the rate of tumour growth in the control group being almost 1.6-fold higher than in the combination group. Interestingly animals receiving zoledronic acid monotherapy had slightly increased tumour volume compared to control tumours.

To our knowledge only two recent studies have been published investigating combination treatment on lung cancer despite the good response reported in studies using BP monotherapy. Yano *et al.* used a murine model in which natural killer cell-depleted SCID mice were injected intravenously with human SCLC SBC-5 cells, which are known to metastasise to bone and visceral organs including lung, liver and kidney [78]. Mice were administered the topoisomerase II inhibitor VP-16 (200 μg, days 2, 3, 9, 10), minodronate (0.2 μg on day 7) and a combination of the drugs for a total of 5 weeks or until moribund. Minodronate treatment significantly reduced bone tumour burden and osteoclast numbers, but did not affect visceral tumour burden (lungs, liver, lymph nodes, kidneys). In contrast, monotherapy with VP-16 resulted in the inhibition of visceral metastases in lungs and liver, but not in kidneys or lymph nodes, and in a reduced number of metastatic foci in bone. Combination treatment enhanced the anti-metastatic effects in bone, reduced osteoclast numbers and reduced lung and liver metastases (compared to control and single treatments) and also prolonged survival significantly ($p<0.05$). In conclusion, combination therapy with minodronate and VP-16 appears to be superior to single treatments at bone, lung and liver tumours in this lung cancer model.

Hyaluron is a major ECM component and has been shown to exhibit stimulatory effects on tumour growth migration and invasion and that the levels of HA in malignant tissues correlate with lung and breast cancer. 4-Methylumbelliferone (MU) inhibits HA synthesis and anti-tumour effects on a variety of cancers have been reported through the inhibition of HA synthesis. In this study the authors assessed the anti-tumour effects of MU in combination with zoledronic acid on progression of murine lung cancer bone metastases [79]. Lewis lung cancer cells were injected intratibially followed by initiation of treatment (daily or weekly vehicle 0.4% carboxymethyl cellulose sodium (CMC) solution, daily MU at 10 mg/body in 0.4% CMC, weekly zoledronic acid 2 μg/body in PBS and the combination of MU and zoledronic acid) 14 days after implantation when animals had established osteolytic disease. Both Mu and zoledronic acid protected bone although the bisphosphonate showed stronger anti-resorptive activity which was accompanied by an increase in TUNEL positive tumour cells in zol treated mice *vs* control animals with the strongest increase in cell death detected in animals receiving combination treatment. The studies therefore suggest that combination treatment may be a potential treatment regimen for patients with lung cancer bone metastases.

There has been one recent study investigating the effect of zoledronic acid in combination with the cytotoxic agent gemcitabine (GEM), the first-line treatment for pancreatic cancer, in mouse models of pancreatic and liver tumour growth [80]. Animals orthotopically (pancreas) injected with the human pancreatic tumour cell line SUIT-2 develop liver metastases. When mice were treated every 7 days starting from day 3 to 31 with zol (0.08 mg/kg), GEM (40 mg/kg), the combination of both or PBS showed that only GEM+zol completely inhibited liver metastases and inhibited peritoneal dissemination, which was accompanied by a significant reduction in pancreatic tumour volume. These effects were reflected by a significant inhibition of the percentage of Ki67-positive cells, increase in apoptosis and a reduction in microvascular density with the most pronounced effects detected in the combination group. In addition the group assessed the effects of zol on liver metastases after intrasplenic SUIT-2 cell implantation. Animals were treated 3 days after tumour cell injection with 0.08, 0.16 and 0.32 mg/kg of zol or PBS on day 3, 10, 17, 24 and the experiment was terminated on day 28. Assessment of the number of liver metastatic nodules and liver weight showed a significant decrease by zoledronic acid treatment in a dose dependent manner. The data from the study confirm findings form other groups that zoledronic acid induced anti-tumour effects are not limited to bone metastases and that combination with a cytotoxic agent increases the anti-tumour effects also in visceral organs.

Most studies using combination treatment have chosen to use agents targeting different pathways. The combined effects of NBPs and statin treatment, both of which inhibit enzymes in the mevalonate pathway, were assessed in two studies investigating anti-tumour effects on subcutaneous prostatic neuroendocrine carcinoma [81] and breast cancer metastases in bone [82]. Interestingly, the studies showed that treatment with either somatostatin analogues [81] or fluvastatin [82] in combination with zoledronic acid did not induce synergistic or additive anti-tumour effects when given in combination suggesting that combination treatment targeting the same pathway is not an effective treatment strategy in this setting. However, statins specifically target the liver, similar to the exclusive localisation of Bps to bone, and thus the concentration of statins in bone and other soft tissues may not be high enough to exert sufficient anti-tumour effects.

As shown in Table **3**, the main body of combination studies have been performed using models of breast cancer, using zoledronic acid in combination with UFT [67], doxycyclin [68] and doxorubicin [71-74]. All studies reported a significant reduction in bone tumour burden following combination therapy, compared to using the single agents. The reported effects on visceral tumours or cancer cells in bone-associated soft tissue are more conflicting, with some studies showing no beneficial effects of drug combinations. These differences may be due to the various models used, but may also be influenced by the different dosing schedules of zoledronic acid, and the different combination regimens tested. Three studies in prostate cancer [75-77], one study in lung [78, 79] and one recent study in pancreatic cancer [80] have reported increased anti-tumour effects of combination therapy with zoledronic acid. Further investigations are required to confirm these promising results and to establish the cellular and molecular processes involved.

BISPHOSPHONATES ALONE AND IN COMBINATION – SUMMARY OF FINDINGS

There is strong evidence that bisphosphonate treatment does reduce tumour growth in bone and inhibits the associated bone disease in a range of different cancer types. The effects on tumours spreading from the bone marrow cavity to the surrounding soft tissue, and on visceral tumours, are less conclusive. The preclinical studies investigating the effects of bisphosphonates on visceral tumours often involved use of very high dosing regimens compared to those used in clinical practice. While some studies reported positive effects on extra-osseous tumour growth and an increase in survival following bisphosphonate treatment, others did not observe effects on tumour growth. The most prominent anti-tumour effects are generated by regimens that include frequent drug administration, possibly due to the resulting high cumulative dose. Also, the need for repeated dosing indicates that bisphosphonates are unable to completely abolish cancer cell growth and merely cause a slowdown of the process. The most potent inhibition of tumour growth is seen when bisphosphonates are given in combination with

Table 3: Effects of Bisphosphonates in Combination with Cytotoxic Drugs

Tumour Type	Cells	BP in Combination	Effect on Visceral Tumour	Effect on Osseous Tumour	Effect on Survival	Refs.
Breast cancer	4T1	UFT: 20 mg/kg/d Zol: 250 μg/kg	No effect	UFT: reduced Zol: reduced Combi: reduced	—	[67]
Breast cancer	MDA-MB-231	Doxycycline: 15 mg/kg/d Zol: 0.2 μg/m every 2 days	—	Combi>single: reduced (intra- & extraosseous)	—	[68]
Breast cancer	MDA-231-B/luc+	Zol: 37.5, 75, 150 μg/kg, 5x/w Ris: 150 μg/kg, 5x/w Docetaxel: 2, 4, 8 mg/kg, 2x/w Combi: Ris 150 μg/kg, 5x/w + docetaxel 4 mg/kg, 2x/w	—	Combi>docetaxel: reduced Zol, ris: no effect	—	[69]
Breast cancer	MDA-MB-231 clone 1833/TGL	Tivantinib: 300 mg/kg/d, Zol: 100 mg/kg, every 3 d. P: d3, T: d13	—	Combi: reduced P>T	Combi: increased	[70]
Breast cancer	MDA-G8	Dox: 2 mg/kg, Zol: 100 μg/kg, dox+zol, dox→zol, zol→dox 1x/w	Single, zol→dox: no effect Dox→zol > Dox+zol: reduced	—	—	[71]
Breast cancer	PyMT	Dox: 2 mg/kg, Zol: 100 μg/kg, dox→zol, 1x/w, 6 weeks	Combi: reduced	—	—	[72]
Breast cancer	B02	Dox: 2 mg/kg, Zol: 100 μg/kg, dox+zol, dox→zol	Extra-osseous tumour growth: No effect	Zol, dox+zol, dox→zol: reduced	Zol, dox+zol dox→zol: increased	[73]
Breast cancer	MDA-MB-231	Dox: 2 mg/kg, Zol: 100 μg/kg, dox→zol 1x, day 3	—	Combi: reduced	—	[74]
Prostate cancer	PC-3MM2	Paclitaxel: 8 mg/kg, 1x/w STI571: 50 mg/kg/d Zol: 25 μg/kg 2x/d for 5 weeks	Paclitaxel, zol: no effect STI571: reduced Combi: reduced	Paclitaxel, zol: no effect STI571: reduced Combi: reduced	—	[75]
Prostate cancer	LuCap	Zol: 0.1 mg/kg 2x/w Docataxel: 20 mg/kg, every 2 weeks	Docataxel: reduced	Combi & zol: reduced	—	[76]

(Table 3) contd.....

Tumour Type	Cells	BP in Combination	Effect on Visceral Tumour	Effect on Osseous Tumour	Effect on Survival	Refs.
Prostate cancer	DU145	Panobinostat: 15 mg/kg 5 d/w, Zol: 0.1 mg/kg 3 days/w	Combi: reduced Zol: slight increase	—	—	[77]
SCLC	SBC-5	VP-16: 200 µg, days 2,3,9,10 Minodronate: 0.2 µg, day 7, 5 weeks	Minodronate: no effect VP-16, combi: reduced	Minodronate, VP-16, combi: reduced	Combi: increased Mino, VP-16: no effect	[78]
Lung cancer	Lewis lung cancer	MU:10 mg/m/d Zol: 2 µg/m/w	—	Combi: reduced	—	[79]
Pancreatic cancer	SUIT-2	Zol: 0.08 mg/kg/w, GEM: 40 mg/kg/w	Combi: reduced Zol: reduced	—	—	[80]

Zol: zoledronic acid, Dox: doxorubicin, Combi: combination treatment, w = week, d = day, m = mouse.

cytotoxic drugs, suggesting that a similar approach may be utilized in the clinical setting. Although still to be firmly established, the suggested possible mechanisms of action involved in the anti-tumour effects of bisphosphonates include induction of apoptosis, inhibition of proliferation and anti-angiogenic effects but more recent studies also imply that alterations to the tumour microenvironment may affect tumour growth. In addition, the often reported increased efficacy of preventive strategies could suggest that the main components of the metastatic niche in bone may be altered by bisphosphonate treatment thus potentially affecting specifically early stages of tumour growth, however, this remains to be investigated.

CONCLUSION – LESSONS LEARNED

The clinical relevance of bisphosphonates as anti-cancer agents has been subject to considerable debate, and results relating to anti-tumour effects from clinical trials of bisphosphonates have been somewhat conflicting. Direct anti-tumour effects on visceral tumours as well as reduction of tumour burden in bone and prolonged survival has been reported in a study investigating the effects of adjuvant oral clodronate administration in breast cancer patients [63, 64]. In contrast, Saarto *et al.* [65] reported no decrease in skeletal tumour burden but an increase in visceral tumours, which was associated with reduced disease free survival when administering oral clodronate. The data from these trials reflect the variable responses generated in the *in vivo* studies reviewed in this article, with the majority reporting anti-tumour effects whereas others found either no effect or increased cancer cell growth. The effects appear to be highly dependent on tumour type, treatment protocol and model system used. While most of the studies have reported the involvement of bone in the anti-cancer activity of bisphosphonates, there is some evidence of direct effects using tumour models independent of bone. Despite this, more detailed trials are required to elucidate whether bisphosphonates exert their anti-cancer activity *via* direct, indirect or a combination of both mechanisms, and it remains to be established which molecular and cellular effects are responsible for the effects of combination treatments. In addition, the relevance of the modification of cells of the tumour microenvironment and the metastatic niche by bisphosphonates in and outside of bone requires further investigation. A greater effect of early compared to late initiation of bisphosphonate treatment was shown by a number of the preclinical studies discussed in this review. The AZURE trial (Adjuvant Zoledronic acid to Reduce Recurrence) furthermore showed that adjuvant zoledronic acid reduced breast cancer bone metastases in postmenopausal women [15], suggesting that early treatment may be beneficial at least for a subset of patients. Collectively the preclinical data show that some cancer types may be more susceptible to the anti-tumour effects of bisphosphonates, and that the effects may be enhanced when used in combination with anti-cancer agents.

ABBREVIATIONS

ApppI	=	I-adenosin-5'-yl ester 3-(3-methylbut-3-enyl) ester
ATP	=	Adenosine-5'-triphosphate
AZURE	=	Adjuvant Zoledronic acid to Reduce Recurrence
BP	=	Bisphosphonate
CIN	=	Cervical intraepithelial neoplasia
i.p.	=	Intraperitoneal

i.v.	=	Intravenous
IPP	=	Isopentenyl pyrophosphate
MMP	=	Matrix metalloproteinase
NBP	=	Nitrogen–containing Bisphosphonate
NSCLC	=	Non-small-cell lung cancer
PBS	=	Phosphate buffered saline
PSA	=	Prostate specific antigen
s.c.	=	Subcutaneous
SCLC	=	Small-cell lung cancer
VEGF	=	Vascular endothelial growth factor

ACKNOWLEDGEMENTS

None declared.

CONFLICT OF INTEREST

The authors confirm that this chapter contents have no conflict of interest.

DISCLOSURE

The chapter submitted for the eBook Series entitled **"Advances in Cancer Drug Targets, Volume 2"** is an update of our article in **Current Cancer Drug Targets, Volume 9, Issue 7, 2009, pp. 807-823,** with additional text and references.

REFERENCES

[1] Coleman RE. Metastatic bone disease: clinical features, pathophysiology and treatment strategies. Cancer Treat Rev 2001 Jun; 27(3): 165-76.

[2] Kohno N, Aogi K, Minami H, Nakamura S, Asaga T, Iino Y, *et al.* Zoledronic acid significantly reduces skeletal complications compared with placebo in Japanese women with bone metastases from breast cancer: a randomized, placebo-controlled trial. J Clin Oncol 2005 May 20; 23(15): 3314-21.

[3] Rosen LS, Gordon DH, Dugan W, Jr., Major P, Eisenberg PD, Provencher L, *et al.* Zoledronic acid is superior to pamidronate for the treatment of bone metastases in breast carcinoma patients with at least one osteolytic lesion. Cancer 2004 Jan 1; 100(1): 36-43.

[4] Benford HL, McGowan NW, Helfrich MH, Nuttall ME, Rogers MJ. Visualization of bisphosphonate-induced caspase-3 activity in apoptotic osteoclasts *in vitro*. Bone. [Research Support, Non-U.S. Gov't] 2001 May; 28(5): 465-73.

[5] Hiroi-Furuya E, Kameda T, Hiura K, Mano H, Miyazawa K, Nakamaru Y, *et al.* Etidronate (EHDP) inhibits osteoclastic-bone resorption, promotes apoptosis and disrupts actin rings in isolate-mature osteoclasts. Calcif Tissue Int 1999 Mar; 64(3): 219-23.

[6] Ito M, Amizuka N, Nakajima T, Ozawa H. Ultrastructural and cytochemical studies on cell death of osteoclasts induced by bisphosphonate treatment. Bone 1999 Oct; 25(4): 447-52.

[7] Bergstrom JD, Bostedor RG, Masarachia PJ, Reszka AA, Rodan G. Alendronate is a specific, nanomolar inhibitor of farnesyl diphosphate synthase. Arch Biochem Biophys 2000 Jan 1; 373(1): 231-41.

[8] Fisher JE, Rogers MJ, Halasy JM, Luckman SP, Hughes DE, Masarachia PJ, *et al.* Alendronate mechanism of action: geranylgeraniol, an intermediate in the mevalonate pathway, prevents inhibition of osteoclast formation, bone resorption, and kinase activation *in vitro*. Proceedings of the National Academy of Sciences of the United States of America 1999 Jan 5; 96(1): 133-8.

[9] van Beek E, Pieterman E, Cohen L, Lowik C, Papapoulos S. Farnesyl Pyrophosphate Synthase Is the Molecular Target of Nitrogen-Containing Bisphosphonates. Biochemical and Biophysical Research Communications 1999 14 October 1999; 264(1): 108-11.

[10] Frith JC, Monkkonen J, Auriola S, Monkkonen H, Rogers MJ. The molecular mechanism of action of the antiresorptive and antiinflammatory drug clodronate: evidence for the formation *in vivo* of a metabolite that inhibits bone resorption and causes osteoclast and macrophage apoptosis. Arthritis Rheum 2001 Sep; 44(9): 2201-10.

[11] Coleman RE, Body JJ, Gralow JR, Lipton A. Bone loss in patients with breast cancer receiving aromatase inhibitors and associated treatment strategies. Cancer Treat Rev 2008; 34 Suppl 1: S31-42.

[12] Conte P, Frassoldati A. Aromatase inhibitors in the adjuvant treatment of postmenopausal women with early breast cancer: Putting safety issues into perspective. Breast J 2007 Jan-Feb; 13(1): 28-35.

[13] Chen T, Berenson J, Vescio R, Swift R, Gilchick A, Goodin S, *et al.* Pharmacokinetics and pharmacodynamics of zoledronic acid in cancer patients with bone metastases. J. Clin Pharmacol. [Clinical Trial Comparative Study Randomized Controlled Trial Research Support, Non-U.S. Gov't] 2002 Nov; 42(11): 1228-36.

[14] Sato M, Grasser W, Endo N, Akins R, Simmons H, Thompson DD, *et al.* Bisphosphonate action. Alendronate localization in rat bone and effects on osteoclast ultrastructure. J Clin Invest 1991 Dec; 88(6): 2095-105.

[15] Coleman RE HS, Bell R, Camreon D, Dodwell D, Liversedge V, Burkinshaw R, Keane M, Gil, M, Marshall H Adjuvant therapy for stage II/III breast cancer with or without zoledronic acid. Final efficacy analysis of the AZURE trial. Cancer and Bone Society, Miami, Florida 2013.

[16] Caraglia M, Santini D, Marra M, Vincenzi B, Tonini G, Budillon A. Emerging anti-cancer molecular mechanisms of aminobisphosphonates. Endocr Relat Cancer 2006 Mar; 13(1): 7-26.

[17] Clezardin P. Anti-tumour activity of zoledronic acid. Cancer Treat Rev 2005; 31 Suppl 3: 1-8.

[18] Holen I, Coleman RE. Anti-tumour activity of bisphosphonates in preclinical models of breast cancer. Breast Cancer Research: BCR. [Review] 2010; 12(6): 214.

[19] Winter MC, Holen I, Coleman RE. Exploring the anti-tumour activity of bisphosphonates in early breast cancer. Cancer Treat Rev 2008 Aug; 34(5): 453-75.

[20] Thudi NK, Martin CK, Nadella MV, Fernandez SA, Werbeck JL, Pinzone JJ, *et al.* Zoledronic acid decreased osteolysis but not bone metastasis in a nude mouse model of canine prostate cancer with mixed bone lesions. Prostate 2008 Jul 1; 68(10): 1116-25.

[21] Hung TT, Chan J, Russell PJ, Power CA. Zoledronic acid preserves bone structure and increases survival but does not limit tumour incidence in a prostate cancer bone metastasis model. PloS One. [Research Support, Non-U.S. Gov't] 2011; 6(5): e19389.

[22] Dallas SL, Garrett IR, Oyajobi BO, Dallas MR, Boyce BF, Bauss F, *et al.* Ibandronate reduces osteolytic lesions but not tumor burden in a murine model of myeloma bone disease. Blood 1999 Mar 1; 93(5): 1697-706.

[23] Shipman CM, Vanderkerken K, Rogers MJ, Lippitt JM, Asosingh K, Hughes DE, *et al.* The potent bisphosphonate ibandronate does not induce myeloma cell apoptosis in a murine model of established multiple myeloma. Br J Haematol 2000 Oct; 111(1): 283-6.

[24] Hortobagyi GN, Theriault RL, Porter L, Blayney D, Lipton A, Sinoff C, *et al.* Efficacy of pamidronate in reducing skeletal complications in patients with breast cancer and lytic bone metastases. Protocol 19 Aredia Breast Cancer Study Group. N Engl J Med 1996 Dec 12; 335(24): 1785-91.

[25] Theriault R. Pamidronate in the treatment of osteolytic bone metastases in breast cancer patients. Br J Clin Pract Suppl 1996 Sep; 87: 8-12; discussion 3-4.

[26] Kostenuik PJ, Orr FW, Suyama K, Singh G. Increased growth rate and tumor burden of spontaneously metastatic Walker 256 cancer cells in the skeleton of bisphosphonate-treated rats. Cancer Res 1993 Nov 15; 53(22): 5452-7.

[27] Yang M, Burton DW, Geller J, Hillegonds DJ, Hastings RH, Deftos LJ, *et al.* The bisphosphonate olpadronate inhibits skeletal prostate cancer progression in a green fluorescent protein nude mouse model. Clin Cancer Res 2006 Apr 15; 12(8): 2602-6.

[28] Burton DW, Geller J, Yang M, Jiang P, Barken I, Hastings RH, *et al.* Monitoring of skeletal progression of prostate cancer by GFP imaging, X-ray, and serum OPG and PTHrP. Prostate 2005 Feb 15; 62(3): 275-81.

[29] Corey E, Brown LG, Quinn JE, Poot M, Roudier MP, Higano CS, *et al.* Zoledronic acid exhibits inhibitory effects on osteoblastic and osteolytic metastases of prostate cancer. Clin Cancer Res 2003 Jan; 9(1): 295-306.

[30] Li X, Liao J, Park SI, Koh AJ, Sadler WD, Pienta KJ, *et al.* Drugs which inhibit osteoclast function suppress tumor growth through calcium reduction in bone. Bone. [Research Support, N.I.H., Extramural] 2011 Jun 1; 48(6): 1354-61.

[31] Neudert M, Fischer C, Krempien B, Bauss F, Seibel MJ. Site-specific human breast cancer (MDA-MB-231) metastases in nude rats: model characterisation and *in vivo* effects of ibandronate on tumour growth. Int J Cancer 2003 Nov 10; 107(3): 468-77.

[32] Mundy GR, Yoneda T, Hiraga T. Preclinical studies with zoledronic acid and other bisphosphonates: impact on the bone microenvironment. Semin Oncol 2001 Apr; 28(2 Suppl 6): 35-44.

[33] Hiraga T, Williams PJ, Mundy GR, Yoneda T. The bisphosphonate ibandronate promotes apoptosis in MDA-MB-231 human breast cancer cells in bone metastases. Cancer Res 2001 Jun 1; 61(11): 4418-24.

[34] Fournier PG, Daubine F, Lundy MW, Rogers MJ, Ebetino FH, Clezardin P. Lowering bone mineral affinity of bisphosphonates as a therapeutic strategy to optimize skeletal tumor growth inhibition *in vivo*. Cancer Research. [Research Support, Non-U.S. Gov't] 2008 Nov 1; 68(21): 8945-53.

[35] Fournier PG, Stresing V, Ebetino FH, Clezardin P. How do bisphosphonates inhibit bone metastasis *in vivo*? Neoplasia. [Research Support, Non-U.S. Gov't] 2010 Jul; 12(7): 571-8.

[36] Hirbe AC, Roelofs AJ, Floyd DH, Deng H, Becker SN, Lanigan LG, *et al.* The bisphosphonate zoledronic acid decreases tumor growth in bone in mice with defective osteoclasts. Bone. [Research Support, N.I.H., Extramural Research Support, Non-U.S. Gov't] 2009 May; 44(5): 908-16.

[37] Daubine F, Le Gall C, Gasser J, Green J, Clezardin P. Antitumor effects of clinical dosing regimens of bisphosphonates in experimental breast cancer bone metastasis. J Natl Cancer Inst 2007 Feb 21; 99(4): 322-30.

[38] van der Pluijm G, Que I, Sijmons B, Buijs JT, Lowik CW, Wetterwald A, *et al.* Interference with the microenvironmental support impairs the de novo formation of bone metastases *in vivo*. Cancer Res 2005 Sep 1; 65(17): 7682-90.

[39] Croucher PI, De Hendrik R, Perry MJ, Hijzen A, Shipman CM, Lippitt J, *et al.* Zoledronic acid treatment of 5T2MM-bearing mice inhibits the development of myeloma bone disease: evidence for decreased osteolysis, tumor burden and angiogenesis, and increased survival. J Bone Miner Res 2003 Mar; 18(3): 482-92.

[40] Zhang H, Yano S, Miki T, Goto H, Kanematsu T, Muguruma H, *et al.* A novel bisphosphonate minodronate (YM529) specifically inhibits osteolytic bone metastasis produced by human small-cell lung cancer cells in NK-cell depleted SCID mice. Clin Exp Metastasis 2003; 20(2): 153-9.

[41] Krempien B, Manegold C. Prophylactic treatment of skeletal metastases, tumor-induced osteolysis, and hypercalcemia in rats with the bisphosphonate Cl2MBP. Cancer 1993 Jul 1; 72(1): 91-8.

[42] Sasaki A, Boyce BF, Story B, Wright KR, Chapman M, Boyce R, *et al.* Bisphosphonate risedronate reduces metastatic human breast cancer burden in bone in nude mice. Cancer Res 1995 Aug 15; 55(16): 3551-7.

[43] Sasaki A, Kitamura K, Alcalde RE, Tanaka T, Suzuki A, Etoh Y, *et al.* Effect of a newly developed bisphosphonate, YH529, on osteolytic bone metastases in nude mice. Int J Cancer 1998 Jul 17; 77(2): 279-85.

[44] Luo KW, Ko CH, Yue GG, Lee MY, Siu WS, Lee JK, *et al.* Anti-tumor and anti-osteolysis effects of the metronomic use of zoledronic acid in primary and metastatic breast cancer mouse models. Cancer Lett 2013 Oct 1; 339(1): 42-8.

[45] Yaccoby S, Pearse RN, Johnson CL, Barlogie B, Choi Y, Epstein J. Myeloma interacts with the bone marrow microenvironment to induce osteoclastogenesis and is dependent on osteoclast activity. Br J Haematol 2002 Feb; 116(2): 278-90.

[46] Gao L, Deng H, Zhao H, Hirbe A, Harding J, Ratner L, *et al.* HTLV-1 Tax transgenic mice develop spontaneous osteolytic bone metastases prevented by osteoclast inhibition. Blood 2005 Dec 15; 106(13): 4294-302.

[47] Rogers TL, Holen I. Tumour macrophages as potential targets of bisphosphonates. J Translat Medicine. [Research Support, Non-U.S. Gov't Review] 2011; 9: 177.

[48] Rogers TL, Wind N, Hughes R, Nutter F, Brown HK, Vasiliadou I, *et al.* Macrophages as potential targets for zoledronic acid outside the skeleton-evidence from *in vitro* and *in vivo* models. Cellular Oncol. [Research Support, Non-U.S. Gov't] 2013 Dec; 36(6): 505-14.

[49] Matsumoto S, Kimura S, Segawa H, Kuroda J, Yuasa T, Sato K, *et al.* Efficacy of the third-generation bisphosphonate, zoledronic acid alone and combined with anti-cancer agents against small cell lung cancer cell lines. Lung Cancer 2005 Jan; 47(1): 31-9.

[50] Li YY, Chang JW, Chou WC, Liaw CC, Wang HM, Huang JS, *et al.* Zoledronic acid is unable to induce apoptosis, but slows tumor growth and prolongs survival for non-small-cell lung cancers. Lung Cancer 2008 Feb; 59(2): 180-91.

[51] Stathopoulos GT, Moschos C, Loutrari H, Kollintza A, Psallidas I, Karabela S, *et al.* Zoledronic acid is effective against experimental malignant pleural effusion. Am J Respir Crit Care Med 2008 Jul 1; 178(1): 50-9.

[52] Giraudo E, Inoue M, Hanahan D. An amino-bisphosphonate targets MMP-9-expressing macrophages and angiogenesis to impair cervical carcinogenesis. J Clin Invest 2004 Sep; 114(5): 623-33.

[53] Wakchoure S, Merrell MA, Aldrich W, Millender-Swain T, Harris KW, Triozzi P, *et al.* Bisphosphonates inhibit the growth of mesothelioma cells *in vitro* and *in vivo*. Clin Cancer Res 2006 May 1; 12(9): 2862-8.

[54] Okamoto S, Kawamura K, Li Q, Yamanaka M, Yang S, Fukamachi T, *et al.* Zoledronic acid produces antitumor effects on mesothelioma through apoptosis and S-phase arrest in p53-independent and Ras prenylation-independent manners. J Thorac Oncol: Official Publication of the International Association for the Study of Lung Cancer. [Research Support, Non-U.S. Gov't] 2012 May; 7(5): 873-82.

[55] Ory B, Heymann MF, Kamijo A, Gouin F, Heymann D, Redini F. Zoledronic acid suppresses lung metastases and prolongs overall survival of osteosarcoma-bearing mice. Cancer 2005 Dec 1; 104(11): 2522-9.

[56] Hiraga T, Williams PJ, Ueda A, Tamura D, Yoneda T. Zoledronic acid inhibits visceral metastases in the 4T1/luc mouse breast cancer model. Clin Cancer Res 2004 Jul 1; 10(13): 4559-67.

[57] Monkkonen H, Auriola S, Lehenkari P, Kellinsalmi M, Hassinen IE, Vepsalainen J, *et al.* A new endogenous ATP analog (ApppI) inhibits the mitochondrial adenine nucleotide translocase (ANT) and is responsible for the apoptosis induced by nitrogen-containing bisphosphonates. Br J Pharmacol. [Research Support, Non-U.S. Gov't] 2006 Feb; 147(4): 437-45.

[58] Monkkonen H, Ottewell PD, Kuokkanen J, Monkkonen J, Auriola S, Holen I. Zoledronic acid-induced IPP/ApppI production *in vivo*. Life Sci. [Research Support, Non-U.S. Gov't] 2007 Sep 8; 81(13): 1066-70.

[59] Benzaid I, Monkkonen H, Stresing V, Bonnelye E, Green J, Monkkonen J, *et al.* High phosphoantigen levels in bisphosphonate-treated human breast tumors promote Vgamma9Vdelta2 T-cell chemotaxis and cytotoxicity *in vivo*. Cancer Res. [Research Support, Non-U.S. Gov't] 2011 Jul 1; 71(13): 4562-72.

[60] Benzaid I, Monkkonen H, Bonnelye E, Monkkonen J, Clezardin P. *In vivo* phosphoantigen levels in bisphosphonate-treated human breast tumors trigger Vgamma9Vdelta2 T-cell

antitumor cytotoxicity through ICAM-1 engagement. Clin Cancer Res: J Am Assoc Cancer Res. [Research Support, Non-U.S. Gov't] 2012 Nov 15; 18(22): 6249-59.

[61] Misso G, Porru M, Stoppacciaro A, Castellano M, De Cicco F, Leonetti C, *et al.* Evaluation of the *in vitro* and *in vivo* antiangiogenic effects of denosumab and zoledronic acid. Cancer Biol Ther. [Research Support, Non-U.S. Gov't] 2012 Dec; 13(14): 1491-500.

[62] Michigami T, Hiraga T, Williams PJ, Niewolna M, Nishimura R, Mundy GR, *et al.* The effect of the bisphosphonate ibandronate on breast cancer metastasis to visceral organs. Breast Cancer Res Treat 2002 Oct; 75(3): 249-58.

[63] Diel IJ, Jaschke A, Solomayer EF, Gollan C, Bastert G, Sohn C, *et al.* Adjuvant oral clodronate improves the overall survival of primary breast cancer patients with micrometastases to the bone marrow: a long-term follow-up. Ann Oncol 2008 Dec; 19(12): 2007-11.

[64] Diel IJ, Solomayer EF, Costa SD, Gollan C, Goerner R, Wallwiener D, *et al.* Reduction in new metastases in breast cancer with adjuvant clodronate treatment. N Engl J Med 1998 Aug 6; 339(6): 357-63.

[65] Saarto T, Blomqvist C, Virkkunen P, Elomaa I. Adjuvant clodronate treatment does not reduce the frequency of skeletal metastases in node-positive breast cancer patients: 5-year results of a randomized controlled trial. J Clin Oncol 2001 Jan 1; 19(1): 10-7.

[66] Jagdev SP, Coleman RE, Shipman CM, Rostami HA, Croucher PI. The bisphosphonate, zoledronic acid, induces apoptosis of breast cancer cells: evidence for synergy with paclitaxel. Br J Cancer 2001 Apr 20; 84(8): 1126-34.

[67] Hiraga T, Ueda A, Tamura D, Hata K, Ikeda F, Williams PJ, *et al.* Effects of oral UFT combined with or without zoledronic acid on bone metastasis in the 4T1/luc mouse breast cancer. Int J Cancer 2003 Oct 10; 106(6): 973-9.

[68] Duivenvoorden WC, Vukmirovic-Popovic S, Kalina M, Seidlitz E, Singh G. Effect of zoledronic acid on the doxycycline-induced decrease in tumour burden in a bone metastasis model of human breast cancer. Br J Cancer 2007 May 21; 96(10): 1526-31.

[69] van Beek ER, Lowik CW, van Wijngaarden J, Ebetino FH, Papapoulos SE. Synergistic effect of bisphosphonate and docetaxel on the growth of bone metastasis in an animal model of established metastatic bone disease. Breast Cancer Res Treat 2008 Nov 7; [Epub ahead of print].

[70] Previdi S, Scolari F, Chila R, Ricci F, Abbadessa G, Broggini M. Combination of the c-Met inhibitor tivantinib and zoledronic acid prevents tumor bone engraftment and inhibits progression of established bone metastases in a breast xenograft model. PloS One 2013; 8(11): e79101.

[71] Ottewell PD, Monkkonen H, Jones M, Lefley DV, Coleman RE, Holen I. Antitumor effects of doxorubicin followed by zoledronic acid in a mouse model of breast cancer. J Natl Cancer Inst 2008 Aug 20; 100(16): 1167-78.

[72] Ottewell PD, Brown HK, Jones M, Rogers TL, Cross SS, Brown NJ, *et al.* Combination therapy inhibits development and progression of mammary tumours in immunocompetent mice. Breast Cancer Res Treat. [Research Support, Non-U.S. Gov't] 2012 Jun; 133(2): 523-36.

[73] Ottewell PD, Deux B, Monkkonen H, Cross S, Coleman RE, Clezardin P, *et al.* Differential effect of doxorubicin and zoledronic acid on intraosseous *versus* extraosseous breast tumor growth *in vivo*. Clin Cancer Res 2008 Jul 15; 14(14): 4658-66.

[74] Brown HK, Ottewell PD, Evans CA, Coleman RE, Holen I. A single administration of combination therapy inhibits breast tumour progression in bone and modifies both osteoblasts and osteoclasts. J Bone Oncol 2012; 1: 47-56.

[75] Kim SJ, Uehara H, Yazici S, He J, Langley RR, Mathew P, *et al.* Modulation of bone microenvironment with zoledronate enhances the therapeutic effects of STI571 and paclitaxel against experimental bone metastasis of human prostate cancer. Cancer Res 2005 May 1; 65(9): 3707-15.

[76] Brubaker KD, Brown LG, Vessella RL, Corey E. Administration of zoledronic acid enhances the effects of docetaxel on growth of prostate cancer in the bone environment. BMC Cancer 2006; 6: 15.

[77] Bruzzese F, Pucci B, Milone MR, Ciardiello C, Franco R, Chianese MI, *et al.* Panobinostat synergizes with zoledronic acid in prostate cancer and multiple myeloma models by increasing ROS and modulating mevalonate and p38-MAPK pathways. Cell Death Dis. [Research Support, Non-U.S. Gov't] 2013; 4: e878.

[78] Yano S, Zhang H, Hanibuchi M, Miki T, Goto H, Uehara H, *et al.* Combined therapy with a new bisphosphonate, minodronate (YM529), and chemotherapy for multiple organ metastases of small cell lung cancer cells in severe combined immunodeficient mice. Clin Cancer Res 2003 Nov 1; 9(14): 5380-5.

[79] Futamura N, Urakawa H, Arai E, Kozawa E, Ishiguro N, Nishida Y. Hyaluronan synthesis inhibitor supplements the inhibitory effects of zoledronic acid on bone metastasis of lung cancer. Clin Experimental Metast. [Research Support, Non-U.S. Gov't] 2013 Jun; 30(5): 595-606.

[80] Zhao M, Tominaga Y, Ohuchida K, Mizumoto K, Cui L, Kozono S, *et al.* Significance of combination therapy of zoledronic acid and gemcitabine on pancreatic cancer. Cancer Sci. [Research Support, Non-U.S. Gov't] 2012 Jan; 103(1): 58-66.

[81] Hashimoto K, Masumori N, Tanaka T, Maeda T, Kobayashi K, Kitamura H, *et al.* Zoledronic acid but not somatostatin analogs exerts anti-tumor effects in a model of murine prostatic neuroendocrine carcinoma of the development of castration-resistant prostate cancer. Prostate 2013 Apr; 73(5): 500-11.

[82] Vintonenko N, Jais JP, Kassis N, Abdelkarim M, Perret GY, Lecouvey M, *et al.* Transcriptome analysis and *in vivo* activity of fluvastatin *versus* zoledronic acid in a murine breast cancer metastasis model. Mol Pharmacol. [Research Support, Non-U.S. Gov't] 2012 Sep; 82(3): 521-8.

CHAPTER 5

Bleomycin and its Role in Inducing Apoptosis and Senescence in Alveolar Epithelial Lung Cells - Modulating Effects of Caveolin-1: An Update

Michael Kasper* **and Kathrin Barth**

Institute of Anatomy, Medical Faculty "Carl Gustav Carus", Technische Universität Dresden, 01307 Dresden, Germany

Abstract: Bleomycin, a widely used anti-tumor agent, is well-known to cause single- and double-strand breaks in cellular DNA *in vivo* and *in vitro* leading finally to genomic instability of damaged cells. Bleomycin causes an increase of reactive oxygen species, resulting in oxidative stress and pulmonary fibrosis. Further, bleomycin induces apoptosis and senescence in epithelial as well as non-epithelial cells of the lung.

Caveolin-1 is a scaffold protein of caveolae, which are particularly abundant in alveolar epithelial type I cells, in endothelial and smooth muscle cells, and in fibroblasts of lung tissue. Caveolin-1 directly interacts with signaling molecules and effects diverse signaling pathways regulating cell proliferation, apoptosis, differentiation, migration and growth.

In this review we discuss aspects of bleomycin resistance. We summarize recent data about the effects of bleomycin in terms of lung cell biology and emphasize that bleomycin-induced injury of lung cells is accompanied by altered expression levels of caveolin-1. Caveolin-1 is involved in bleomycin-induced apoptosis and senescence of normal and lung cancer cells. Investigating the role of caveolin-1 may provide new tools for therapeutic interventions in lung disease and for the understanding of tumor biology.

Keywords: Apoptosis, bleomycin, caveolin-1, lung cancer, pulmonary fibrosis, resistance, senescence.

INTRODUCTION

Bleomycin, the anticancer drug, is well known for its side effect to induce severe interstitial pulmonary fibrosis and there is experimental evidence of a marked

***Corresponding Author Michael Kasper:** Institute of Anatomy, Medical Faculty "Carl Gustav Carus", Technische Universität Dresden, 01307 Dresden, Germany; Tel: +49351 4586080; Fax: +49351 4586303; E-mail: michael.kasper@tu-dresden.de

Atta-ur-Rahman (Ed)

increase in the incidence of lung cancer in people with pulmonary fibrosis [1]. Further, bleomycin-induced chromosomal instability is associated with an increased risk for the development of lung cancer [2]. Bleomycin induces apoptosis as well as cellular senescence in pulmonary epithelial cells *in vivo* and *in vitro* [3-7]. Both events are involved in remodeling processes during fibrogenesis and in cancer development (Fig. **1**). Both apoptosis and senescence contribute to the suppression of tumors.

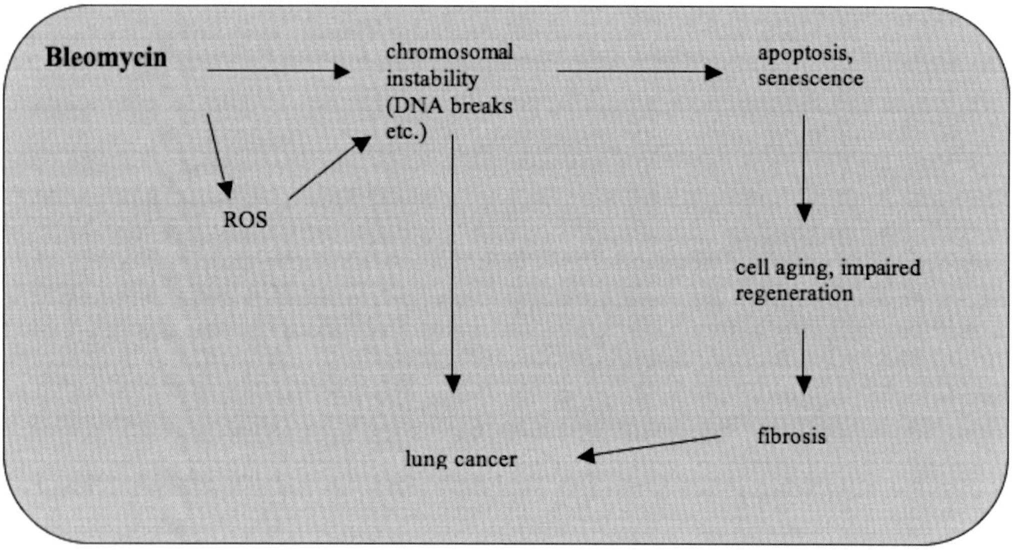

Fig. (1): Bleomycin effects in lung tissues.

Caveolin-1, a 21 kDa integral membrane protein, is a principal component of caveolae, which are the site of important dynamic and regulatory events at the plasma membrane, particular abundant in alveolar epithelial type I (ATI) cells, in endothelial and muscle cells of the lung [8]. Cells of caveolin-1 knockout mice show increased proliferation [9, 10]. The lung of these animals exhibits a pathologic phenotype with signs of fibrosis [9]. Bleomycin-induced fibrosis is accompanied by a loss of caveolin-1 in alveolar epithelial and other lung cells [8, 11]. Moreover, evidence for a role of caveolin-1 in cancer has been well documented, wherein caveolin-1 was suggested to be a tumor suppressor [12]. A loss of caveolin-1 accelerates tumorigenesis [13]. These and other data (reviewed in [14]) provide strong evidence for an association of caveolar dysfunction with human disease.

Below, we review cell biological aspects of senescence and apoptosis after bleomycin treatment of lung cells or tissues and discuss the role of caveolin-1 in modulating of both processes. In order to investigate the bleomycin effects on normal and cancer cells, the review preferably focuses on the (alveolar) epithelial compartment of lung parenchyma *e.g.* on alveolar ATI cells which have in abundance ultrastructurally detectable caveolae including their structural proteins caveolin-1 and -2. There is a controversy in the literature about the presence of caveolin in ATII cells (reviewed in [15, 16]). ATII cells, to the best of our knowledge, do not have morphologically detectable caveolae. Caveolin-1 is also present in other inflammatory cells of the lung such as monocytes, alveolar macrophages, lymphocytes and mast cells. Its exact subcellular distribution is, however, not yet clear, since these cells do not form classical caveolae. There is also no evidence that caveolae are the most important sites of action for caveolin-1 in the regulation of disease processes which are described in the following review. For a more comprehensive review of the role of caveolin-1 in fibrotic disease in general see [17].

BLEOMYCIN, LUNG DISEASE AND CAVEOLIN-1

Caveolae are flask-shaped plasmalemmal invaginations present in most mammalian cell types with a diameter of 50-100 nm. Fig. (**2**) shows a representative microphotograph of the distribution of caveolae in the alveolar epithelial and capillary endothelial cells of the lung.

There exist a group of 21-24-kDa integral membrane proteins in caveolae, called caveolins. Caveolin-1 and caveolin-2 are present in non-muscle cells such as, for example, in endothelial and ATI cells, whereas caveolin-3 occurs preferably in smooth-muscle and other muscle cells.

Caveolin-1 is the prototypical member of the caveolin family. Therefore, it has been the primary focus of many biochemical studies dealing with caveolins. Caveolin-1 has two isoforms, termed α and β, with the α-isoform consisting of residues 1-178 and the β-isoform containing residues 32-178, resulting in a protein which is 3 kDa smaller in size [18]. As known, caveolin-1 expression is sufficient and necessary to drive the formation of caveolae [19]. In addition, caveolin-1 expression is necessary for the stable expression and membrane localization of caveolin-2. Caveolin-2 alone is insufficient to induce caveolae biogenesis [20]. The NH_2 and COOH termini of caveolin-1 face the cytoplasm with an intervening hydrophobic domain inserted into the membrane. Cholesterol binds caveolin-1 and seems to be necessary for maintaining caveolae and their signalling and trafficking function [21].

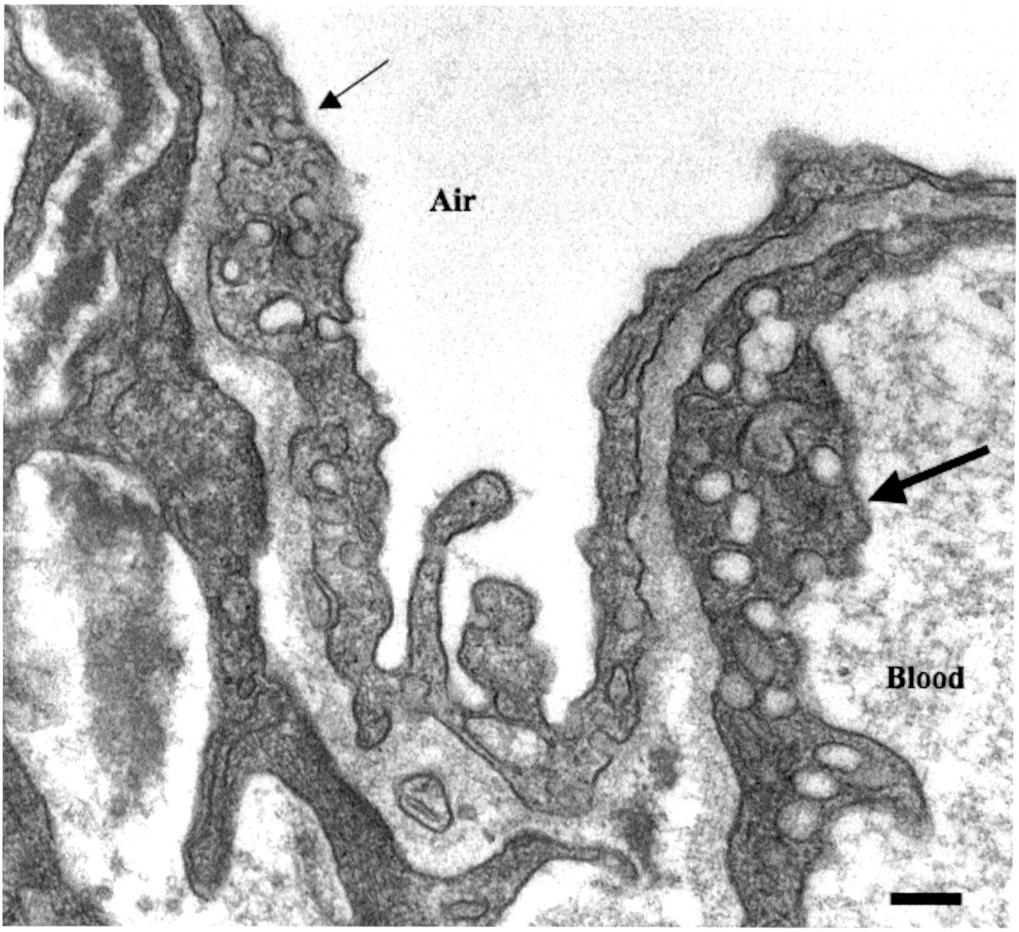

Fig. (2): Ultrastructural demonstration of caveolae in the mouse lung. Thick arrow indicates the capillary endothelium, thin arrow indicates the alveolar epithelium (ATI cell). Note the numerous caveolae in both cell types. Scale bar = 120 mm.

Many cellular functions have been addressed to caveolae: endocytosis (entry of pathogens), transcytosis, calcium signaling, lipid metabolism, and signal transduction in cellular proliferation and apoptosis [14] (see below). Caveolae may act as organized transducing centres which concentrate key signaling molecules compartments. In this way the proper proximity is created for rapid, efficient and specific propagation of signals from the cell surface to the inside of the cell.

Caveolae share similarities with plasmamembrane microdomain forming lipid rafts. Like caveolae, lipid rafts are detergent-resistent microdomains that are enriched in cholesterol and glycosphingolipids. They also can function as specialized signaling platforms [22]. Unlike caveolae, which have a distinct invaginated form, lipid rafts are very small, plasmalemmal microdomains that are enriched in various glycosylphosphatidylinositol-anchored proteinsand devoid of caveolin.

First evidence for the involvement of caveolin-1 in lung disease was provided from the study of radiation-induced fibrosis in rat and mini-pig lungs [8]. Indirect immunoperoxidase staining with polyclonal anti-caveolin 1-3 antibodies, confirmed by double fluorescence studies with ATI cell-specific lectins, revealed a selective expression of caveolin 1-3 (isotype-specific antibodies were to that time not available!) in ATI but not in ATII cells and also not in alveolar macrophages of normal lung tissues of rats and mini pigs. Furthermore, a dramatic loss of caveolin immunoreactivity was found in ATI cells of injured lungs in both fibrosis models. This downregulation of caveolin seems to be rather a pathophysiological event than the result of a necrotic or other type of destruction of ATI cells, since the corresponding ATI cell marker *Lycopersicon esculentum* lectin histochemically indicated in this study an intact alveolar lining layer. The alveolar epithelial loss of caveolin-1 has been later shown in bleomycin-induced fibrosis models [11, 23, 24]. In our experience, endothelial caveolin-1 was never changed or rather enhanced applying immunohistochemistry in different fibrotic lung samples of different animal models (bleomycin-, radiation-induced; [8, 23]). The reasons are not understood so far.

Other reports on pulmonary fibrosis after bleomycin-induced injury have been described a loss of caveolin-1 from other lung cell such as from fibroblasts [11], from leukocytes [25] and from bronchiolar epithelial cells [26]. The loss of caveolin-1 from endothelial cells in plexiform lesions of patients with pulmonary hypertension [27] and in experimental models of pulmonary hypertension [28, 29] is not the focus of this review, also not the impact of downregulated caveolin-1 in inflammatory cells such as monocytes and lymphocytes for the development of fibrosis (reviewed by [25, 30]).

To address the role of caveolin-1 in the development of pulmonary fibrosis, we investigated the phenotype of caveolin-1 knockout mice [9]. Mice deficient in caveolin-1 or caveolin-2 develop a lung pathology that resembles fibrosis [9, 10, 20]. Specifically knockout mice show smaller air-spaces and thickened alveolar walls showing hypercellularity and increased deposition of extracellular matrix proteins (Fig. **3A-C**).

Since caveolin-1 knockout mice contain no caveolin-2 protein in the lung [9] and caveolin-2 knockout mice develop similar pulmonary alterations [20], a specific pathogenetic role of caveolin-2 has to take in account. Investigations in this direction were not done for a long time. Very recently, de Almeida *et al.* [31] demonstrated that caveolin-2 is also involved in modulation of fibrotic response and that bleomycin decreased the expression of caveolin-2 and its phosphorylation at tyrosine 19. In contrast to caveolin-1 (see below), mechanisms of fibrotic alterations in the caveolin-2 knockout mice did not include alterations in the TGF-β signaling pathway.

Wang *et al.* conducted an excellent study to demonstrate the important function of caveolin-1 during fibrogenesis [11]. They used an adenovirus-mediated caveolin-1 gene transfer for the suppression of bleomycin-induced pulmonary fibrosis in mice and demonstrated *in vitro* that caveolin-1 suppresses the TGF-β1-induced production of collagen type I and other matrix proteins *via* the c-jun N-terminal kinase pathway in pulmonary fibroblasts and that caveolin-1 modulates the TGF-β1-induced smad signaling. Further extensive observations linking caveolin-1 to the regulation of extracellular matrix overproduction *in vitro* and the progression

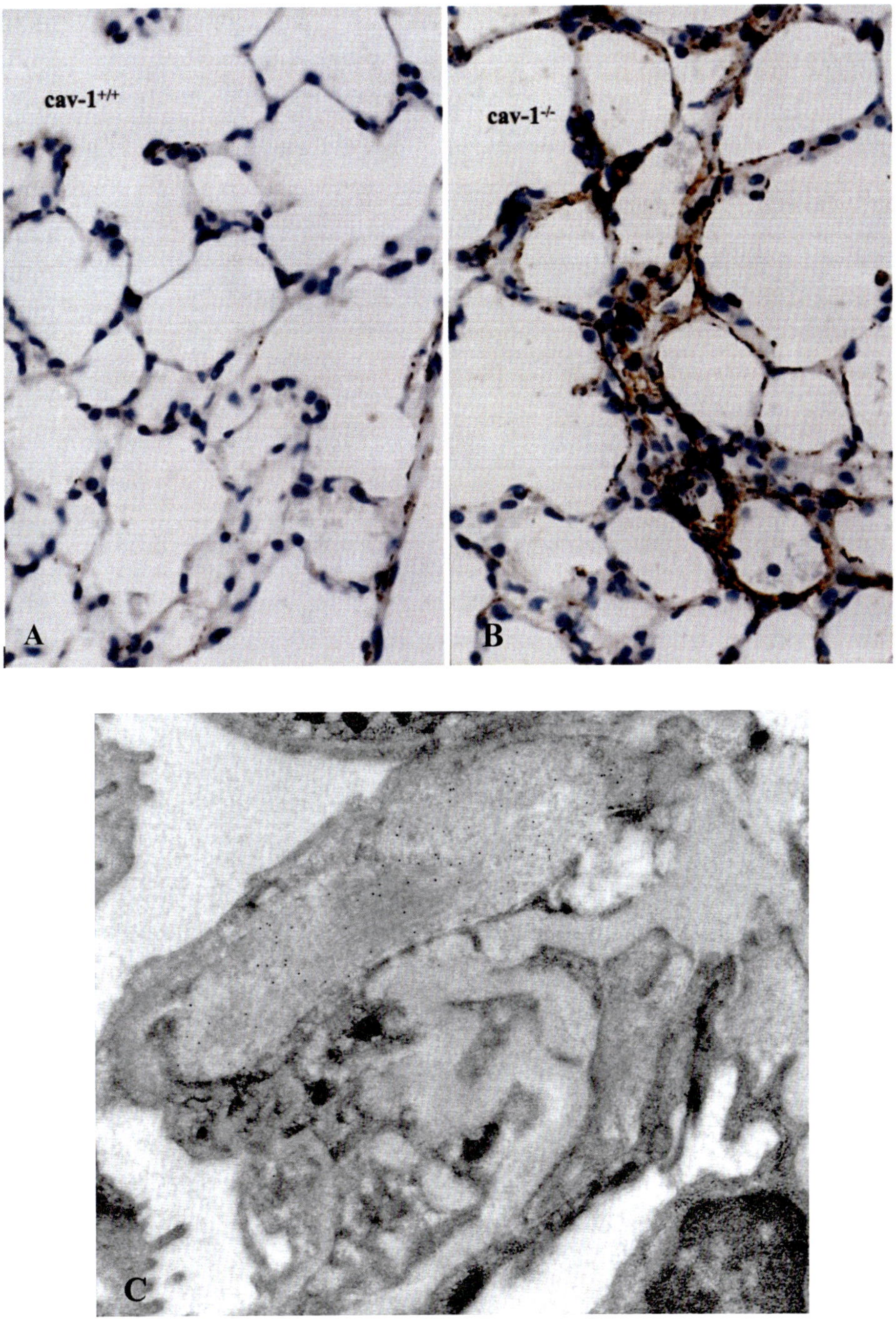

Fig. (3): (**A**, **B**) Immunperoxidase detection of collagen type I on paraffin sections of mouse lung tissue. (**C**) Lowicryl HM20 post-embedding. Immunogold detection of collagen type I in caveolin$^{-/-}$ mouse.

of bleomycin-induced fibrosis *in vivo* were provided by Tourkina *et al.* [32]. Using a peptide equivalent to the caveolin-1 scaffolding domain (CSD peptide) the authors were able to suppress the extent of fibrosis *via* inhibition of collagen, tenascin and alpha smooth muscle cell actin. Further, the administration of this peptide to bleomycin-treated mice was leading to a reduction of the extent of apoptosis in alveolar epithelial cells [32]. To the same time Del Galdo *et al.* [33] showed that increasing caveolin-1 expression markedly improved bleomycin-induced pulmonary fibrosis. Systemic administration of penetratin-caveolin-1 peptide (CSD peptide) to mice with bleomycin-induced lung fibrosis reduced fibrosis. Recent data of Bhandary *et al.* [34] provided further evidence that increased epithelial apoptosis due to bleomycin exposure of mice as well as of isolated ATII cells could be reversed by treatment with CSD peptide.

The CSD peptide directly affects eNOS, PKC, RAS, EGF receptors and various MAP kinases by restoring caveolin-1 function and thereby reversing the hyperactivation of the mentioned signaling molecules [15]. In general, TGF-β inhibits the expression of caveolin-1 in fibroblast and other lung cells. In alveolar epithelial cells caveolin-1 regulates the TGF-β signaling *via* its effects on the internalization of the TGF-β ligand-receptor complex [35]. It has been shown recently that pyridine agents, such as pirfenidone, are effective drugs with anti-inflammatory and antifibrotic properties can prevent bleomycin-induced lung fibrosis [36, 37]. Pirfenidone restores caveolin-1 protein and mRNA expression and inhibits mitogen-activated protein kinase (MAPK) signaling pathways. It is further well accepted that the (bleomycin-induced) modulation of TGF-β-related signal transduction has an impact on processes of apoptosis and senescence in lung cells [38-40], see below.

It is noteworthy to mention that caveolin-1 has previously been shown to be involved in other kind of lung injury. For example, deletion of caveolin-1 protects against hyperoxia-induced epithelial cell death *via* upregulation of cytoprotective genes, such as hemeoxygenase and survivin [41-43].

BLEOMYCIN

Bleomycin is a group of glycopeptides (molecular weight approximately 1500 dalton) isolated from Streptomyces verticillus by Umezawa *et al.* [44]. The commercial preparation is a mixture of different bleomycins which differ in their terminal amine moiety, consisting predominantly of bleomycin A2 (55-70%) and B2 (20-30%) [45]; (Fig. **4**). Bleomycin as a cytotoxic drug is widely used in cancer therapy, particular in therapy of testicular and ovarian germ cell neoplasms, Hodgkin's and non-Hodgkin's lymphomas and various squamous cell carcinomas (for review see [46, 47]). Several case-control studies have also shown that bleomycin sensitivity is an independent risk factor for tobacco-related cancers (for review see [2]). It causes extensive damage to DNA (single and double strand breaks) similar to that generated by ionizing radiation (radiomimetic drug). DNA damage is both oxygen and metal-ion dependent, with the preference for iron which includes the N-terminus with the metal-binding region [48]. The Bleomycin-Fe^{II} has been shown to bind O_2 to form an Bleomycin-Fe^{III}-superoxide complex that accepts an additional electron thus forming Bleomycin-Fe^{III}-OOH, called "activated bleomycin" [49]. The C-terminus domain is responsible for the DNA binding affinity and plays a critical role in pulmonary toxicity due to its ability of producing of hydroxyl free radicals [50]. Other domains of bleomycin such as the carbohydrate domain and the linker domain should increase the efficiency of the DNA cleavage. Recent work of Regulus *et al.* describes bleomycin-induced double strand breaks likely arising from the formation of two vicinal DNA strand breads, initiated by oxidation of the sugar moiety leading to the formation of 2'-deoxycytidine adducts [51]. According to previous data [52, 53] bleomycin cleaves also RNA and DNA-RNA-hybrids. Degradation of RNA should have implications for an inhibition of protein biosynthesis. The biological importance of this reactivity is still undefined [48]. "Activated bleomycin" is also able to oxidize lipids [54].

Bleomycins are hydrophilic molecules that cannot cross the cell membrane by free diffusion. The mechanism of its uptake is not clear. There is one single evidence that bleomycin binds to a receptor on the plasma membrane [55]. *In vitro* investigations revealed that bleomycin-induced DNA damage is cell-cycle dependent [45, 56]. The cellular response to bleomycin can be summarized as apoptosis and senescence (see below).

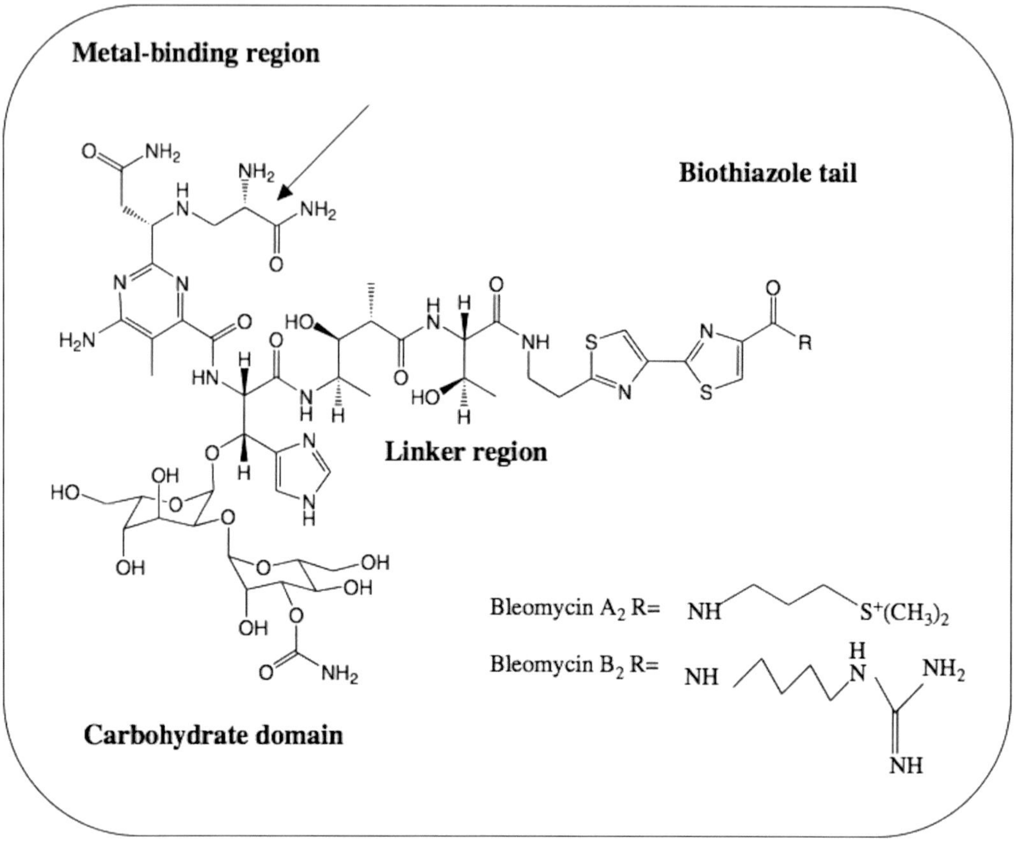

Fig. (4): Chemical structure of bleomycin, modified from [49]. Arrow indicates the β-aminoalanine moiety.

BLEOMYCIN RESISTANCE AND SENSITIVITY

Some prokaryotic as well as eukaryotic cells have a system to protect themselves from bleomycin-induced toxicity. The derminants of bleomycin resistance have been the topic of excellent and comprehensive reviews (for example [57]). Bleomycin can be metabolically inactivated in normal and cancer cells by the enzyme bleomycin hydrolase [58]. This enzyme has an aminopeptidase activity and hydrolyzes the amide in the ß-aminoalanine moiety of bleomycin [59] (arrow in Fig. **4**). The natural substrates of this enzyme are unknown.

Bleomycin hydrolase knockout mice are healthy and fertile but more sensitive to bleomycin [60]. Normal tissues with low levels of hydrolase, such as lung and skin tissue are less resistant to bleomycin, whereas tumor cells that acquire resistance to bleomycin express high levels of hydrolase activity [57]. High levels of hydrolase mRNA are also observed in human cancer cell lines [61, 62]. Functional studies of bleomycin hydrolase activity indicate that this enzyme affects bleomycin-induced pulmonary fibrosis [63]. There exist, however, no data about bleomycin hydrolase activity in the alveolar epithelium. It is tempting to speculate that ATI and ATII cells differ in their hydrolase content and therefore in their resistance to bleomycin.

A more recent addition to the explanation of bleomycin resistance has been the discovery that mice deficient in inducible nitric oxidase synthase [64], in neutrophil elastase [65], in the receptor for advanced glycation end products (RAGE) [66], the nuclear factor, erythroid 2 related factor (Nrf2) [67], the $p47^{phox}$ subunit of NADPH-oxidase [68], and CXC chemokine receptor 3 [69] are resistant to bleomycin-induced pulmonary fibrosis.

There is broad evidence in the literature that sensitivity to mutagens can increase the risk of developing cancer (for review see [70]). Bleomycin-induced DNA damage induces DNA repair genes as is the case for human 8-oxoguanine DNA glycosylase [71]. Knockdown of this gene in human lung cancer cell lines alters the cellular sensitivity to bleomycin. Increased sensitivity to bleomycin and other chemotherapeutic agents were recently found in cancer cells lacking the human telomerase reverse transcriptase (hTERT) after si-RNA-based inhibtion of hTERT [72]. The precise molecular mechansism of this effect is unknwon. For the discussion of the involvement of the telomerase system in processes of apoptosis see below.

LUNG CELL TYPES INVOLVED IN APOPTOSIS AFTER BLEOMYCIN EXPOSURE

Table **1** only summarizes apoptosis data related to the normal cell types in the lung, which are injured by bleomycin. There is, however, also evidence that bleomycin sensitivity is consistently associated with an increased risk of lung cancer [2, 73]. Bleomycin-induced genomic changes and changes of the apoptotic rate of lung cancer cells may have tumorigenic potential [74]. The intracellular cell death pathways that are activated on direct exposure of bleomycin to epithelial lung cancer cells, however, remain to be clarified.

Table 1: Different Lung Cell Types Involved in Apoptotic Events After Bleomycin-Induced Lung Injury

Cell Type	References
Alveolar epithelial cells, lymphocytes	[82, 83]
AM	[171]
Alveolar epithelial cells	[172]
ATII	[173]
AM	[174]
Alveolar and bronchial epithelial cells, AM, infiltrating inflammatory cells	[5, 175, 176]
AM	[176, 177]
Alveolar epithelial cells	[109, 178, 179]
Endothelial cells	[180, 181]
Myofibroblasts	[182, 183]
Alveolar epithelial cells	[86]
ATII	[184]

AM: alveolar macrophages; ATII: alveolar epithelial type II cells.

Histological studies from bleomycin-inducedlung fibrosis in animals as well as in humans (after cancer therapy) showed that bleomycin treatment results in damage to endothelial cells in lung blood vessels, to inflammatory cells (alveolar macrophages, granulocytes, and lymphocytes) and myofibroblasts which accumulate during fibrogenesis and importantly in damage to epithelial cells of the bronchial and the alveolar epithelium (compare Table **1**). There is consens in the literature that in the epithelial part of lung parenchyma the alveolar type II cells are the main target of bleomycin-induced apoptosis (Table **1**). It is, however, not known, how ATI cells are affected by bleomycin. Previous data favour a necrotic cell death [75]. It is still an open question, whether ATI cells choose the apoptotic pathway after severe injury [76]. Interestingly, there is also no evidence that ATI cells undergo programmed cell death during postnatal lung development, a process of structural lung maturation, which is characterized by the selective reduction of fibroblasts and ATII cells *via* apoptosis [77].

MECHANISMS OF BLEOMYCIN-INDUCED APOPTOSIS IN LUNG CELLS

Two principal pathways of apoptosis are known: One is a direct (extrinsic) pathway which includes the ligation of death receptors such as Fas (which binds Fas ligand) or tumor-necrosis factor (TNF) receptor (which binds TNF) at the cell membrane, the subsequent activation of the caspase cascade over an activated caspase-8, and an irreversible cell injury and cell death. The second pathway is induced by infectious agents such as viruses and bacteria, genotoxic drugs, radiation and by other free radical-mediated oxidative stress. This (intrinsic) pathway starts in mitochondria with a release of cytochrome c into the cytosol, leading to its binding to Apafl and ATP, followed by activation of caspase-9, and subsequently to execution of apoptosis. Both pathways are at least in part activated under certain circumstances to the same time in the same cell [78]. Using a mouse lung epithelial (MLE) cell line for the study of bleomycin-induced apoptosis, the authors demonstrated accumulation of free radicals, apoptosis, increased caspase-8 and -9 activity and increased cell surface expression of Fas and FasL.

THE Fas-FasL PATHWAY

The most representative example for a death receptor-mediated pathway is the Fas-FasL induced apoptosis of lung cells after treatment with bleomycin *in vivo* and *in vitro*. Fas antigen (CD95) is a differentiation antigen expressed on a variety of cell lines and known to regulate peripheral immune responses. The Fas receptor is activated by FasL, a member of the TNF family and predominantly expressed on activated lymphocytes but also on pulmonary epithelial and other lung cells or by a soluble form of FasL (sFasL), which can be cleaved from cell membranes by the action of specific serine proteinases such as metalloproteinases 7 and 3 (MMP-7, MMP-3) [79, 80]. The membrane Fas is clustered by FasL, specialized docking proteins (including Fas-associated death domain (FADD) which aggregate around the intracellular tails of clustered Fas molecules. This death-initiating complex (DISC) recruits procaspase 8 molecules, which undergo activation by autocatalytic cleavage, resulting in the activation of a cascade of downstream intracellular caspases [81]. In animal models of bleomycin-induced fibrosis FasL mRNA was upregulated in infiltrating lymphocytes, and Fas was elevated in pulmonary epithelial cells with signs of apoptosis [82]. They demonstrated that bleomycin firstly damaged DNA of epithelial cells immediately after intratracheal instillation *in vivo*, but DNA damage was repaired within 3 days, followed by epithelial cell apoptosis, which is Fas-dependent, from 5 to 14 days. Later on, the same group demonstrated the induction of excessive apoptosis after ligation of Fas by inhalation of anti-Fas antibody thus mimicking Fas-FasL crosslinking [83]. Furthermore, soluble FasL has been detected in the bronchoalveolar lavage (BAL) from patients with acute lung injury (ARDS) [84] and Fas and FasL are upregulated in pulmonary edema fluid and coexpressed in inflammatory and slaughed epithelial cells of lung tissue from ARDS patients [85]. From this Kuwano *et al.* expect the Fas-mediated apoptotic pathway as essential for pulmonary fibrosis, including bleomycin-induced fibrosis [83]. Interestingly, Golan-Gerstl *et al.* [86] provided direct evidence for bleomycin-induced Fas^+ epithelial cell apoptosis during fibrogenesis. FasL is overexpressed on alpha smooth muscle actin-positive myofibroblasts and in human lungs with interstitial fibrosis. FasL-positive myofibroblasts killed Fas-positive epithelial cells *in vitro*, whereas FasL-deficient myofibroblasts were not cytotoxic for epithelial lung cells in co-culture experiments. Opposite data presented Aoshiba *et al.* [87] performing experiments with Fas-deficient and FasL-deficient mice exposed to bleomycin. Intratracheal instillation of bleomycin revealed no differences in the lung pathology between the wild-type and knockout animals. In this case, however, differences in the mice strain used for the experiments have to take in account. Data of Wallach-Dayabn *et al.* [78] argue against a solely Fas/FasL concept in bleomycin induced apoptosis. Bleomycin-treated mouse MLE cells showed increased reactive oxygen species (ROS) resulting in oxidative stress, mitochondrial leakage and apoptosis. They found an upregulation of caspases-8 and -9 and solely Fas antigen, but anti FasL treatment did not change the apoptotic effects. The situation *in vitro*, however, seems to be different and not reasonable to compare with animal models of bleomycin-induced fibrosis.

Considerable experimental evidence indicates that the Fas receptors are either localized in or recruited to lipid rafts as an initial step necessary for the induction of apoptosis. Lipid rafts are enriched in sphingomyelin, a precursor of ceramide and sphingomyelinase, the enzyme responsible for generating ceramide [88]. The sphingolipid ceramide has been implicated to manage the clustering of Fas in ceramide-rich rafts [89]. Schenk *et al.* [90] reported that receptor clustering mediated by ceramide seems to function as a general mechanism to amplify signals generated upon ligand binding but does not seem to be a specific event of the receptor-initiated signaling cascade. No clear cut data are available about a direct interaction between caveolin-1 and the Fas receptors. Zhang *et al.* [91] reported that caveolin-1 regulates hyperoxia/ROS-induced apoptosis through interactions with Fas and BID, probably *via* Fas palmitoylation and caveolin-1 Y14 phosphorylation, respectively. By this it mediates the communication between extrinsic and intrinsic pathways. Fas pathways require also caveolin-1 for interaction with hyperoxia-induced factors in epithelial lung cell death [92].

THE ROS AS APOPTOSIS FACTORS

ROS induce apoptosis in lung epithelial and lung cancer cells *via* the intrinsic pathway. Bleomycin consists of an oxygen activating domain and a DNA binding domain and induces DNA-breaks by oxygen activation [93]. The bleomycin-induced ROS production is based on intracellular iron-binding. The bleomycin-iron complex reduces molecular oxygen to superoxide (O_2^-) and hydroxy radical (OH*). Free radicals causing strand cleavage of DNA and lipid peroxidation [94]. Bleomycin can also utilize H_2O_2 to cleave DNA in the presence of ferric ions [49]. Free iron is able to participate in several deleterious oxidation reactions. The steps in iron-mediated free radical generation can be summarized as follows:

$$Fe^{2+} + O_2 \longleftrightarrow Fe^{3+} + O_2^-$$

$$Fe^{2+} + O_2^- + 2H+ \longleftrightarrow Fe^{3+} + H_2O_2$$

$$Fe^{2+} + H_2O_2 \longleftrightarrow Fe^{3+} + \bullet OH + - OH^-$$

The cellular store of iron is usually not free available and iron must be detached from iron binding proteins such as cytochromes, transferrin and ferritin. Also free radicals have the potential to release iron from proteins [95, 96].

Foreign compounds responsible for ROS-induced lung injury are different drugs such as paraquat, nitrofurantoin, and bleomycin, furthermore, cigarette smoke, diesel exhaust, ozone, nitrogen dioxide, silica, asbestos fibers and other particles from air pollutions. Excessive generation of ROS can induce direct cell injury *via* secretion of chemotactic factors, proteolytic enzymes, lipogenases, cyclooxygenases and activation of transcription factors (reviewed in [97]). The formation of ROS induces further an antioxidant cascade, which includes ROS scavenger enzymes such as gluthatione peroxidases and superoxide dismutases [98].

There is some but not overall evidence that bleomycin-induced apoptosis is mediated by the mitochondrial death pathway caused by the generation of iron-derived free radicals [99]. These authors tested the interaction between iron chelators and oxidative stress-mediated cytotoxicity of bleomycin and have shown that the ability to chelate iron as such is not the sole determinant to prevent bleomycin-induced apoptosis. Very recently, it was shown that Edavarone, a free radical scavenger known to inhibit the generation of both hydroxyl radicals and iron-induced peroxidative injuries, significantly attenuated both the apoptosis and TGF-β expression induced by bleomycin [100]. Furthermore, there is evidence that ROS regulate caspases of the extrinsic pathway. Bleomycin induces caspase-8 in MLE cells independently from death receptor induction [78]. The mechanism is still unclear.

Final evidence for the importance of ROS in regulation of bleomycin-induced apoptosis comes from experiments using mice deficient for the $p47^{phox}$ subunit of NADPH-oxidase [68]. The absence of ROS production in these animals protects against bleomycin-induced pulmonary fibrosis.

Functional studies substantiated that caveolin-1 is a sensitive target to oxidative stress. Caveolin-1 is subject of two types of post-translational modification, phosphorylation and palmitoylation that might be critical for regulating its intracellular activity and localization. Recent studies indicate that both phosphorylation [101] and palmitoylation of caveolin-1 can be regulated by ROS. Treatment of endothelial cells with ROS caused a release of caveolin-1 from membranes and also a decrease in the number of caveolae detected by electron microscopy [102]. After bleomycin treatment of normal R3/1 lung cells the caveolin-1 expression is decreased [103]. In contrast to untreated cells, caveolin-1 was remarkably excluded from the caveolae-enriched fractions in bleomycin treated cells. The data imply that caveolin-1 is not targeted to caveolae under these conditions.

ROS and caveolin-1 also play an essential role in lung cancer motility and tumor progression [104]. *In vitro* studies with lung cancer cells revealed that caveolin-1 attenuates hydrogen-peroxide induced oxidative damage [105] and anoikis resistance [106].

THE ANGIOTENSIN MECHANISM OF BLEOMYCIN-INDUCED APOPTOSIS

Angiotensin II induces apoptosis in human and rat alveolar epithelial cells [107] and is synthesized and released from alveolar epithelial cells undergoing apoptosis regardless of the initiating stimulus (*e.g.* FasL, bleomycin or TNF) in an autocrine fashion from the precursor angiotensinogen [108]. A prerequisite for this process is the binding of angiotensin II (Ang II) to the G-protein-coupled Ang II type 1 receptor (AT_1-R). AT_1-R blockers such as losartan and saralasin prevent alveolar epithelial apoptosis and fibrosis [109]. Furthermore, knockout mice deficient in the receptor AT_1 are resistant to bleomycin-induced lung fibrosis [110]. To explain the involvement of angiotensin II in apoptotic pathways we have to understand its function as potent activator of NAD(P)H oxidase (for review see [111]).

Although abundant evidence suggests that angiotensin II mediates apoptosis, little information is available towards the subsequent steps leading to the activation of the apoptotic cascade.

NAD(P)H oxidase activation by angiotensin II induces ROS in endothelial cells [111]. There is earlier experimental evidence that NAD(P)H oxidase-produced ROS are required for downstream activation of the transcription factors IRF and STAT in virus-infected airway epithelial cells [112] and that NAD(P)H derived ROS contribute to alveolar epithelial cell death [113]. Wyse *et al.* [114]

investigated the role of caveolin-1 in AT_1-R localization and trafficking in kidney cells. They found that the AT_1-R is not concentrated in caveolae. Further studies show that the inactive receptor is clustered in both cyclodextrin-resistant and cyclodextrin-sensitive microdomains. Activation of the AT_1-R results in an increased degree of clustering that is completely sensitive to cyclodextrin treatment. The interpretation of these results was that activation of AT_1-R is accompanied by a migration of the receptor in lipid rafts. A role for caveolin-1 in AT_1-R transport to the cell surface is also strongly supported by the observation that in cells lacking caveolin-1 and caveolin-3; AT_1-R remains in the endoplasmic reticulum unless caveolin-1 or caveolin-3 are ectopically expressed. Endogenous renal AT_1-R levels are lower in caveolin-1 null mice compared with wild type controls.

In vascular smooth muscle cells, it was shown that Ang II promotes association of AT_1-R with caveolin-1 and AT_1-R trafficking into caveolin-enriched /lipid rafts. Nothing is known about the function of caveolin-1 for AT_1-R localization in lung cells and the effects of bleomycin on AT_1-R [115].

INCREASED TELOMERASE ACTIVITY AND BLEOMYCIN-INDUCED APOPTOSIS

Early events during the induction of apoptosis are the modulation of telomere length and telomerase activity and telomere loss can also be a consequence of apoptosis [116]. There is evidence that bleomycin and other cytostatics are responsible for genomic instability of cells *via* damage of the telomere–telomerase system [117]. Fridlander *et al.* [118] found that bleomycin causes an initial increase and then a reduction in telomerase activity in lung epithelial cells *in vitro* and *in vivo* in lung epithelial cells isolated from bleomycin-treated mice. Stabilizing telomerase activity decreases epithelial cell apoptosis. From this the authors suggest that apoptosis may be the trigger for the induction of telomerase as a defense mechanism from bleomycin-induced apoptosis. Interestingly, recent data provide evidence that mutation in genes encoding telomerase are present in familial interstitial fibrosis [119].

Furthermore, telomerase reverse transcriptase (TERT) deficient mice showed attenuated lung fibrosis after treatment with bleomycin [120]. Moreover, isolated fibroblasts from bleomycin treated TERT-deficient animals showed a higher rate of apoptosis. The role of alveolar epithelial apoptosis was not investigated in this context.

MicroRNAs, CAVEOLIN-1 AND THE REGULATION OF BLEOMYCIN-INDUCED FIBROSIS

MicroRNAs (miRNAs) represent a class of small (20-23 nucleotides), non-coding RNAs that regulate protein levels post-transcriptionally *via* binding to the 3' UTR of target genes mRNAs and on this way impair their translation or induce their degradation. miRNAs play important regulatory roles in many cellular processes, including differentiation, neoplastic transformation, and cell replication and regeneration. In pulmonary fibrosis approximately 10% of the microRNAs are significantly changed. Downregulated miRNAs were found in processes related to epithelial mensenchymal transition (EMT), whereas upregulated miRNAs (for example miR-21 and miR-155) could be detected in bleomycin-induced fibrosis models (for review see [121, 122]). TGF-β1, a central pathological mediator of fibrotic diseases, enhanced miR-21 expression in primary pulmonary fibroblasts [123]. miR-29 is negatively regulated by TGF-β/Smad3 and has a therapeutic potential for pulmonary fibrosis [124]. miR-155 serum levels were used for monitoring the fibrotic disease in patients [125]. miRNA can be detected in all cell types of lung and may be also exported *via* microvesicles and exosomes to realize intercellular functions [126]. Very recently, it was shown that miR-199 activates pulmonary fibrosis by regulating caveolin-1 and by this the TGF-β signaling in lung fibroblasts [127]. It remains open, how miRNAs directly or indirectly decrease the caveolin-1 expression in epithelial AT1 cells, a hallmark of disease in different fibrosis models [23, 24, 127].

Further pulmonary miRNA profiling, particularly in alvolar epithelial cells, may contribute to the understanding of the complex transcriptional program of lung fibrosis and to provide potential therapeutic tools.

MECHANISMS OF BLEOMYCIN (STRESS)-INDUCED SENESCENCE IN EPITHELIAL LUNG AND LUNG CANCER CELLS

Caveolin-1 was found to play a greater role in epithelial cell senescence than regulating apoptosis in bleomycin-induced lung injury models [30]. Senescence, a kind of permanent growth arrest, is associated with characteristic morphologic alterations (flattening, swelling, increased granularity, increase in vacuoles), enzyme activities (SA-β-galactosidase), and changes in chromatin architecture (senescence associated heterochromatin foci), reviewed in [128]. Normal cells undergo replicative (intrinsic senescence, *e.g.* they finish proliferation after a finite number of cell divisions ("Hayflick limit" [129]). Responsible for this process is the shortening of telomeres- the repetitive sequence and specialized proteins that cap the ends of eukaryotic linear chromosomes (for review see [116]). Telomerase, a reverse transcriptase containing an RNA template, contributes to the maintenance of telomere structure. In contrast to normal cells, embryonic stem cells, immortalized cell lines and tumor cells have an indefinitive replicative capacity and display telomerase activity (reviewed in [130]). Increased telomerase activity has further been reported during fibrogenesis in the lung, during tissue regeneration and during wound healing in other organ systems [131, 132]. Replicative senescence is difficult to distinguish from a more general process, called cellular or stress-induced premature (extrinsic or acutely inducible [128]) senescence, whereby cells underwent growth arrest in response to genotoxic and non-genotoxic stresses [7]. Bleomycin-induced lung injury is a characteristic example for increased oxidative damage resulting in stress-induced senescence. Mechanisms that acutely lead to an irreversible cell-cycle arrest may include ROS and unresolved DNA damage or suboptimal culture conditions *in vitro* [133].

A probably telomere-independent form of senescence is represented by an epigenetic derepression of the INK4a/ARF locus (comprehensively reviewed in [130]). The INK4a/ARF locus (encoding $p16^{INK4a}$, ARF) can be activated by oncogenes leading to oncogene-induced senescence [130]. However, oncogenes are believed to trigger also the premature senescence program [128]. INK4a/ARF-related senescence as well as telomerase-coupled senescence have an impact on remodelling processes *via* accumulation of senescent cells in tissues due to impaired stem cell functions [130].

Since genomic instability is a driving force for the development of cancer, drug-inducible senescence may be of importance. Bleomycin induces G_2/M arrest in A549 lung cancer cells [3, 4] and in other tumor cell lines [134-136]. How does bleomycin interfere with the cell cycle? Microarray analysis of bleomycin-exposed lymphoblastoid cells led to the identification of aberrantly expressed genes which have been reported to be involved in cell cycle control and proliferation, for example CDKN1A (encoding p21), DNA repair genes, CCNB2 (encoding cyclin B2) and CCNA2 (encoding cyclin A2] [137]. Bleomycin exposure of normal fibroblasts induces $p16^{INK4a}$ [138]. Microarray analysis of bleomycin- treated mouse and human cells revealed a comprehensive list of genes that are involved in DNA repair, cell cycle regulation, oxidative stress response processes and apoptosis [139]. Other bleomycin data in terms of molecular changes directly relevant to pulmonary fibrosis including cell cycle pathways were examined in detail and summarized by Peng *et al.* [140].

THE INVOLVEMENT OF CAVEOLIN-1 IN BLEOMYCIN-INDUCED SENESCENCE

Caveolin-1 is acting not only as a critical regulator of pulmonary fibrosis [11], caveolin-1 plays a role in senescence-associated signal transduction [141-143], and in controlling cellular senescence (replicative and stress-induced premature senescence [7]). Caveolin-1 influences the process of cellular senescence in human diploid fibroblasts, for example by suppressing the activation of ERK1/2 upon EGF stimulation [142]. Previous studies have demonstrated that mouse embryonic fibroblasts transgenically overexpressing caveolin-1 show a senescent-like morphology and a reduced lifespan. Overexpression of caveolin-1 was sufficient to arrest the fibroblasts in the G_0/G_1 phase of the cell cycle through activation of the p53/p21-dependent pathway [144]. The importance of caveolin-1 in replicative senescence was also supported by data describing higher levels of caveolin-1 in older cells or in tissues of older animals and of aged humans (reviewed [7]).

First report of Volonte *et al.* [145] using subcytotoxic level of hydrogen peroxide has shown that caveolin-1 is mainly involved in stress-induced premature senescence. Signaling upstream of caveolin-1 include p38 MAPK, Sp1, NF-κB, phosphatidylcholine-specific phospholipase C and cyclooxygenase-2 [7]. Signaling downstream of caveolin-1 include p53/p21 pathway, epidermal growth factor receptor, focal adhesion kinase and small Rho GTPase pathways. Caveolin-1 regulates a large number of single steps in these pathways listed in detail in the review of Zou *et al.* [7].

To investigate the potential role of caveolin-1 in stress-induced premature senescence in pulmonary epithelial cells, we have studied its behaviour in A549 lung cancer cells after treatment with bleomycin before and after knockdown of caveolin-1 [4]. Bleomycin, when added to cycling cells, blocks both the G_1/S and G_2/M transitions [146]. p53 is stabilized in response to genotoxic stress and controls the upregulation of several genes implicated in both the G_1/S and G_2/M transitions [147]. Expression of p21 is transcriptionally regulated by p53 upon DNA damage or cellular senescence and it is known to induce cell cycle arrest both at G_1/S and G_2/M check-points [148, 149]. In this study, we demonstrated that bleomycin treated A549 cells exhibited increased caveolin-1 expresssion but also senescence-like cell morphology, senescence-associated increase in SA-β-galactosidase activity, cell cycle arrest and up-regulation of p53 and p21 [4]. Interestingly, senescence associated cell cycle arrest *via* p21 and SA-β-galactosidase activity was greatly prevented in A549 cells when short hairpin RNA specific for caveolin-1 was applied before bleomycin treatment. The caveolin-1 downregulation following bleomycin exposure influenced the bleomycin-induced growth arrest in the G_2/M phase and, in addition the p53 and p21 expresssion. The mechanism, how caveolin-1 influences the expression of p21 protein remains unclear. A possible association is the involvement of the STAT3 transcription factor, which recruits cyclin D1 to the p21 promoter (reviewed in [150]), and caveolin-1 inhibits cell proliferation by suppressing the activation of STAT3. Such down-stream effects have been described recently, where caveolin-1 silencing arrests the proliferation of metastatic lung cancer cells *via* inhibition of STAT3 [151].

Another important aspect of caveolin-1 expression concerns its tumor suppressor function (reviewed in [152]). The level of caveolin-1 expression is low in most (but not all) cancer cells [153]. Clinical studies showed that caveolin-1 levels were inversely correlated with metastatic potential in breast adenocarcinoma cells. Simultaneously, however, evidence for an oncogenic role of caveolin-1 also began to accumulate. Such evidence included the demonstration that caveolin-1 levels are increased in drug-resistant variants of human lung carcinoma, and other carcinoma cell lines cell lines (reviewed in [154]). In addition, lung adenocarcinoma cells selected for a highly invasive phenotype had elevated caveolin-1 levels [155]. There is evidence that certain genetic silencing mechanisms exist for caveolin-1 downregulation. For example, repression of the caveolin-1 promoter can be achieved by oncogenes myc and ras [156, 157]. In other cases, the observed induction of caveolin-1 expression during the development of a multidrug-resistant (MDR) phenotype in breast cancer cells [158] may represent one but not the only mechanism of tumor survival. The exact relationship between caveolin-1 and MDR or p-glycoprotein has not been established.

To gain a better understanding of the molecular basis of this phenomenon, caveolin-1-enriched microdomains of untreated and bleomycin-treated growth-arrested A549 cells were analyzed for differential protein expression using 2-D DIGE followed by LC-MS/MS. One of these differentially expressed proteins was found to be the multidrug resistance-associated protein (MGr1-Ag). We show that MGr1-Ag becomes partly localised in lipid rafts following bleomycin treatment, and that MGr1-Ag and caveolin-1 occur in a common protein complex *in vivo* using co-immunoprecipitation studies. GST pull-down assays demonstrated an increased interaction between MGr1-Ag and caveolin-1 following bleomycin treatment *in vitro*. Our results reveal MGr1-Ag as a novel lipid raft protein. Its increased association with caveolin-1 in bleomycin-induced cell cycle arrest and subsequent cellular senescence might contribute to the success of chemotherapy [159].

There is evidence that the caveolin-1-dependent cholesterol metabolism is somehow connected with the efflux of lipophilic chemotherapeutic drugs [153].

Noteworthy to mention that bleomycin is not lipophilic and therefore, not a substrate of p-glycoprotein [160].

Otherpotent tumor suppressor mechanisms might be apoptosis as well as senescence [161] (see above). Senescence and apoptosis prevent damaged cells from undergoing neoplastic transformation [162] and senescence can contribute to the success of chemotherapy [130].

A further aspect of caveolin-1 expression concerns its effects on lung cancer cell migration. Caveolin-1 knockdown inhibited cell proliferation and reduced focal adhesion kinase (Fak) phosphorylation in H1299 lung cancer cells [163]. Increased migratory properties of lung cancer cells were found to be connected with an increased caveolin-1 expression after long-term nitric oxide (NO) exposure. NO treatment enhanced cell motility *via* Fak- and ATP-dependent tyrokinase (Akt)-dependent mechanisms [164].

CAVEOLIN-1 DEFICIENCY PROTECTS FROM BLEOMYCIN-INDUCED PULMONARY FIBROSIS BY MODULATING EPITHELIAL CELL SENESCENCE

There were several reasons to investigate the phenotype of caveolin-1 knockout mice in the bleomycin-induced lung injury models: i: the current paradigm of a role of caveolin-1 in inhibiting profibrogenic signaling; ii: *in vitro* data about the involvement of caveolin-1 in epithelial senescence in the context of bleomycin-related stress-induced senescence [4], and iii: reports about the resistance of ATI cell-specific antigen-deficient mice against bleomycin (for example the RAGE knockout mice [165]).

From the involvement of caveolin-1 in the regulation of inflammation and fibrosis [30] we expected an increased fibrogenic effect of bleomycin in caveolin-1 knockout mice. Caveolin-1 knockout animals show a dramatical reduction in life span [166] but no signs of progression of pulmonary fibrosis which includes the presence of active myofibroblasts in the alveolar wall, occurrence of fibroblastic foci and honeycombing (own unpublished data). Concluding, the caveolin-1 knockout is not a fibrosis model.

Our results, moreover, indicated that caveolin-1 deficiency protects the animals from fibrotic injury caused by bleomycin and that this protection was related to reduced epithelial senescence and apoptosis during the early phase of lung injury [167]. Important to note that challenge of caveolin-1 knockout mice with endotoxin, showed a resistance to LPS-induced injury and the contribution of caveolin-1 to regulate immune functions in the non-epithelial compartment of the lung [168]. To understand the complex role of caveolin-1 during pulmonary fibrogenesis we have to expect probably different cell-specific effects of caveolin-1 in the lung which results in a separate interaction of caveolin-1 with inflammatory and epithelial pathways [17, 169]. Recent experiments using CSD subdomains instead of full-length CSD indicate the heterogeneity of caveolin-1 dependent signaling pathways in different cell types involved in the specific disease process [170].

SUMMARY

Immunohistochemical and biochemical analysis of lung tissues from experimental animals with pulmonary fibrosis and *in vitro* investigations have shown that bleomycin modulates the expression of caveolin-1 in alveolar epithelial and other lung cells. On one side the bleomycin-induced loss of caveolin-1 seems to initiate several signaling events leading to the fibrotic phenotype of lung cells. On the other side the bleomycin-induced increase of caveolin-1 in cancer cells *in vitro* seems to be connected with the modulation of the cell cycle and influencing by this way the proliferation, migration, apoptosis and senescence of cancer cells. Importantly, administration of cavcolin-1 scaffolding domain peptide or transgenic overexpression of caveolin-1 can reverse the effects of bleomycin-induced injury.

Therapeutic interference with different caveolin-1 functions may provide new tools for influencing bleomycin-induced effects in normal and lung cancer cells.

ACKNOWLEDGEMENTS

None declared.

CONFLICT OF INTEREST

The authors confirm that this chapter contents have no conflict of interest.

DISCLOSURE

The chapter submitted for the eBook Series entitled **"Advances in Cancer Drug Targets, Volume 2"** is an update of our article in **Current Cancer Drug Targets, Volume 9, Issue 3, 2009, pp. 341-353,** with additional text and references.

REFERENCES

[1] Le Jeune I, Gribbin J, West J, Smith C, Cullinan P, Hubbard R. The incidence of cancer in patients with idiopathic pulmonary fibrosis and sarcoidosis in the UK. Respir Med 2007 Dec; 101(12): 2534-40.

[2] Zheng YL, Loffredo CA, Yu Z, Jones RT, Krasna MJ, Alberg AJ, *et al.* Bleomycin-induced chromosome breaks as a risk marker for lung cancer: a case-control study with population and hospital controls. Carcinogenesis 2003 Feb; 24(2): 269-74.

[3] Aoshiba K, Tsuji T, Nagai A. Bleomycin induces cellular senescence in alveolar epithelial cells. Eur Respir J 2003 Sep; 22(3): 436-43.

[4] Linge A, Weinhold K, Blasche R, Kasper M, Barth K. Downregulation of caveolin-1 affects bleomycin-induced growth arrest and cellular senescence in A549 cells. Int J Biochem Cell Biol 2007; 39(10): 1964-74.

[5] Kuwano K, Kunitake R, Maeyama T, Hagimoto N, Kawasaki M, Matsuba T, *et al.* Attenuation of bleomycin-induced pneumopathy in mice by a caspase inhibitor. Am J Physiol Lung Cell Mol Physiol 2001 Feb; 280(2): L316-25.

[6] Aoshiba K, Tsuji T, Kameyama S, Itoh M, Semba S, Yamaguchi K, *et al.* Senescence-associated secretory phenotype in a mouse model of bleomycin-induced lung injury. Exp Toxicol Pathol 2013 Nov; 65(7-8): 1053-62.

[7] Zou H, Stoppani E, Volonte D, Galbiati F. Caveolin-1, cellular senescence and age-related diseases. Mech Ageing Dev 2011 Nov-Dec; 132(11-12): 533-42.

[8] Kasper M, Reimann T, Hempel U, Wenzel KW, Bierhaus A, Schuh D, *et al.* Loss of caveolin expression in type I pneumocytes as an indicator of subcellular alterations during lung fibrogenesis. Histochem Cell Biol 1998 Jan; 109(1): 41-8.

[9] Drab M, Verkade P, Elger M, Kasper M, Lohn M, Lauterbach B, *et al.* Loss of Caveolae, Vascular Dysfunction, and Pulmonary Defects in Caveolin-1 Gene-Disrupted Mice. Science 2001; 9: 9.

[10] Razani B, Engelman JA, Wang XB, Schubert W, Zhang XL, Marks CB, *et al.* Caveolin-1 null mice are viable but show evidence of hyperproliferative and vascular abnormalities. J Biol Chem 2001 Oct 12; 276(41): 38121-38.

[11] Wang XM, Zhang Y, Kim HP, Zhou Z, Feghali-Bostwick CA, Liu F, *et al.* Caveolin-1: a critical regulator of lung fibrosis in idiopathic pulmonary fibrosis. J Exp Med 2006 Dec 25; 203(13): 2895-906.

[12] Razani B, Schlegel A, Liu J, Lisanti MP. Caveolin-1, a putative tumour suppressor gene. Biochem Soc Trans 2001 Aug; 29(Pt 4): 494-9.

[13] Koleske AJ, Baltimore D, Lisanti MP. Reduction of caveolin and caveolae in oncogenically transformed cells. Proc Natl Acad Sci U S A 1995 Feb 28; 92(5): 1381-5.

[14] Parton RG, Simons K. The multiple faces of caveolae. Nat Rev Mol Cell Biol 2007 Mar; 8(3): 185-94.

[15] Tourkina E, Hoffman S. Caveolin-1 signaling in lung fibrosis. Open Rheumatol J 2012; 6: 116-22.

[16] Maniatis NA, Kardara M, Hecimovich D, Letsiou E, Castellon M, Roussos C, *et al.* Role of caveolin-1 expression in the pathogenesis of pulmonary edema in ventilator-induced lung injury. Pulm Circ 2012 Oct; 2(4): 452-60.

[17] Gvaramia D, Blaauboer ME, Hanemaaijer R, Everts V. Role of caveolin-1 in fibrotic diseases. Matrix Biol 2013 Aug 8; 32(6): 307-15.

[18] Scherer PE, Tang Z, Chun M, Sargiacomo M, Lodish HF, Lisanti MP. Caveolin isoforms differ in their N-terminal protein sequence and subcellular distribution. Identification and epitope mapping of an isoform-specific monoclonal antibody probe. J Biol Chem 1995 Jul 7; 270(27): 16395-401.

[19] Li S, Song KS, Lisanti MP. Expression and characterization of recombinant caveolin. Purification by polyhistidine tagging and cholesterol-dependent incorporation into defined lipid membranes. J Biol Chem 1996 Jan 5; 271(1): 568-73.

[20] Razani B, Wang XB, Engelman JA, Battista M, Lagaud G, Zhang XL, *et al.* Caveolin-2-deficient mice show evidence of severe pulmonary dysfunction without disruption of caveolae. Mol Cell Biol 2002 Apr; 22(7): 2329-44.

[21] Murata M, Peranen J, Schreiner R, Wieland F, Kurzchalia TV, Simons K. VIP21/caveolin is a cholesterol-binding protein. Proc Natl Acad Sci U S A 1995 Oct 24; 92(22): 10339-43.

[22] Simons K, Toomre D. Lipid rafts and signal transduction. Nat Rev Mol Cell Biol 2000 Oct; 1(1): 31-9.

[23] Gabazza EC, Kasper M, Ohta K, Keane M, D'Alessandro-Gabazza C, Fujimoto H, *et al.* Decreased expression of aquaporin-5 in bleomycin-induced lung fibrosis in the mouse. Pathol Int 2004 Oct; 54(10): 774-80.

[24] Wang XM, Zhang Y, Kim HP, Zhou Z, Feghali-Bostwick CA, Liu F, *et al.* Caveolin-1: a critical regulator of lung fibrosis in idiopathic pulmonary fibrosis. J Exp Med 2006 Dec 25; 203(13): 2895-906.

[25] Tourkina E, Richard M, Oates J, Hofbauer A, Bonner M, Gooz P, *et al.* Caveolin-1 regulates leucocyte behaviour in fibrotic lung disease. Ann Rheum Dis 2010 Jun; 69(6): 1220-6.

[26] Odajima N, Betsuyaku T, Nasuhara Y, Nishimura M. Loss of caveolin-1 in bronchiolization in lung fibrosis. J Histochem Cytochem 2007 Sep; 55(9): 899-909.

[27] Achcar RO, Demura Y, Rai PR, Taraseviciene-Stewart L, Kasper M, Voelkel NF, *et al.* Loss of caveolin and heme oxygenase expression in severe pulmonary hypertension. Chest 2006 Mar; 129(3): 696-705.

[28] Jasmin JF, Mercier I, Hnasko R, Cheung MW, Tanowitz HB, Dupuis J, *et al.* Lung remodeling and pulmonary hypertension after myocardial infarction: pathogenic role of reduced caveolin expression. Cardiovasc Res 2004 Sep 1; 63(4): 747-55.

[29] Tarasevicienc-Stewart L, Scerbavicius R, Choe KH, Cool C, Wood K, Tuder RM, *et al.* Simvastatin causes endothelial cell apoptosis and attenuates severe pulmonary hypertension. Am J Physiol Lung Cell Mol Physiol 2006 Oct; 291(4): L668-76.

[30] Jin Y, Lee SJ, Minshall RD, Choi AM. Caveolin-1: a critical regulator of lung injury. Am J Physiol Lung Cell Mol Physiol 2011 Feb; 300(2): L151-60.

[31] de Almeida CJ, Jasmin JF, Del Galdo F, Lisanti MP. Genetic ablation of caveolin-2 sensitizes mice to bleomycin-induced injury. Cell Cycle.2013 Jul 15; 12(14): 2248-54.

[32] Tourkina E, Richard M, Gooz P, Bonner M, Pannu J, Harley R, *et al.* Anti-fibrotic properties of caveolin-1 scaffolding domain *in vitro* and *in vivo*. Am J Physiol Lung Cell Mol Physiol 2008 Jan 18.

[33] Del Galdo F, Sotgia F, de Almeida CJ, Jasmin JF, Musick M, Lisanti MP, *et al.* Decreased expression of caveolin 1 in patients with systemic sclerosis: crucial role in the pathogenesis of tissue fibrosis. Arthritis Rheum 2008 Sep; 58(9): 2854-65.

[34] Bhandary YP, Shetty SK, Marudamuthu AS, Gyetko MR, Idell S, Gharaee-Kermani M, *et al.* Regulation of alveolar epithelial cell apoptosis and pulmonary fibrosis by coordinate expression of components of the fibrinolytic system. Am J Physiol Lung Cell Mol Physiol 2012 Mar 1; 302(5): L463-73.

[35] Shi Y, Gochuico BR, Yu G, Tang X, Osorio JC, Fernandez IE, *et al.* Syndecan-2 exerts antifibrotic effects by promoting caveolin-1-mediated transforming growth factor-beta receptor I internalization and inhibiting transforming growth factor-beta1 signaling. Am J Respir Crit Care Med 2013 Oct 1; 188(7): 831-41.

[36] Meng J, Zou Y, Hu C, Zhu Y, Peng Z, Hu G, *et al.* Fluorofenidone attenuates bleomycin-induced pulmonary inflammation and fibrosis in mice *via* restoring caveolin 1 expression and inhibiting mitogen-activated protein kinase signaling pathway. Shock 2012 Nov; 38(5): 567-73.

[37] Togami K, Kanehira Y, Tada H. Possible involvement of pirfenidone metabolites in the antifibrotic action of a therapy for idiopathic pulmonary fibrosis. Biol Pharm Bull 2013; 36(10): 1525-7.

[38] Zeng G, McCue HM, Mastrangelo L, Millis AJ. Endogenous TGF-beta activity is modified during cellular aging: effects on metalloproteinase and TIMP-1 expression. Exp Cell Res 1996 Nov 1; 228(2): 271-6.

[39] Ehata S, Hanyu A, Hayashi M, Aburatani H, Kato Y, Fujime M, *et al.* Transforming growth factor-beta promotes survival of mammary carcinoma cells through induction of antiapoptotic transcription factor DEC1. Cancer Res 2007 Oct 15; 67(20): 9694-703.

[40] Kang HR, Cho SJ, Lee CG, Homer RJ, Elias JA. Transforming growth factor (TGF)-beta1 stimulates pulmonary fibrosis and inflammation *via* a Bax-dependent, bid-activated pathway that involves matrix metalloproteinase-12. J Biol Chem 2007 Mar 9; 282(10): 7723-32.

[41] Jin Y, Kim HP, Cao J, Zhang M, Ifedigbo E, Choi AM. Caveolin-1 regulates the secretion and cytoprotection of Cyr61 in hyperoxic cell death. Faseb J 2009 Feb; 23(2): 341-50.

[42] Jin Y, Kim HP, Chi M, Ifedigbo E, Ryter SW, Choi AM. Deletion of caveolin-1 protects against oxidative lung injury *via* up-regulation of heme oxygenase-1. Am J Respir Cell Mol Biol 2008 Aug; 39(2): 171-9.

[43] Zhang M, Lin L, Lee SJ, Mo L, Cao J, Ifedigbo E, *et al.* Deletion of caveolin-1 protects hyperoxia-induced apoptosis *via* survivin-mediated pathways. Am J Physiol Lung Cell Mol Physiol 2009 Nov; 297(5): L945-53.

[44] Umezawa H. Bleomycin and other antitumor antibiotics of high molecular weight. Antimicrob Agents Chemother (Bethesda) 1965; 5: 1079-85.

[45] Sikic BI. Biochemical and cellular determinants of bleomycin cytotoxicity. Cancer Surv 1986; 5(1): 81-91.

[46] Galm U, Hager MH, Van Lanen SG, Ju J, Thorson JS, Shen B. Antitumor antibiotics: bleomycin, enediynes, and mitomycin. Chem Rev 2005 Feb; 105(2): 739-58.

[47] Froudarakis M, Hatzimichael E, Kyriazopoulou L, Lagos K, Pappas P, Tzakos AG, *et al.* Revisiting bleomycin from pathophysiology to safe clinical use. Crit Rev Oncol Hematol 2013 Jul; 87(1): 90-100.

[48] Chen J, Stubbe J. Bleomycins: towards better therapeutics. Nat Rev Cancer 2005 Feb; 5(2): 102-12.

[49] Kumar D, Hirao H, Shaik S, Kozlowski PM. Proton-shuffle mechanism of O-O activation for formation of a high-valent oxo-iron species of bleomycin. J Am Chem Soc 2006 Dec 20; 128(50): 16148-58.

[50] Xu ZD, Wang M, Xiao SL, Liu CL, Yang M. Synthesis, biological evaluation and DNA binding properties of novel bleomycin analogues. Bioorg Med Chem Lett 2003 Aug 4; 13(15): 2595-9.

[51] Regulus P, Duroux B, Bayle PA, Favier A, Cadet J, Ravanat JL. Oxidation of the sugar moiety of DNA by ionizing radiation or bleomycin could induce the formation of a cluster DNA lesion. Proc Natl Acad Sci U S A 2007 Aug 28; 104(35): 14032-7.

[52] Magliozzo RS, Peisach J, Ciriolo MR. Transfer RNA is cleaved by activated bleomycin. Mol Pharmacol 1989 Apr; 35(4): 428-32.

[53] Vorobjev PE, Smith JB, Pyshnaya IA, Levina AS, Zarytova VF, Wickstrom E. Site-specific cleavage of RNA and DNA by complementary DNA--bleomycin A5 conjugates. Bioconjug Chem 2003 Nov-Dec; 14(6): 1307-13.

[54] Ekimoto H, Takahashi K, Matsuda A, Takita T, Umezawa H. Lipid peroxidation by bleomycin-iron complexes *in vitro*. J Antibiot (Tokyo) 1985 Aug; 38(8): 1077-82.

[55] Pron G, Mahrour N, Orlowski S, Tounekti O, Poddevin B, Belehradek J, Jr., *et al.* Internalisation of the bleomycin molecules responsible for bleomycin toxicity: a receptor-mediated endocytosis mechanism. Biochem Pharmacol 1999 Jan 1; 57(1): 45-56.

[56] Olive PL, Banath JP. Detection of DNA double-strand breaks through the cell cycle after exposure to X-rays, bleomycin, etoposide and 125IdUrd. Int J Radiat Biol 1993 Oct; 64(4): 349-58.

[57] Sugiyama M, Kumagai T. Molecular and structural biology of bleomycin and its resistance determinants. J Biosci Bioeng 2002; 93(2): 105-16.

[58] Umezawa H, Takeuchi T, Hori S, Sawa T, Ishizuka M. Studies on the mechanism of antitumor effect of bleomycin of squamous cell carcinoma. J Antibiot (Tokyo) 1972 Jul; 25(7): 409-20.

[59] Akiyama S, Ikezaki K, Kuramochi H, Takahashi K, Kuwano M. Bleomycin-resistant cells contain increased bleomycin-hydrolase activities. Biochem Biophys Res Commun 1981 Jul 16; 101(1): 55-60.

[60] Schwartz DR, Homanics GE, Hoyt DG, Klein E, Abernethy J, Lazo JS. The neutral cysteine protease bleomycin hydrolase is essential for epidermal integrity and bleomycin resistance. Proc Natl Acad Sci U S A 1999 Apr 13; 96(8): 4680-5.

[61] Bromme D, Rossi AB, Smeekens SP, Anderson DC, Payan DG. Human bleomycin hydrolase: molecular cloning, sequencing, functional expression, and enzymatic characterization. Biochemistry 1996 May 28; 35(21): 6706-14.

[62] Jakubowski H. Metabolism of homocysteine thiolactone in human cell cultures. Possible mechanism for pathological consequences of elevated homocysteine levels. J Biol Chem 1997 Jan 17; 272(3): 1935-42.

[63] Haston CK, Wang M, Dejournett RE, Zhou X, Ni D, Gu X, *et al.* Bleomycin hydrolase and a genetic locus within the MHC affect risk for pulmonary fibrosis in mice. Hum Mol Genet 2002 Aug 1; 11(16): 1855-63.

[64] Genovese T, Cuzzocrea S, Di Paola R, Failla M, Mazzon E, Sortino MA, *et al.* Inhibition or knock out of inducible nitric oxide synthase result in resistance to bleomycin-induced lung injury. Respir Res 2005; 6: 58.

[65] Chua F, Dunsmore SE, Clingen PH, Mutsaers SE, Shapiro SD, Segal AW, *et al.* Mice lacking neutrophil elastase are resistant to bleomycin-induced pulmonary fibrosis. Am J Pathol 2007 Jan; 170(1): 65-74.

[66] He M, Kubo H, Ishizawa K, Hegab AE, Yamamoto Y, Yamamoto H, *et al.* The role of the receptor for advanced glycation end-products in lung fibrosis. Am J Physiol Lung Cell Mol Physiol 2007 Dec; 293(6): L1427-36.

[67] Cho HY, Reddy SP, Yamamoto M, Kleeberger SR. The transcription factor NRF2 protects against pulmonary fibrosis. Faseb J 2004 Aug; 18(11): 1258-60.

[68] Manoury B, Nenan S, Leclerc O, Guenon I, Boichot E, Planquois JM, *et al.* The absence of reactive oxygen species production protects mice against bleomycin-induced pulmonary fibrosis. Respir Res 2005; 6: 11.

[69] Gao JM, Lu B, Guo ZJ. CXC chemokine receptor 3 modulates bleomycin-induced pulmonary injury *via* involving inflammatory process. Chin Med Sci J 2006 Sep; 21(3): 152-6.

[70] Chao DL, Maley CC, Wu X, Farrow DC, Galipeau PC, Sanchez CA, *et al.* Mutagen sensitivity and neoplastic progression in patients with Barrett's esophagus: a prospective analysis. Cancer Epidemiol Biomarkers Prev 2006 Oct; 15(10): 1935-40.

[71] Mei W, Zunzhen Z, Wangjun C. Suppression of a DNA base excision repair gene, hOGG1, increases bleomycin sensitivity of human lung cancer cell line. Toxicol Appl Pharmacol 2007 Dec 27.

[72] Nakamura M, Masutomi K, Kyo S, Hashimoto M, Maida Y, Kanaya T, *et al.* Efficient inhibition of human telomerase reverse transcriptase expression by RNA interference sensitizes cancer cells to ionizing radiation and chemotherapy. Hum Gene Ther 2005 Jul; 16(7): 859-68.

[73] Wu X, Kemp B, Amos CI, Honn SE, Zhang W, Walsh GL, *et al.* Associations among telomerase activity, p53 protein overexpression, and genetic instability in lung cancer. Br J Cancer 1999 May; 80(3-4): 453-7.

[74] Lucattelli M, Fineschi S, Geppetti P, Gerard NP, Lungarella G. Neurokinin-1 receptor blockade and murine lung tumorigenesis. Am J Respir Crit Care Med 2006 Sep 15; 174(6): 674-83.

[75] Bachofen M, Weibel ER. Structural alterations of lung parenchyma in the adult respiratory distress syndrome. Clin Chest Med 1982 Jan; 3(1): 35-56.

[76] Brown RF, White DE. Ultrastructure of rat lung following inhalation of ricin aerosol. Int J Exp Pathol 1997 Aug; 78(4): 267-76.

[77] Schittny JC, Djonov V, Fine A, Burri PH. Programmed cell death contributes to postnatal lung development. Am J Respir Cell Mol Biol 1998 Jun; 18(6): 786-93.

[78] Wallach-Dayan SB, Izbicki G, Cohen PY, Gerstl-Golan R, Fine A, Breuer R. Bleomycin initiates apoptosis of lung epithelial cells by ROS but not by Fas/FasL pathway. Am J Physiol Lung Cell Mol Physiol 2006 Apr; 290(4): L790-L6.

[79] Wang WS, Chen PM, Wang HS, Liang WY, Su Y. Matrix metalloproteinase-7 increases resistance to Fas-mediated apoptosis and is a poor prognostic factor of patients with colorectal carcinoma. Carcinogenesis 2006 May; 27(5): 1113-20.

[80] Matsuno H, Yudoh K, Watanabe Y, Nakazawa F, Aono H, Kimura T. Stromelysin-1 (MMP-3) in synovial fluid of patients with rheumatoid arthritis has potential to cleave membrane bound Fas ligand. J Rheumatol 2001 Jan; 28(1): 22-8.

[81] Martin TR, Hagimoto N, Nakamura M, Matute-Bello G. Apoptosis and epithelial injury in the lungs. Proc Am Thorac Soc 2005; 2(3): 214-20.

[82] Hagimoto N, Kuwano K, Nomoto Y, Kunitake R, Hara N. Apoptosis and expression of Fas/Fas ligand mRNA in bleomycin-induced pulmonary fibrosis in mice. Am J Respir Cell Mol Biol 1997 Jan; 16(1): 91-101.

[83] Kuwano K, Hagimoto N, Kawasaki M, Yatomi T, Nakamura N, Nagata S, *et al.* Essential roles of the Fas-Fas ligand pathway in the development of pulmonary fibrosis. J Clin Invest 1999 Jul; 104(1): 13-9.

[84] Matute-Bello G, Liles WC, Steinberg KP, Kiener PA, Mongovin S, Chi EY, *et al.* Soluble Fas ligand induces epithelial cell apoptosis in humans with acute lung injury (ARDS). J Immunol 1999 Aug 15; 163(4): 2217-25.

[85] Albertine KH, Soulier MF, Wang Z, Ishizaka A, Hashimoto S, Zimmerman GA, *et al.* Fas and fas ligand are up-regulated in pulmonary edema fluid and lung tissue of patients with acute lung injury and the acute respiratory distress syndrome. Am J Pathol 2002 Nov; 161(5): 1783-96.

[86] Golan-Gerstl R, Wallach-Dayan SB, Amir G, Breuer R. Epithelial cell apoptosis by fas ligand-positive myofibroblasts in lung fibrosis. Am J Respir Cell Mol Biol 2007 Mar; 36(3): 270-5.

[87] Aoshiba K, Yasui S, Tamaoki J, Nagai A. The Fas/Fas-ligand system is not required for bleomycin-induced pulmonary fibrosis in mice. Am J Respir Crit Care Med 2000 Aug; 162(2 Pt 1): 695-700.

[88] Liu P, Anderson RG. Compartmentalized production of ceramide at the cell surface. J Biol Chem 1995 Nov 10; 270(45): 27179-85.

[89] Fanzo JC, Lynch MP, Phee H, Hyer M, Cremesti A, Grassme H, *et al.* CD95 rapidly clusters in cells of diverse origins. Cancer Biol Ther 2003 Jul-Aug; 2(4): 392-5.

[90] Schenck M, Carpinteiro A, Grassme H, Lang F, Gulbins E. Ceramide: physiological and pathophysiological aspects. Arch Biochem Biophys 2007 Jun 15; 462(2): 171-5.

[91] Zhang M, Lee SJ, An C, Xu JF, Joshi B, Nabi IR, *et al.* Caveolin-1 mediates Fas-BID signaling in hyperoxia-induced apoptosis. Free Radic Biol Med 2011 May 15; 50(10): 1252-62.

[92] Tanaka A, Jin Y, Lee SJ, Zhang M, Kim HP, Stolz DB, *et al.* Hyperoxia-induced LC3B interacts with the Fas apoptotic pathway in epithelial cell death. Am J Respir Cell Mol Biol 2012 Apr; 46(4): 507-14.

[93] Umezawa K, Otsuka M. [Molecular design of apoptosis inducing agents derived from bleomycin]. Gan To Kagaku Ryoho 1997 Feb; 24(4): 412-7.

[94] Droge W, Schipper HM. Oxidative stress and aberrant signaling in aging and cognitive decline. Aging Cell 2007 Jun; 6(3): 361-70.

[95] Bannister JV, Bannister WH, Hill HA, Thornalley PJ. Enhanced production of hydroxyl radicals by the xanthine-xanthine oxidase reaction in the presence of lactoferrin. Biochim Biophys Acta 1982 Mar 15; 715(1): 116-20.

[96] Motohashi N, Mori I. Superoxide-dependent formation of hydroxyl radical catalyzed by transferrin. FEBS Lett 1983 Jun 27; 157(1): 197-9.

[97] Vallyathan V, Shi X. The role of oxygen free radicals in occupational and environmental lung diseases. Environ Health Perspect 1997 Feb; 105 Suppl 1: 165-77.

[98] Quinlan TR, Marsh JP, Janssen YM, Borm PA, Mossman BT. Oxygen radicals and asbestos-mediated disease. Environ Health Perspect 1994 Dec; 102 Suppl 10: 107-10.

[99] Kaiserova H, den Hartog GJ, Simunek T, Schroterova L, Kvasnickova E, Bast A. Iron is not involved in oxidative stress-mediated cytotoxicity of doxorubicin and bleomycin. Br J Pharmacol 2006 Dec; 149(7): 920-30.

[100] Asai T, Ohno Y, Minatoguchi S, Funaguchi N, Yuhgetsu H, Sawada M, *et al.* The specific free radical scavenger edaravone suppresses bleomycin-induced acute pulmonary injury in rabbits. Clin Exp Pharmacol Physiol 2007 Jan-Feb; 34(1-2): 22-6.

[101] Vepa S, Scribner WM, Natarajan V. Activation of protein phosphorylation by oxidants in vascular endothelial cells: identification of tyrosine phosphorylation of caveolin. Free Radic Biol Med 1997; 22(1-2): 25-35.

[102] Peterson TE, Poppa V, Ueba H, Wu A, Yan C, Berk BC. Opposing effects of reactive oxygen species and cholesterol on endothelial nitric oxide synthase and endothelial cell caveolae. Circ Res 1999 Jul 9; 85(1): 29-37.

[103] Barth K, Gentsch M, Blasche R, Pfuller A, Parshyna I, Koslowski R, *et al.* Distribution of caveolin-1 and connexin43 in normal and injured alveolar epithelial R3/1 cells. Histochem Cell Biol 2005 Mar; 123(3): 239-47.

[104] Luanpitpong S, Talbott SJ, Rojanasakul Y, Nimmannit U, Pongrakhananon V, Wang L, *et al.* Regulation of lung cancer cell migration and invasion by reactive oxygen species and caveolin-1. J Biol Chem.2010 Dec 10; 285(50): 38832-40.

[105] Suchaoin W, Chanvorachote P. Caveolin-1 attenuates hydrogen peroxide-induced oxidative damage to lung carcinoma cells. Anticancer Res 2012 Feb; 32(2): 483-90.

[106] Songserm T, Pongrakhananon V, Chanvorachote P. Sub-toxic cisplatin mediates anoikis resistance through hydrogen peroxide-induced caveolin-1 up-regulation in non-small cell lung cancer cells. Anticancer Res 2012 May; 32(5): 1659-69.

[107] Wang R, Zagariya A, Ibarra-Sunga O, Gidea C, Ang E, Deshmukh S, *et al.* Angiotensin II induces apoptosis in human and rat alveolar epithelial cells. Am J Physiol 1999 May; 276(5 Pt 1): L885-9.

[108] Uhal BD. Epithelial apoptosis in the initiation of lung fibrosis. Eur Respir J Suppl 2003 Sep; 44: 7s-9s.

[109] Li X, Zhang H, Soledad-Conrad V, Zhuang J, Uhal BD. Bleomycin-induced apoptosis of alveolar epithelial cells requires angiotensin synthesis *de novo*. Am J Physiol Lung Cell Mol Physiol 2003 Mar; 284(3): L501-7.

[110] Li X, Rayford H, Uhal BD. Essential roles for angiotensin receptor AT1a in bleomycin-induced apoptosis and lung fibrosis in mice. Am J Pathol 2003 Dec; 163(6): 2523-30.

[111] Hitomi H, Kiyomoto H, Nishiyama A. Angiotensin II and oxidative stress. Curr Opin Cardiol 2007 Jul; 22(4): 311-5.

[112] Liu T, Castro S, Brasier AR, Jamaluddin M, Garofalo RP, Casola A. Reactive oxygen species mediate virus-induced STAT activation: role of tyrosine phosphatases. J Biol Chem 2004 Jan 23; 279(4): 2461-9.

[113] Pantano C, Anathy V, Ranjan P, Heintz NH, Janssen-Heininger YM. Nonphagocytic oxidase 1 causes death in lung epithelial cells *via* a TNF-RI-JNK signaling axis. Am J Respir Cell Mol Biol 2007 Apr; 36(4): 473-9.

[114] Wyse BD, Prior IA, Qian H, Morrow IC, Nixon S, Muncke C, *et al.* Caveolin interacts with the angiotensin II type 1 receptor during exocytic transport but not at the plasma membrane. J Biol Chem 2003 Jun 27; 278(26): 23738-46.

[115] Ushio-Fukai M, Alexander RW. Caveolin-dependent angiotensin II type 1 receptor signaling in vascular smooth muscle. Hypertension 2006 Nov; 48(5): 797-803.

[116] Mondello C, Scovassi AI. Telomeres, telomerase, and apoptosis. Biochem Cell Biol 2004 Aug; 82(4): 498-507.

[117] Rubio MA, Davalos AR, Campisi J. Telomere length mediates the effects of telomerase on the cellular response to genotoxic stress. Exp Cell Res 2004 Aug 1; 298(1): 17-27.

[118] Fridlender ZG, Cohen PY, Golan O, Wallach-Dayan S, Breuer R. Telomerase activity in bleomycin-induced epithelial cell apoptosis and lung fibrosis. Eur Respir J 2007 May 15.

[119] Armanios MY, Chen JJ, Cogan JD, Alder JK, Ingersoll RG, Markin C, *et al.* Telomerase mutations in families with idiopathic pulmonary fibrosis. N Engl J Med 2007 Mar 29; 356(13): 1317-26.

[120] Liu T, Chung MJ, Ullenbruch M, Yu H, Jin H, Hu B, *et al.* Telomerase activity is required for bleomycin-induced pulmonary fibrosis in mice. J Clin Invest 2007 Dec; 117(12): 3800-9.

[121] Pandit KV, Milosevic J, Kaminski N. MicroRNAs in idiopathic pulmonary fibrosis. Transl Res 2011 Apr; 157(4): 191-9.

[122] Vettori S, Gay S, Distler O. Role of MicroRNAs in Fibrosis. Open Rheumatol J 2012; 6: 130-9.

[123] Liu G, Friggeri A, Yang Y, Milosevic J, Ding Q, Thannickal VJ, *et al.* miR-21 mediates fibrogenic activation of pulmonary fibroblasts and lung fibrosis. J Exp Med 2010 Aug 2; 207(8): 1589-97.

[124] Xiao J, Meng XM, Huang XR, Chung AC, Feng YL, Hui DS, *et al.* miR-29 inhibits bleomycin-induced pulmonary fibrosis in mice. Mol Ther 2012 Jun; 20(6): 1251-60.

[125] Li P, Zhao GQ, Chen TF, Chang JX, Wang HQ, Chen SS, *et al.* Serum miR-21 and miR-155 expression in idiopathic pulmonary fibrosis. J Asthma 2013 Nov; 50(9): 960-4.

[126] Etheridge A, Gomes CP, Pereira RW, Galas D, Wang K. The complexity, function and applications of RNA in circulation. Front Genet 2013; 4: 115.

[127] Lino Cardenas CL, Henaoui IS, Courcot E, Roderburg C, Cauffiez C, Aubert S, *et al.* miR-199a-5p Is upregulated during fibrogenic response to tissue injury and mediates TGFbeta-induced lung fibroblast activation by targeting caveolin-1. PLoS Genet 2013; 9(2): e1003291.

[128] Schmitt CA. Cellular senescence and cancer treatment. Biochim Biophys Acta 2007 Jan; 1775(1): 5-20.

[129] Hayflick L, Moorhead PS. The serial cultivation of human diploid cell strains. Exp Cell Res 1961 Dec; 25: 585-621.

[130] Collado M, Blasco MA, Serrano M. Cellular senescence in cancer and aging. Cell 2007 Jul 27; 130(2): 223-33.

[131] Gonzalez-Suarez E, Samper E, Ramirez A, Flores JM, Martin-Caballero J, Jorcano JL, *et al.* Increased epidermal tumors and increased skin wound healing in transgenic mice overexpressing the catalytic subunit of telomerase, mTERT, in basal keratinocytes. Embo J 2001 Jun 1; 20(11): 2619-30.

[132] Wege H, Muller A, Muller L, Petri S, Petersen J, Hillert C. Regeneration in pig livers by compensatory hyperplasia induces high levels of telomerase activity. Comp Hepatol 2007; 6: 6.

[133] Balin AK, Fisher AJ, Anzelone M, Leong I, Allen RG. Effects of establishing cell cultures and cell culture conditions on the proliferative life span of human fibroblasts isolated from different tissues and donors of different ages. Exp Cell Res 2002 Apr 1; 274(2): 275-87.

[134] Holgersson A, Heiden T, Castro J, Edgren MR, Lewensohn R, Meijer AE. Different G2/M accumulation in M059J and M059K cells after exposure to DNA double-strand break-inducing agents. Int J Radiat Oncol Biol Phys 2005 Mar 1; 61(3): 915-21.

[135] Taron M, Plasencia C, Abad A, Martin C, Guillot M. Cytotoxic effects of topotecan combined with various active G2/M-phase anticancer drugs in human tumor-derived cell lines. Invest New Drugs 2000 May; 18(2): 139-47.

[136] Sullivan GF, Garcia-Welch A, White E, Lutzker S, Hait WN. Augmentation of apoptosis by the combination of bleomycin with trifluoperazine in the presence of mutant p53. J Exp Ther Oncol 2002 Jan-Feb; 2(1): 19-26.

[137] Cloos J, de Boer WP, Snel MH, van den Ijssel P, Ylstra B, Leemans CR, *et al.* Microarray analysis of bleomycin-exposed lymphoblastoid cells for identifying cancer susceptibility genes. Mol Cancer Res 2006 Feb; 4(2): 71-7.

[138] Robles SJ, Adami GR. Agents that cause DNA double strand breaks lead to p16INK4a enrichment and the premature senescence of normal fibroblasts. Oncogene 1998 Mar 5; 16(9): 1113-23.

[139] Islaih M, Li B, Kadura IA, Reid-Hubbard JL, Deahl JT, Altizer JL, *et al.* Comparison of gene expression changes induced in mouse and human cells treated with direct-acting mutagens. Environ Mol Mutagen 2004; 44(5): 401-19.

[140] Peng R, Sridhar S, Tyagi G, Phillips JE, Garrido R, Harris P, *et al.* Bleomycin induces molecular changes directly relevant to idiopathic pulmonary fibrosis: a model for "active" disease. PLoS One 2013; 8(4): e59348.

[141] Dai SM, Shan ZZ, Nakamura H, Masuko-Hongo K, Kato T, Nishioka K, *et al.* Catabolic stress induces features of chondrocyte senescence through overexpression of caveolin 1: possible involvement of caveolin 1-induced down-regulation of articular chondrocytes in the pathogenesis of osteoarthritis. Arthritis Rheum 2006 Mar; 54(3): 818-31.

[142] Park WY, Park JS, Cho KA, Kim DI, Ko YG, Seo JS, *et al.* Up-regulation of caveolin attenuates epidermal growth factor signaling in senescent cells. J Biol Chem 2000 Jul 7; 275(27): 20847-52.

[143] Cho KA, Ryu SJ, Oh YS, Park JH, Lee JW, Kim HP, *et al.* Morphological adjustment of senescent cells by modulating caveolin-1 status. J Biol Chem 2004 Oct 1; 279(40): 42270-8.

[144] Volonte D, Zhang K, Lisanti MP, Galbiati F. Expression of caveolin-1 induces premature cellular senescence in primary cultures of murine fibroblasts. Mol Biol Cell 2002 Jul; 13(7): 2502-17.

[145] Volonte D, Zhang K, Lisanti MP, Galbiati F. Expression of caveolin-1 induces premature cellular senescence in primary cultures of murine fibroblasts. Mol Biol Cell 2002 Jul; 13(7): 2502-17.

[146] Kaufmann WK, Kies PE. DNA signals for G2 checkpoint response in diploid human fibroblasts. Mutat Res 1998 May 25; 400(1-2): 153-67.

[147] Taylor WR, Stark GR. Regulation of the G2/M transition by p53. Oncogene 2001 Apr 5; 20(15): 1803-15.

[148] Sherr CJ, Roberts JM. Inhibitors of mammalian G1 cyclin-dependent kinases. Genes Dev 1995 May 15; 9(10): 1149-63.

[149] Barboule N, Lafon C, Chadebech P, Vidal S, Valette A. Involvement of p21 in the PKC-induced regulation of the G2/M cell cycle transition. FEBS Lett 1999 Feb 5; 444(1): 32-7.

[150] Mathew R, Huang J, Shah M, Patel K, Gewitz M, Sehgal PB. Disruption of endothelial-cell caveolin-1alpha/raft scaffolding during development of monocrotaline-induced pulmonary hypertension. Circulation 2004 Sep 14; 110(11): 1499-506.

[151] Pancotti F, Roncuzzi L, Maggiolini M, Gasperi-Campani A. Caveolin-1 silencing arrests the proliferation of metastatic lung cancer cells through the inhibition of STAT3 signaling. Cell Signal 2012 Jul; 24(7): 1390-7.

[152] Burgermeister E, Xing X, Rocken C, Juhasz M, Chen J, Hiber M, *et al.* Differential expression and function of caveolin-1 in human gastric cancer progression. Cancer Res 2007 Sep 15; 67(18): 8519-26.

[153] Nakatani K, Wada T, Nakamura M, Uzawa K, Tanzawa H, Fujita S. Expression of caveolin-1 and its correlation with cisplatin sensitivity in oral squamous cell carcinoma. J Cancer Res Clin Oncol 2005 Jul; 131(7): 445-52.

[154] Lloyd PG, Hardin CD. Caveolae in cancer: two sides of the same coin? Focus on "Hydrogen peroxide inhibits non-small cell lung cancer cell anoikis through the inhibition of caveolin-1 degradation". Am J Physiol Cell Physiol. [Comment Editorial] 2011 Feb; 300(2): C232-4.

[155] Ho CC, Huang PH, Huang HY, Chen YH, Yang PC, Hsu SM. Up-regulated caveolin-1 accentuates the metastasis capability of lung adenocarcinoma by inducing filopodia formation. Am J Pathol. [Comparative Study Research Support, Non-U.S. Gov't] 2002 Nov; 161(5): 1647-56.

[156] Park DS, Razani B, Lasorella A, Schreiber-Agus N, Pestell RG, Iavarone A, *et al.* Evidence that Myc isoforms transcriptionally repress caveolin-1 gene expression *via* an INR-dependent mechanism. Biochemistry 2001 Mar 20; 40(11): 3354-62.

[157] Engelman JA, Zhang XL, Razani B, Pestell RG, Lisanti MP. p42/44 MAP kinase-dependent and -independent signaling pathways regulate caveolin-1 gene expression. Activation of Ras-MAP kinase and protein kinase a signaling cascades transcriptionally down-regulates caveolin-1 promoter activity. J Biol Chem 1999 Nov 5; 274(45): 32333-41.

[158] Lavie Y, Fiucci G, Liscovitch M. Upregulation of caveolin in multidrug resistant cancer cells: functional implications. Adv Drug Deliv Rev 2001 Jul 28; 49(3): 317-23.

[159] Linge A, Meleady P, Henry M, Clynes M, Kasper M, Barth K. Bleomycin treatment of A549 human lung cancer cells results in association of MGr1-Ag and caveolin-1 in lipid rafts. Int J Biochem Cell Biol 2011 Jan; 43(1): 98-105.

[160] Chen G, Jaffrezou JP, Fleming WH, Duran GE, Sikic BI. Prevalence of multidrug resistance related to activation of the mdr1 gene in human sarcoma mutants derived by single-step doxorubicin selection. Cancer Res 1994 Sep 15; 54(18): 4980-7.

[161] Bandyopadhyay D, Gatza C, Donehower LA, Medrano EE. Analysis of Cellular Senescence in Culture *In Vivo*: The Senescence-Associated beta-Galactosidase Assay. Curr Protoc Cell Biol 2005 Jul; Chapter 18: Unit18 9.

[162] Rodier F, Campisi J, Bhaumik D. Two faces of p53: aging and tumor suppression. Nucleic Acids Res 2007; 35(22): 7475-84.

[163] Shatz M, Lustig G, Reich R, Liscovitch M. Caveolin-1 mutants P132L and Y14F are dominant negative regulators of invasion, migration and aggregation in H1299 lung cancer cells. Exp Cell Res 2010 Jun 10; 316(10): 1748-62.

[164] Sanuphan A, Chunhacha P, Pongrakhananon V, Chanvorachote P. Long-term nitric oxide exposure enhances lung cancer cell migration. Biomed Res Int 2013; 2013: 186972.

[165] Englert JM, Kliment CR, Ramsgaard L, Milutinovic PS, Crum L, Tobolewski JM, *et al.* Paradoxical function for the receptor for advanced glycation end products in mouse models of pulmonary fibrosis. Int J Clin Exp Pathol 2011 Mar; 4(3): 241-54.

[166] Park DS, Cohen AW, Frank PG, Razani B, Lee H, Williams TM, *et al.* Caveolin-1 null (-/-) mice show dramatic reductions in life span. Biochemistry. [Research Support, Non-U.S. Gov't Research Support, U.S. Gov't, P.H.S.] 2003 Dec 30; 42(51): 15124-31.

[167] Shivshankar P, Brampton C, Miyasato S, Kasper M, Thannickal VJ, Le Saux CJ. Caveolin-1 deficiency protects from pulmonary fibrosis by modulating epithelial cell senescence in mice. Am J Respir Cell Mol Biol.2012 Jul; 47(1): 28-36.

[168] Garrean S, Gao XP, Brovkovych V, Shimizu J, Zhao YY, Vogel SM, *et al.* Caveolin-1 regulates NF-kappaB activation and lung inflammatory response to sepsis induced by lipopolysaccharide. J Immunol 2006 Oct 1; 177(7): 4853-60.

[169] King TE, Jr., Pardo A, Selman M. Idiopathic pulmonary fibrosis. Lancet. [Review] 2011 Dec 3; 378(9807): 1949-61.

[170] Reese C, Dyer S, Perry B, Bonner M, Oates J, Hofbauer A, *et al.* Differential regulation of cell functions by CSD peptide subdomains. Respir Res 2013; 14(1): 90.

[171] Ortiz LA, Moroz K, Liu JY, Hoyle GW, Hammond T, Hamilton RF, *et al.* Alveolar macrophage apoptosis and TNF-alpha, but not p53, expression correlate with murine response to bleomycin. Am J Physiol 1998 Dec; 275(6 Pt 1): L1208-18.

[172] Wang R, Ibarra-Sunga O, Verlinski L, Pick R, Uhal BD. Abrogation of bleomycin-induced epithelial apoptosis and lung fibrosis by captopril or by a caspase inhibitor. Am J Physiol Lung Cell Mol Physiol 2000 Jul; 279(1): L143-51.

[173] Nici L, Calabresi P. Amifostine modulation of bleomycin-induced lung injury in rodents. Semin Oncol 1999 Apr; 26(2 Suppl 7): 28-33.

[174] Davis DW, Weidner DA, Holian A, McConkey DJ. Nitric oxide-dependent activation of p53 suppresses bleomycin-induced apoptosis in the lung. J Exp Med 2000 Sep 18; 192(6): 857-69.

[175] Kuwano K, Hagimoto N, Tanaka T, Kawasaki M, Kunitake R, Miyazaki H, *et al.* Expression of apoptosis-regulatory genes in epithelial cells in pulmonary fibrosis in mice. J Pathol 2000 Feb; 190(2): 221-9.

[176] Hong JS, Ko HH, Han ES, Lee CS. Inhibition of bleomycin-induced cell death in rat alveolar macrophages and human lung epithelial cells by ambroxol. Biochem Pharmacol 2003 Oct 1; 66(7): 1297-306.

[177] Zhao HW, Hu SY, Barger MW, Ma JK, Castranova V, Ma JY. Time-dependent apoptosis of alveolar macrophages from rats exposed to bleomycin: involvement of tnf receptor 2. J Toxicol Environ Health A 2004 Sep 10; 67(17): 1391-406.

[178] Inoshima I, Kuwano K, Hamada N, Hagimoto N, Yoshimi M, Maeyama T, *et al.* Anti-monocyte chemoattractant protein-1 gene therapy attenuates pulmonary fibrosis in mice. Am J Physiol Lung Cell Mol Physiol 2004 May; 286(5): L1038-44.

[179] Li X, Rayford H, Shu R, Zhuang J, Uhal BD. Essential role for cathepsin D in bleomycin-induced apoptosis of alveolar epithelial cells. Am J Physiol Lung Cell Mol Physiol 2004 Jul; 287(1): L46-51.

[180] Day RM, Yang Y, Suzuki YJ, Stevens J, Pathi R, Perlmutter A, *et al.* Bleomycin upregulates gene expression of angiotensin-converting enzyme *via* mitogen-activated protein kinase and early growth response 1 transcription factor. Am J Respir Cell Mol Biol 2001 Nov; 25(5): 613-9.

[181] Burdick MD, Murray LA, Keane MP, Xue YY, Zisman DA, Belperio JA, *et al.* CXCL11 attenuates bleomycin-induced pulmonary fibrosis *via* inhibition of vascular remodeling. Am J Respir Crit Care Med 2005 Feb 1; 171(3): 261-8.

[182] Mizuno S, Matsumoto K, Li MY, Nakamura T. HGF reduces advancing lung fibrosis in mice: a potential role for MMP-dependent myofibroblast apoptosis. Faseb J 2005 Apr; 19(6): 580-2.

[183] Avivi-Green C, Singal M, Vogel WF. Discoidin domain receptor 1-deficient mice are resistant to bleomycin-induced lung fibrosis. Am J Respir Crit Care Med 2006 Aug 15; 174(4): 420-7.

[184] Young LR, Pasula R, Gulleman PM, Deutsch GH, McCormack FX. Susceptibility of Hermansky-Pudlak mice to bleomycin-induced type II cell apoptosis and fibrosis. Am J Respir Cell Mol Biol 2007 Jul; 37(1): 67-74.

CHAPTER 6

Biomarkers for Risk Assessment and Prevention of Breast Cancer

Massimiliano Cazzaniga[*,1], Andrea Decensi[2], Bernardo Bonanni[1], Alberto Luini[3] and Oreste Gentilini[3]

[1]Division of Cancer Prevention and Genetics, European Institute of Oncology, Milan, Italy; [2]Medical Oncology, E.O. Ospedali Galliera, Genoa, Italy; and [3]Division of Breast Surgery, European Institute of Oncology, Milan, Italy

Abstract: Breast carcinogenesis is a multistep and multipath disease process which occurs in the epithelium lining of the ductal system in the vast majority of cases. Several studies have shown that the relative risk of breast cancer increases in every step of this progression and many tumour associated antigens or biomarkers appear during each phase of carcinogenesis. However, their ability to predict for a substantial likelihood of developing breast cancer remains unclear. The acquisition of breast tissue samples, representative of an individual's cellular stability and subcellular biochemical and molecular state could lead to definition of surrogates for risk, early detection, pharmacodynamic determination and finally chemopreventive intervention. The intraductal approach includes nipple aspiration fluid (NAF), ductal lavage (DL) and mammary ductoscopy (MD). These techniques together with random periareolar fine needle aspiration (RPFNA) represent the available techniques for the sampling of breast fluid and exfoliated epithelial cells. At the moment, these procedures are not considered a screening procedure for early breast cancer detection but might provide a powerful research tool for studying breast carcinogenesis *in vivo*.

We summarize the current knowledge regarding the vast array of molecules involved at all stages of carcinogenesis and the possibility to utilize them as candidate biomarkers to refine risk assessment, and their possible use in prevention strategies.

Keywords: Biomarkers, prevention and breast cancer, risk assessment.

INTRODUCTION

Despite major diagnostic and therapeutic innovations, breast cancer is a major cause of morbidity and mortality in both pre- and postmenopausal women. One of the factors contributing to this limited success is our relative lack of

***Corresponding Author Massimiliano Cazzaniga:** Division of Cancer Prevention and Genetics, European Institute of Oncology, Via Ripamonti 435, 20141, Milan, Italy; Tel: +39 2 57489892; Fax: +39 2 57489809; E-mail: massimiliano.cazzaniga@ieo.it

Atta-ur-Rahman (Ed)

understanding about the natural history of the disease. To date it is accepted that breast carcinogenesis is a multistep, multiyear and multipath disease process involving progressive phenotypic changes from normal histology to early precancerous to superficial cancer and finally to invasive disease [1]. Thus the long latency offers a major scientific opportunity to interfere with the progression. In recent decades the major challenge for physicians was to accurately define risk profiles for individual patients in order to create new opportunities for more targeted approaches to the prevention and treatment of breast cancer (Fig. **1**). Over the past several decades a variety of statistical models have been designed to either estimate a woman's risk of developing breast cancer or an estimation of the likelihood of harboring a heritable genetic mutation such as the BRCA gene. The goal of this accurate individualized risk assessment was to have the ability to assess a particular woman's individual risk and then to appropriately tailor preventive strategies to those that will have maximal benefit with least harm. The

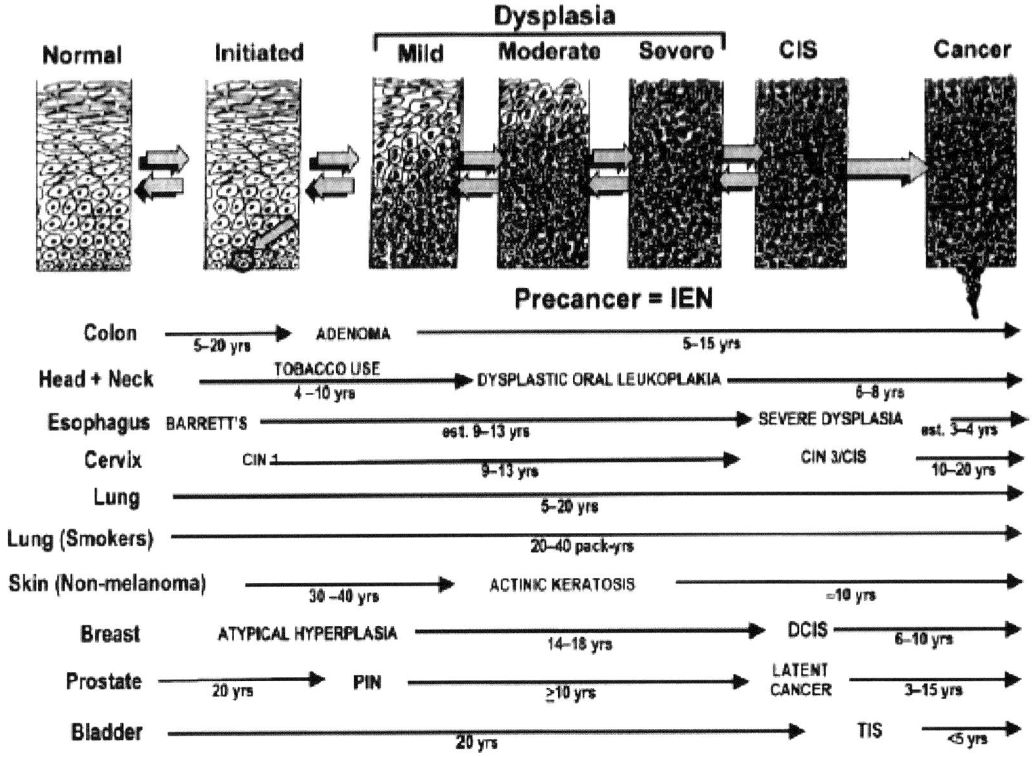

Fig. (1). Human carcinogenesis is a multistep, multiyear and multipath disease (Taken from O'Shaughnessy *et al.* Clin Cancer Res 2002).

epidemiologic models used for breast cancer risk assessment, of which the most commonly used is the Gail model, are well-calibrated for screening populations but have suboptimal discriminatory accuracy because they only hold modest value for individual women and thus may prove partially helpful in individual risk assessment and decision making [2]. However, to estimating a woman's future risk of breast cancer, risk-assessment models may be used to determine eligibility for clinical trials, chemoprevention, genetic testing and magnetic resonance imaging (MRI) screening.

Recently, the use of intraductal approach (IA) techniques has increased the ability to recruit breast tissue and ductal fluid in order to improve our understanding of the pathophysiologic mechanism of breast carcinogenesis [3, 4] which begins with an unbalanced, but still reversible, change in normal cellular metabolism creating new pathological pathways in the cell. In particular, thousands of tumour associated antigens or "biomarkers" appear expressed during the different stage of disease progression [5] and increasing attention is being devoted to these risk biomarkers, which may improve short-term predictive accuracy for the individual woman. Biomarkers might be particularly useful in helping women who are identified as being at increased risk from epidemiologic models, in order to make decisions about medical or surgical prevention options. This review summarizes the current knowledge of the main groups of biomarkers and their possible use for refining breast cancer risk assessment, prevention strategies and drug testing in chemoprevention trials.

SOURCE OF BREAST BIOMARKERS

Histological and cytological features of breast epithelial cells and the subsequent risk of breast cancer have been investigated for several years [6, 7]. Breast tissue and ductal fluid provide a rich source of biomarkers [8] and the ability to utilize them as a surrogate endpoint in breast precancer treatment trials has been significantly hampered by our current inability to measure the extent of atypical tissue in the breast. IA techniques seem to be a promising way to solve this issue. Nipple aspiration (NAF) obtained by a manual pomp or with the use of a device like the Halo® Breast Pap Test (FDA approved) [9, 10], ductal lavage (DL) [11] and mammary ductoscopy (MD) [12] are able to recruit material to contributing to the understanding of the biology of breast cancer and hopefully in the future to its early detection. Moreover another kind of approach defined "transcutaneous", such as random periareolar fine needle aspiration (RPFNA), is currently utilized to collect breast epithelial cells with the same endpoint [13].

However the meaning of their biologic features in relation to risk of breast cancer development remains controversial. Several potential biomarkers have been associated with increased risk [14], including for example growth factors and their binding proteins [15], hormone levels [16] and intraepithelial neoplasia associated biomarkers of dysregulated proliferation [17] but several others remains with an unspecified role in carcinogenesis. IA methods could be used to study biomarker expression profile of precancerous lesions and to compare them with those of non-proliferative and overtly malignant lesions with the objective of exploring the possibility that some of these markers or combination of them could be used as a potential surrogate endpoint for future chemoprevention trials.

In particular this approach could permit us to refine individual risk assessment in order to have the possibility of preventing or arresting the carcinogenesis process, and of developing new chemoprevention agents which exert fewer side effects and/or are effective in the prevention setting.

BREAST BIOMARKERS

In general, an appropriate biomarker should be able to define risks and to identify the early stages of carcinogenesis. In addition it should:

- Be closely linked to the causal pathway for cancer.
- Permit stratification of patients, their treatments and be modulated by chemopreventive agents.
- Have a differential expression in low- and high-risk populations.
- Should be present in a reasonable proportion of the high-risk population.
- Have an association with cancer in prospective studies.
- Have an expression minimally influenced by normal physiologic processes.

Moreover it is important to be able to obtain the markers by minimally invasive techniques with an assessment method that provides reproducible results. Finally biomarkers have the potential to make drug development more rational, thereby optimizing preclinical and clinical efforts and ultimately delivering timely benefits to patients. Key features of appropriate biomarkers are summarized in Tables **1a** and **1b**.

Table 1a. Characteristics of Ideal Biomarkers

- Differentially expressed in normal and high-risk tissue
- Biologic plausibility and closely linked to causal pathway for cancer (*e.g.*, expression increases/decreases with severity of dysplasia)
- Modulated by chemopreventive agents
- Latency is short compared with cancer
- Expression minimally influenced by normal physiologic processes
- Assay for biomarker standardized and validated
- Dose-related response to the chemopreventive agent is observed
- Statistically significant difference observed between levels in treatment groups and controls
- Obtained by noninvasive or relatively noninvasive techniques and not technically difficult
- Reproducible results
- Modulation correlates to decreased cancer incidence

Table 1b. Characteristics of Biomarkers for a Chemopreventive Drug Development Process

- Identify and validate therapeutic and optimal targets populations
- Optimize agents
- Enhance mechanistic understanding of drugs, predict response and toxicity

Thus, we could recognize several molecules having these features in every step of mammary cancer genesis and progression. However, no single biomarker seems at the moment to be able to identify an individual predictive breast cancer risk. This limitation in sensitivity and specificity of individual markers could be partially overcome by considering a panel of molecules and their co-expression in precancerous lesions. Anyway, the key for identifying potential biomarkers of risk is to understand the pathophysiologic mechanism of carcinogenesis and consequently obtain and tested targeted chemopreventive agents able to inhibit this initiation

In this review we divided the most important pathways or groups of proteins and biological markers associated with the known correspondent drugs into different categories: hormonal and nuclear receptors, membrane receptors and signal transduction, anti-inflammatory and antioxidant, apoptosis and angiogenesis markers, proliferation antigens, epigenetic modulation, cellular inducible enzymes and cell cycle regulators. They are summarized in Table **2**.

Table 2. Pathways, Biomarkers and Relative Drugs

Class	Biomarkers	Drugs or Agents
Hormonal and Nuclear Receptors	Estrogen And Progesterone Receptors (ER And PgR) Circulating estrogens and their metabolites	Tamoxifen, Roaloxifene, Toremifene, Arzoxifene, Indole-3-Carbinol, 3,3diindoylmethane, Rosveratrol, Soy Isoflavones
	PPRγ	Rosiglitazone, Pioglitazone
	Retinoic Acid Receptor, RxR	Fenretinide (4-HPR), 9cis-Retinoic Acid, Targretin
	Aromatase	AIs: Examestane, Letrozole, Anastrazole
	VDR	Vit D3 Analogues
Membrane Receptors and Signal Transduction	HMGCoA	Statins
	Tyrosine Kinase, Map-Kinase	Gefitinib
	HER-1, HER-2/Neu	Trastuzumab (Herceptin)
	EGFR	Lapatinib,Gefitinib, Erlotinib
	TGFα,TGFβ Receptors	?
	Mammary-Type Apomucin Heregulin α	?
	C Kit Ras Family	?
	IGF-Receptors, IGF-1 IGFBP-3	Metformin
Anti-Inflammatory and Antioxidant	COX-2	Celecoxib,Rofecoxib,NSAIDs
	Metallothionein(Mt) Matrix Metalloproteases (Mmps)	Protease Inhibitors
	Topoisomerase	Topoisomerase Inhibitors
	Prostaglandine (1-4)	Ono 8711
	Upa/Pai	?
	Nf-Kb	Curcumin, Statins, NSAIDs, Tea Polyphenols
	E-Cadherin	?

(Table 2) contd.....

Class	Biomarkers	Drugs or Agents
Apoptosis	Survivin, Bcl2 Protein, P53, Tnf Family, IAPs, Caspase	Pro-Apoptotic Drugs ?
Angiogenesis	VEGF	Bevacizumab
Proliferation Antigens	Ki 67, PCNA, MIB-1	Antiproliferative Agents
Epigenetic Modulation	DNA Methylation	Folic Acid, Azacytidine
	Histone Deacetylase	SAHA
	LOH	?
	Polymorphisms	?
Cellular Inducible, Enzymes	Telomerase Activity, Topoisomerase	Telomerase Inhibitors
Cell Cycle Regulators	Cyclins, Cathepsine D, Heat Shock Protein 27, CDK	CDK Inhibitors
Microenvironment	CAF and Angiogenesis	Anti-VEGFs and TKinhibitors
Metabolism	(PI3K)/Akt/mTOR system hyperinsulinemia and HIF-1	Metformin
Genomics	miRNA	?

Before the analysis of the current knowledge of all these biomarkers we describe the importance of the biomarkers of risk that are related to the hypothesized first critical step in the initiation of breast cancer, namely, the reaction of catechol estrogen quinone metabolites with DNA (CE-3,4-Q) and the importance of presence of the intraepithelial neoplasia (IEN), which is considered an independent risk factor and both also a great source of biomarkers [18].

Circulating Estrogens and Their Metabolites

An association between breast cancer risk and persistently elevated blood levels of estrogen has been found consistently in many studies [19]. The mechanisms of carcinogenesis in the breast caused by estrogen include the metabolism of hormones to genotoxic, mutagenic metabolites and the stimulation of tissue growth. Together, these processes cause initiation, promotion and progression of carcinogenesis. The classic mechanism of direct action of estrogen on nuclear DNA involves the binding of the hormone to an important group of proteins as nuclear estrogens receptors (ER) analyzed below as risk biomarkers. However, recently, some investigations need to develop beyond the stochastic model based on the paradigm that estrogens bind the correspondent receptors and stimulate the transcription of genes involved in cell proliferation and creating potential mutation [20]. Laboratory and epidemiological data also suggest that non-receptor mediated mechanisms resulting from the genotoxic effects of estrogen metabolites are involved in breast cancer development and clarify the presence of both ER-dependent and -independent mechanisms and the weight of evidence supports the possibility that both mechanisms are involved in breast cancer development. Moreover, discovery that specific oxidative metabolites of estrogens can react with DNA [18] led to and has confirmed the hypothesis that these metabolites can become endogenous chemical carcinogens. Mutations generated by this specific DNA damage can result in the start of cancer process in hormone-dependent and independent tissues and in particular, the reaction of specific estrogens metabolites, namely, catechol estrogens-3,4-quinones (CE-3,4-Q) can generate the critical mutations that initiate breast cancer [21]. Moreover, an important study [22] found that estrogens metabolites, conjugates and depurinating DNA adducts differ between healthy women and women with breast cancer or at high risk of breast cancer. These results confirm that the depurinating estrogen-DNA adducts are possible biomarkers for early detection of breast cancer risk and response to preventive treatment. In this setting it's important to consider how breast cancer preventative agents as anti-estrogens block only receptor mediated pathways whereas the aromatase inhibitors block both.

Intraepithelial Neoplasia (IEN)

Subjects with **IEN**, which spans the continuum from simple hyperplasia without atypia to *in situ* neoplasia, are at significantly higher risk than the general population for developing invasive cancer especially in presence of atypical cells [23, 24] (Fig. **2**). Presence of IEN represents the highest risk of developing breast cancer with the exception of germ-line mutations that occur in genetic syndromes [25]. The relative risk (RR) of invasive breast cancer increases twofold in the presence of proliferative disease or simple hyperplasia without atypical cells (*i.e.*, papillomas and fibroadenomas), four- to fivefold in cases of atypical hyperplasia (AH) but without family history tenfold in the presence of family history or LCIS and twentyfold for DCIS [26-28]. Recently the relationship between the presence of atypical hyperplasia and breast cancer risk was analyzed into the Mayo Benign

Breast Disease Cohort. The results obtained shown that women with AH multiple foci of atypia and the presence of histological calcifications may indicate "very high risk" status (> 50% risk at 20 years). Interestingly in this work seems that a positive family history does not further increase risk [29]. However, in recent history several studies, utilizing both intraductal and transcutaneous approaches to recruit adequate material, have provided some data documenting this relationship between the various steps of IEN and breast cancer risk [30-36]. The findings of the historical studies in this setting are summarized in Table **3**.

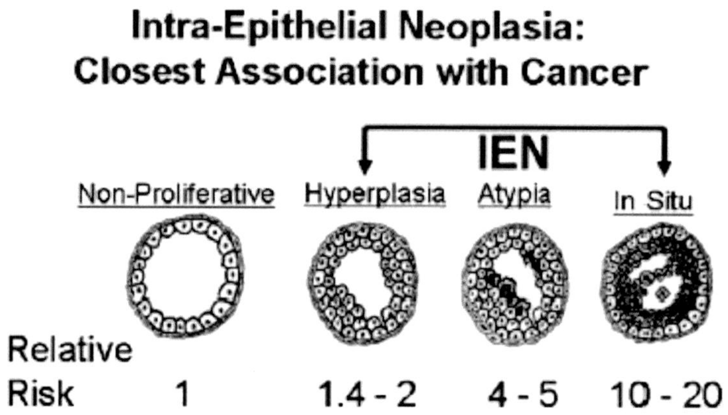

Fig. (2). IEN and RR of BC (Taken from Fabian, *et al.* Clin Cancer Res 2007).

Table 3. **Breast Cancer Risk Associated with Atypia**

Study	Number of Patients	Method of Detection	% of Atypia	Breast Cancer RR (95% CI)
Hutchinson *et al.* 1980	1.053	Surgical biopsy specimens	3.1%	2.85 (0.34-10.28)
Dupont and Page 1985	3.303	Surgical biopsy specimens	3.6%	All: 5.3 (3.1-8.8) With FH: 8.9 (4.8-17) Without FH: 3.5 (2.3-5.5)
Wrensch *et al.* 1992	2.343	Nipple Aspirate Fluid (NAF)	2%	4.9 (1.7-13.9)
Wrensch *et al.* 2001	3.633 (Group 1) 3.271 (Group 2)	Nipple Aspirate Fluid (NAF)	2.4% 0.7%	2.4 (1.6-3.7) 2.8 (1.5-5.5)
Fabian *et al.* 2000	480	Periareolar Fine Needle Aspiration (FNA)	12% (at baseline) 21% (in follow-up)	5.02 (2.01-12.56)
Dupont *et al.* 1999	9.494	Surgical biopsy specimens	3.0%	3.58 (2.6-5.0)

Atypia may therefore provide some temporal measure of breast cancer risk and the relative risks for breast cancer associated with cytological atypia identified by intraductal and percutaneous approach are similar to those conferred by the histopathological findings on breast biopsy.

Moreover, IEN or precancerous lesions could be a significant source of breast cancer risk biomarkers. Recent findings about molecular pathways in determining the malignant potential of premalignant breast lesion have improved our ability to understand the mechanisms and the role of related biomarkers in carcinogenesis. Alteration of DNA methylation levels were monitored during carcinogenesis progression and the methylation of four genomic biomarkers increased significantly during the progressive stages of breast cancer development [37]. This hypermethylation should be considered as predictor biomarkers for malignant transformation. Moreover, diminished expression of a number of tumor suppressor genes and of the expression of estrogen receptors are observed in the early stages of IEN and may also result from a hypermethylation process [38-40]. Increase of growth factors, proliferation antigens, tyrosine kinase receptor activity as well as diminished apoptosis markers are observed in early breast IEN [41-44]. In early IEN there is also an increased expression of p53 mutation [45-46] and LOH (loss of heterozygosity) [47].

Hormonal and Nuclear Receptor Biomarkers

The past decade has seen a remarkable increase in the knowledge of the structures and functions of steroidal and non-steroidal hormone receptors. We describe the most important classes with particular emphasis on estrogen and progesterone receptors (ER and PgR), peroxisome proliferators-activated receptor (PPAR), retinoic acid receptor (RAR) and retinoic X receptor (RXR), Vitamin D receptor (VDR), all members of the nuclear receptor family (NRF) and aromatase activity.

In general the role of the major elements of NRF in breast carcinogenesis is still unclear although their altered expression or activity in breast cancer cells seems to be ascertained.

Estrogen regulates normal growth and differentiation of breast epithelium by interacting with their receptors [48, 49]. They are a potent mitogen for normal breast epithelial cells and are believed to have a major role in the pathogenesis of breast cancer [50]. Thus, the essential role of ER and PgR in the regulation of breast cancer growth has been clearly established [51, 52] and this knowledge has brought to the design of therapeutic strategies directed at the modulation of these elements as well as their validation as prognostic and predictive markers in breast cancer. The proportion of breast epithelial cells expressing ER varies with age, menopausal status and, in pre-menopausal women during the phase of the menstrual cycle, being highest in the follicular phase [53]. However, in healthy women without proliferative disease ERs are expressed in the majority of ductal and lobular tissues [54] and this expression increases according to the presence of IEN up to a 90% of ER positive cells in cases of atypical ductal hyperplasia (ADH) [55]. In general it is possible to say that these kinds of lesions significantly overexpress ER and that progressive modification in receptors value accompanies the transition of normal cells to hyperplastic and carcinoma in situ [56, 57]. Moreover, has been clearly demonstrated that in contrast to normal tissue, almost all cases of ADH and low-grade DCIS and LCIS show a marked increase in ER expression while on the other hand the relation to age and menopausal status is lost [58]. To confirm this, in normal and hyperplastic benign breast tissue there is a scarce concurrent expression of hormonal receptors and proliferation markers such as for example Ki67, but the number of cells co-expressing ER and Ki67 increase with progression of the precursor lesions to cancer [54]. More recently, advances in genomic technologies have provided a global prospective on hormones and their receptors activities and led to a number of significant discoveries, including the role of co-regulatory factors and non-coding RNAs. For example, gene expression profiling studies using microarrays have identified hundreds of oestrogen responsive genes, both transcriptional targets as well as those downstream of ER-regulated signalling pathways, which can be exploited as both markers of oestrogen responsiveness in tumour cells and as targetable genes and gene networks, which specifically regulate tumour cell proliferation [59-61]. Finally, Genomic studies have also highlighted the emerging importance of non-coding RNAs in basic and translational research. Small microRNAs (miRNAs) serve as key regulators of gene expression by targeting genes for degradation or by blocking their translation. ERα-positive breast cancers display a distinct miRNA-expression profile compared with ERα-negative breast cancers [62-65]. Whether ERα directly regulates miRNA is not clear, but miRNA regulations are nonetheless likely to occur indirectly *via* other oestrogen-responsive genes or through ERα interaction with the miRNA processing machinery [66-68] The rapid progress in understanding the roles of RNAs in oestrogen signalling and ER functions suggests the potential of applying RNA therapeutics, singly or in combination with existing chemo- and endocrine therapy drugs, in improving the specificity and efficacy of endocrine therapy in breast cancer prevention and treatment. All these data concerning an increased sensibility to estrogen may play an important role in the development and progression to breast carcinoma and accumulating insights regarding oestrogen signalling and mechanisms of action of ligands and ER provide opportunities for the development of novel markers, targets, and therapeutic strategies.

Peroxisome proliferators-activated receptors (PPARs) is a family of nuclear receptors composed of three members named α, δ and γ [69]. Although PPARs are expressed primarily in adipose tissue and regulate lipid, glucose and amino acid metabolism, they are also expressed in many other tissues and cells including breast cancer cell lines [70]. Interestingly, PPAR-γ synthetic ligands both inhibit proliferation [71] and cause differentiation [72] of human breast cancer cell lines *in vitro* and in general we can say that these receptors are implicated in progression, cellular differentiation and apoptosis of cancer [73, 74]. Consistent with having an antitumorigenic effect, PPAR-γ expression in human tumors was found to be positively associated with an improved clinical outcome of breast carcinoma patients [75]. This pre-clinical and clinical correlative studies suggest that PPAR-γ plays a predominantly anti-tumorigenic role in human breast cancer. There are several known ligands for PPARs including the natural prostaglandin (PGJ2) and some anti-diabetic synthetic drugs like Rosiglitazone, Troglitazone and Pioglitazone which could have the ability to inhibit breast cancer cell growth through modulation of cell cycle regulators [76]. A recent trial examining PPAR-γ expression in tumors from women after rosiglitazone therapy demonstrated that down-regulation of nuclear PPAR-γ expression occurred after PPAR-γ ligand administration [77]. Given the preclinical results suggesting a role for PPAR-γ activation in glandular differentiation, PPAR-γ ligand administration may be useful as a strategy for treating precancerous lesions or much earlier stages of breast cancer. Interestingly some of the growth-inhibitory effects seem to be related to the reduction of the aromatase activity and by inhibition of HER2 tyrosine phosphorylation [78]. Findings suggests that activation of PPARs may play important and likely opposing roles in mammary tumor formation, and that the pharmacological activation of these receptors is likely to have important consequences in breast epithelium Finally compounds influencing PPAR signaling pathways have been shown to reveal chemopreventive potential by mediating tumor suppressive activities in breast cancer and could represent a potential new strategy to inhibit breast carcinogenesis and progression.

Retinoids are the natural and synthetic derivatives of vitamin A and their actions are mediated through two distinct NR families: the **Retinoids nuclear receptors** (RAR-α, RAR-β, and RAR-γ) each of which bind to both all-*trans* retinoic acid (ATRA) or 9-*cis*-retinoic acid (9-*cis*-RA), and the **RXRs** (RXR-α, RXR-β, and RXR-γ), which preferentially bind 9-*cis*-RA [79]. They are known to play a crucial role in cellular and tissue differentiation and can suppress tumour promotion and modify some properties of fully transformed malignant cells by activating and/or repressing specific genes [80]. Retinoid receptors are expressed in normal and malignant epithelial breast cells and are critical for normal development. Although the mechanism underlying breast cell growth inhibition by retinoids has not yet been completely elucidated, experimental evidence suggests that it is likely to involve multiple signal transduction pathways and to result from direct and indirect effects on gene expression. Binding of retinoids to the nuclear receptors leads to regulation of several cellular processes, including growth, differentiation and apoptosis [81]. Interestingly, these compounds might be more active in ER positive than ER negative precancerous tissue [82] and their presence decrease during the malignancy transformation. To confirm this in a series of histological sections of specimens of 70 breast cancer patients that included adjacent normal tissue, DCIS and IDC was observed a significant reduction during carcinogenesis progression of the RAR expression when compared DCIS (83%) with IDC (51%) [83]. Moreover in invasive carcinoma the lower expression was observed in the poorly differentiated tumors. These findings suggest that the loss of RAR may be an important event during breast carcinogenesis.

In the setting of chemoprevention, the synthetic amide of retinoic acid, *N*-(4-hydroxyphenyl) retinamide, or fenretinide (4-HPR), has been widely studied because of its favorable toxicity profile and an historical prospective randomized phase III prevention trial has shown its ability to decrease incidence of contralateral breast cancer in premenopausal women with stage I breast cancer patients undergoing adjuvant treatment [84]. In this trial almost 3000 stage I breast cancer women were randomized to receive for 5 years either 200mg/die of Fenretinide or no treatment, with a significant reduction (38%) of contralateral breast cancer in the premenopausal treatment sub-group. These results were confirmed after fifteen-years of follow-up [85] and the ability of 4-HPR in premenopausal but not in postmenopausal women suggest a hormone-sensitizing effect, in particular on IGF-1, on IGF-binding protein-3 (IGFBP3) and sex hormone binding globulin (SHBG). This hypothesis remains controversial because it was explored in a phase II trial comparing fenretinide with placebo in postmenopausal women receiving HRT [86] and results shown that 4_HPR exerted little modulation on these biomarkers and suggests that the inhibition of circulating IGF-I bioactivity does not represent a major pathway of the preventive effect of fenretinide in this subset of women. 4-HPR was also study in combination with SERMs. A clinical trial with the combination of fenretinide and low-dose tamoxifen was recently conducted at the European Institute of Oncology. Despite favorable effects on plasma IGF-I levels and mammographic density, the combination of low-dose tamoxifen plus fenretinide did not reduce breast neoplastic events compared to placebo, whereas both single agents, particularly fenretinide, showed numerical reduction in annual odds of breast neoplasms [87].

In an attempt to separate the chemopreventive activity of retinoids from their toxic side effects, others receptor-selective ligands have recently been developed In particular a RXR-selective retinoids, (also termed rexinoids) named LGD1069, or bexarotene (Targretin), suppressed both ER-positive and ER-negative tumour development with minimal toxicity [88] in fact recent findings on the mechanisms of ER-negative mammary tumour inhibition by rexinoids suggest that these agents suppress the growth of premalignant mammary epithelial cells, thus preventing their evolution into invasive cancer [89]. Additional investigations, in particular in high risk premenopausal women, are needed in the future, but the receptor-selective retinoids and their evolution rexinoids are realistic promising agents for ER positive or negative breast cancer prevention.

Estrogen, one of the most important risk factors for breast cancer, can be also produced in the breast itself through the conversion of androgens to estrogens, a process catalyzed by the **enzyme aromatase** mostly in post-menopausal women. Aromatase, an enzyme of the cytochrome P-450 super family and the product of the *CYP19* gene, is expressed in several tissues, including subcutaneous fat, liver, muscle, brain, normal breast tissues, and mammary adenocarcinoma [90]. It is responsible for the conversion of the adrenal androgen substrate androstenedione to estrogen in peripheral tissues [91], the predominant source of estrogen in postmenopausal women and obviously, levels of estrogen in the breast tissue increase when aromatase is overexpressed [92]. Several studies have shown that benign and precancerous breast tissue contains aromatase enzyme activity. For example, breast biopsy containing ADH revealed aromatase presence in both stromal and epithelial cells [93]. Although SERMs are currently used for breast cancer prevention and although the particular role of tamoxifen in reducing the relative risk of developing hormone-sensitive breast cancer in chemoprevention trials is universally accepted [94], often the use in prevention setting of compounds able to interfere and inhibit this enzyme action like the aromatase inhibitors (AIs), has been hampered by their long-term toxicity profile especially bone related and the intriguing possibility of utilizing these drugs in chemoprevention settings remains unclear. AIs are classified as first, second, or third generation according to the specificity and potency with which they inhibit the aromatase enzyme. They are further subclassified as type 1 or type 2 inhibitors, according to the reversibility of their inhibitory activity [95] Third-generation AIs (*i.e.*, anastrozole, letrozole, and exemestane) are the most potent, most selective, and least toxic AIs known today and can reduce serum estrogen by more than 95%. Current data indicate that aromatase inhibitors are equivalent or superior to tamoxifen as first-line therapy for metastatic breast cancer and as neoadjuvant treatment for primary breast cancer [96]. In addition, randomized studies have shown that aromatase inhibitors can be administered instead of tamoxifen as a single agent for 5 years or sequentially with tamoxifen for 5 or 10 years [97]. Moreover, theoretically, AIs have a greater potential to prevent the development of cancer by reducing estrogen levels and in turn their damaging metabolites. Their mechanism of action which suppresses plasma estrogen levels by inhibiting or inactivating the enzyme aromatase could be superior to tamoxifen which inhibits estrogen receptor-mediated function only. In randomized trials in the adjuvant setting, AIs are relative safety drugs and they shown an opposite behavior respect SERMs about toxicity with a minor incidence of endometrial cancer and thromboembolic events but with a higher deleterious effects on bone mineral density [98]. This data make them a potentially better chemopreventive agent than tamoxifen in selected postmenopausal high-risk women.

There is increasing interest in Vitamin D, its receptor (**VDR**) and its relationship with several disorders including chronic and cardiovascular diseases, diabetes mellitus and several types of cancer. An important meta-analysis [99] showed that low vitamin D status is associated with higher mortality from life-threatening conditions (including cancer) and that an intake of ordinary doses of Vitamin D supplements seems to be associated with a decrease in total mortality rates. However in prevention setting and especially when we consider the breast cancer incidence results are still controversial as shown in a recent systematic review and meta-analysis on VIT D supplementation which report that vitamin D use seems not to be associated with a reduced risk of breast cancer development in postmenopausal women [100]. In general the active metabolite of vitamin D, 1,25-dihydroxyvitamin D3 [1,25(OH)2-D3], modulates cellular proliferation and differentiation of both normal and malignant cells. The majority of Vitamin D originates from epidermal synthesis in the skin upon exposure to ultraviolet (UV) radiation and this process has considerable individual variation due to skin pigmentation, sunscreen use, age, season, latitude and other lifestyle factors [101]. Although humans can ingest vitamin D (in particular the two naturally occurring forms of Vitamin D named cholecalciferol and ergocalciferol) from food, very few natural nourishments have vitamin D in significant quantities. The vitamin D receptor **(VDR)** and its ligand 1α,25 dihydroxyvitamin D3 (1,25D), exert effects in almost every tissue and there I substantial evidence of VDR involvement in cell differentiation and inhibition of cellular proliferation suggests that vitamin D plays a role in many diseases, cancer included [102]. The level of VDR expression was found to be higher in invasive breast carcinoma than in normal breast tissue and patients with VDR positive tumors had better disease-free survival than those with VDR negative neoplasm [103]. Thus, these observations have prompted studies into the possible role of 1,25D in the treatment of breast cancer, alone or in association with other agents such as tamoxifen (the majority of the studies suggest that the effects of 1,25D are limited to ER positive tumors) [104] or retinoids in the retinoid-sensitive cell lines [105]. However, relevant biomarkers of vitamin D status that could be relevant for cancer prevention remain to be identified. In fact in contrast to the extensive studies demonstrating the effects of 1,25D on transformed mammary cells [106, 107], there has been less emphasis on defining the role of vitamin D in mammary cancerogenesis and in the prevention setting. An hypothesis to support this relationship is that VDR and its ligand 1,25D exert a negative growth regulatory effect on mammary epithelial cells and that they contribute to maintenance of the differentiated phenotype, in particular inhibiting the proliferation. The deletion of this process could alter the balance between proliferation and apoptosis with a relevant susceptibility to carcinogenesis. In fact, *in vitro* studies have shown vitamin D to inhibit hormone driven proliferation and to reduce the number of pre-neoplastic lesions during the initiation and the promotion stages. This data seems to confirm epidemiological findings about the ability of vitamin D to exert an anti-neoplastic effect in several steps of the carcinogenesis process [108, 109]. To further confirm the potential protective effects of vitamin D on breast cancer, well-designed cohort studies and clinical trials are warranted.

Membrane Receptors and Signal Transduction

3 Hydroxy-3-methylglutaryl CoA **(HMGCoA)** reductase inhibitors (statins) are a class of drugs which reduce plasma cholesterol levels and which are currently used to manage and prevent coronary heart disease. Emerging interest in the use of statins as anticancer agents is based on their pleiotropic effects on various cells and tissues. The hypothesis is that inhibition of HMG-CoA reductase by statins leads to reduced levels of mevalonate and its downstream products. This concept is strongly supported by the recent finding that mutant p53, which is present in

more than half of all human cancers, can significantly upregulate mevalonate metabolism and protein prenylation in carcinoma cells [110]. Many of these downstream products play important roles in cellular and subcellular pathways critical for cancer formation and its progression, including membrane integrity, cell signalling, cell cycle progression, immune/inflammatory reactions, stromal-epithelial cell interactions, endogenous energy metabolism, oxidative stress, and intracellular vitamin and steroid content [111]. Alterations of these processes in cancer cells or in the tumour microenvironment may therefore lead to inhibition of tumour initiation, growth, and metastasis. Despite this, the association of this class of agents with various cancers remains controversial and unclear. In preclinical breast cancer models statins carry potent anti-neoplastic activity but epidemiological and randomized trials suggest that statins could be carcinogenic [112] while other laboratory studies showed that statins induce apoptosis and reduce cell invasiveness in various cell lines, including breast carcinoma cells, suggesting a potential role in therapeutic and chemopreventive setting [113-114]. However, an interesting cohort study published in 2007 [115] found no difference in breast cancer risk among statin users compared with non-users. Moreover the risk did not differ according to duration of use or kind of drugs while there is suggestive evidence of increased risk among statin users of $\geq$ 5 years. This study also showed an increased risk of estrogen receptor-negative tumors (ER-) with increasing duration of statin use. A recent meta-analysis on seven large randomized trials and nine observational studies does not support a protective effect against breast cancer but these conclusions are limited by the short follow-up time of the studies and mostly by the presence of both lipophobic and lipophilic statins [116]. Despite these apparently negative findings, researchers have hypothesized that lipophilic statins may have antiproliferative effects on breast cancer cells [117] while on the other hand hydrophilic statins may promote cancer [118]. Further evaluations of longer durations of statin use by type of drug in relation to breast cancer risk are warranted and clinical trials of the effects of statins on breast cancer risk and biological end points, such as breast density, have been suggested.

Signal transduction (a process which regulates the interaction among the extra and intracellular compartments of the cell) works *via* some essential components such as: growth factors, cell surface receptors (*i.e.*, tyrosine kinases) and intracellular signalling pathways. These elements constitute attractive targets for therapy and prevention because their abnormal signalling has been often associated with tumour development and growth. For example over-expression of growth factors, including IGF, EGF, TGF-β, SCF (stem cells factor) and PDGF (platelet-derived growth factor) and their receptors, play pivotal roles in the regulation of epithelial cell growth and differentiation and have been associated with poor prognosis in breast cancer [119]. Therefore, a number of **receptor tyrosine kinase (RTKs)** are already targets for novel designed drugs, which involve tyrosine kinase inhibitors and monoclonal antibodies.

One particular molecular target recently considered in oncology is the **Epidermal Growth Factors Receptor (EGFR)** which is over-expressed, disregulated or mutated in many epithelial malignancies, and its activation appears related to tumor growth and progression [120]. Members of the human EGFR family, especially HER1 and HER2, are frequently implicated in the pathogenesis of breast cancer. There is strong pre-clinical evidence to link EGFR expression and its signaling to de novo and acquired anti-hormone resistance in estrogen receptor positive (ER+) as well as in ER-negative (ER-) breast tumor growth [121]. The most clinically advanced approach to EGFR inhibition includes the use of monoclonal antibodies (mAbs; Trastuzumab or Herceptin) [122] or the use of tyrosine kinase inhibitors (Lapatinib, Gefitinib or Iressa; Erlotinib or Tarceva) [123]. Mechanisms of action for EGFR inhibitors have been investigated in preclinical model systems and safety, activity, pharmacokinetics and pharmacodynamics have been assessed also in clinical trials [124]. The anti-EGFR mAbs and TKIs have partially overlapping toxicity profiles, but distinct routes of administration, serum half-lives and therefore dosing schedules are still under investigation mostly in the prevention setting. Moreover, a more interesting area of recent investigation is the combination of the two kinds of agent or the combinations of these drugs with angiogenesis modulators, in particular research into agents targeting vascular endothelial growth factor (VEGF) is extremely promising.

HER-2 amplification and over-expression is present in almost 30% of breast cancer cases [125] and this presence is actually considered a pivotal clinical information in adjuvant therapy decision making. In fact, HER-2 is a recognized prognostic factor, indicating more aggressive tumors [126], predicting resistance to endocrine therapy in ER+ women [127] and indicating which patients receive more benefit from anthracycline-containing regimens in adjuvant treatment [128]. These information was confirmed also in the recent molecular subtypes classification where the HER 2 positive subtypes exhibit a relatively high histologic grade, frequent multifocal/multicentric disease, positive lymph node and high volume nodal involvement [129].

The humanized monoclonal antibody trastuzumab was the first anti-HER2 drug shown to be active in breast cancer. Its effectiveness was initially shown in treating metastatic HER2-positive breast cancer [130] and subsequently in treating early-stage, HER2- positive breast cancer [131] and in neoadjuvant settings involving HER2-positive disease (before surgical resection). Another anti-HER2 antibodies have been tested clinically with promising results. The evident clinical activity of lapatinib in the metastatic setting led to FDA approval this drug in combination with capecitabine for the treatment of HER2-positive breast cancer and also provided the rationale for testing lapatinib in the clinical setting of early-stage, HER2-positive breast cancer,

In fact, about the approaches for preventing ER negative, and increased prevention of ER-positive breast cancers, a growing body of preclinical and clinical work support targeting the HER family for preventing ER-negative and possibly ER-positive breast cancer.. Clinical trials include a recent placebo-controlled phase IIb presurgical trial [132] of the dual EGFR HER2 inhibitor lapatinib that suppressed growth of breast premalignancy, including atypical ductal hyperplasia (ADH) and DCIS and invasive cancer in patients with early-stage, HER2-overexpressing or -amplified breast cancer. These preclinical and clinical signals provide a compelling rationale for testing HER-targeting drugs for breast cancer prevention in women at moderate-to-high risk, leading perhaps to combinations that prevent ER-negative and ER-positive breast cancer.

Transforming growth factor beta (TGF β) is a regulator of several cellular processes including proliferation, differentiation, migration, cell survival, apoptosis, angiogenesis and immunosurveillance [133]. Alterations of this pathway are frequently observed in human cancer. In fact, TGF β has the potential to function as a tumor suppressor not only with effects on proliferation, replication and apoptosis but also as a tumor promoter with effects on migration, invasion, angiogenesis and the immune system. However the precise mechanism for the dichotomous function remains unclear. In the breast the TGF β plays an important role in normal mammary biology and in particular it is implicated in epithelial proliferation, in ductal and alveolar development and in postlactation involution of the mammary gland [134]. Moreover, the TGF β also plays an important role in breast carcinogenesis [135, 136]. Some important studies showed a decrease of breast cancer formation in patients with elevated levels of TGF β [137] but also a poorer prognosis for human breast cancer patients with elevated levels of TGF β [138]. Further studies are necessary to understand the correct mechanism of action of this molecule, but the evidence that the chemopreventive and therapeutic effects of tamoxifen could be mediated through the induction of TGF β [139] open the possibility of utilizing TGF as a surrogate biomarker in the breast chemoprevention setting.

The **Insulin-like growth factor system (IGF)** and its components (IGF-I and IGF-II) are peptides, which have mitogenic and anti-apoptotic effects and influence the proliferation of various cell types including normal and transformed epithelial breast cells [140]. There is abundant evidence that IGFs affect breast cancer growth and it is currently held that the relationship between circulating IGF levels and breast cancer risk differs by menopausal status [141]. A systematic review [142] and a cumulative meta analysis [143] reported that levels of IGF-I were predictive for pre-menopausal but not for post-menopausal breast cancer risk. In contrast the role of IGF-I binding protein (IGFBP-3) is still unclear. Relationship between circulating levels of IGF-I and breast cancer risk suggest that this pathway could in fact be an appropriate target for chemoprevention. Moreover the evidence of the collaboration between endogenous hormones and growth factors in the proliferation of the normal and altered mammary tissue (IGF increased the response in breast cells to oestrogens), suggest a possibility for a chemopreventive intervention strategy on IGF-I based on anti-oestrogen drugs. A chemoprevention trial of tamoxifen *versus* placebo in healthy high risk women showed that tamoxifen administration reduced circulating levels of IGF-I by

23.5% [144]. Moreover, even a low dose of tamoxifen seems to be effective on modulation of the IGF family relative to the conventional dose [145]. A recent study determined that raloxifene administration is associated with an increase in IGFBP-3 in premenopausal high risk women and that an increase in IGFBP-3 may potentially decrease the activity of IGF-I [146].

The synthetic retinoid fenretinide showed a beneficial effect on second breast cancer in premenopausal women [84] Decensi *et al.* [147] found a long term effect of fenretinide on IGF-I levels and showed a significant reduction of the risk maintained for up to 5 years. Moreover numerous inhibitors of the IGF1 receptor (IGF1R) have been recently developed (monoclonal antibodies and tirosine kinase inhibitors mainly) [148], and they displayed remarkable antineoplastic activity in preclinical models and promising success in early phase clinical trials. However, while responses have been observed in numerous cancer types, breast including, they have occurred in a minority of patients, and serious toxicities have been observed. Identifying patients likely to benefit from anti-IGF1R therapy requires further characterizing the role of IGF1 signaling in various stages of tumorigenesis in order to identify critical downstream factors that may be used as predictors of response, or to serve as novel therapeutic targets.

Finally, there are also several dietary ingredients under investigation regarding their effects on the IGF-I system, such as curcumin, genistein, green tea polyphenols, rosveratrol, lycopene and various other natural agents [149-153]. Dietary agents, which interfere with the IGF pathway, offer the possibility to develop nontoxic agents that override any toxicity of synthetic IGF inhibitors. Although these dietary agents have been shown to modulate IGF-I axis, the correct mechanism is still unclear and as for synthetic compounds, and therefore there is a need for more clinical trials to examine the real effect of natural agents on the IGF pathway and breast cancer development.

Anti-Inflammatory and Antioxidant

Cyclooxygenase 2 (COX-2) is an inducible enzyme, which converts arachidonic acid to prostaglandins. This pathway is involved in the development and growth of several different neoplastic lesions [154]. It is frequently over-expressed not only in invasive breast cancer but also in adjacent intraductal neoplasia and therefore it might be an early event in mammary tumorigenesis. In detail it seems overexpressed in invasive breast cancer but is also implicated in breast cancer progression. The mechanism seems to interest the cancer microenvironment and in particular involve epithelial-to-mesenchymal transition (EMT) and the consequent hypoxia status.

This suggests that non-steroidal anti-inflammatory drugs or better-selective COX-2 inhibitors may be useful not only in therapy but also in chemoprevention of breast cancer especially in an ER negative setting. There are different subtypes which are either COX-2 selective, the so-called coxibs, *e.g.,* celecoxib and rofecoxib, or non-selective, *e.g.,* acetylsalicylic acid, ibuprofen and indomethacin, which block both subtypes of COX. Epidemiological studies support the hypothesis of breast cancer prevention by NSAID administration. A meta-analysis of 14 epidemiological studies showed a decrease in breast cancer risk by 18% after constant NSAID use [155, 156] even reported a reduction of breast cancer risk by 24%, while Harris *et al.* observed a reduction by 40% by NSAID intake [157-158]. A recent case-control study showed that a short window of exposure to selective COX-2 inhibitors produced a significant (71%) reduction of breast cancer risk underlining their strong potential impact for breast cancer chemoprevention [159]. While there are several trials with promising results in adjuvant setting, only few studies reported an analysis of COX-2 expression in DCIS of the breast; however, in comparison to invasive cancer, Half *et al.* hypothesized that COX-2 up-regulation is an early event in carcinogenesis and thus is overexpressed in pre-invasive lesions [160-162] Women with initial DCIS lesions that express COX-2 have a higher risk for developing subsequent invasive cancer in comparison to those with COX-2 negative DCIS [163]. These results were corroborated by systematic review and meta-analysis [164, 165]. Trials are currently ongoing to investigate the possible role of COX-2 inhibitors in limiting the development of precancerous lesions of the breast. Moreover studies are in progress in order to evaluate the use of COX-2 inhibitors in combination with other agents in early breast cancer.

About aspirin, epidemiological evidence from case-control and cohort studies suggests that the risk of breast cancer is reduced by about 10% in individuals taking aspirin [166]. Randomised prevention trials have indicated that these drugs need to be taken long term before a benefit is seen, but after 20 years of follow-up overall cancer mortality was reduced by about 20% in people taking aspirin [167]. Although the effect of aspirin on breast cancer incidence is too small to justify its use solely as a preventive therapy, a larger evaluation taking into account the risk reduction seen for other cancers, particularly gastrointestinal cancers, as well as the effects on the cardiovascular system and gastrointestinal side-effects might prove the usefulness of aspirin in this context [168].

The **matrix-metalloproteinases** (MMPs) are a family of zinc-dependent endopeptidases and recent data showed that these are involved in breast cancer initiation, invasion and metastasis [168]. In fact, Elevated levels of MMP-1-3, MMP-7-9, MMP-11, MMP- 13-15, and MMP-26 are reported in the blood, urine, and/or cancer tissue from breast cancer patients [169-174]. Moreover, In a recent study including 295 breast cancer patients, high mRNA level of MMP-1 was found to be significantly associated with poor patient outcome although it is not an independent prognostic predictor [175]. These results were confirmed also when other MM are involvement In a large study including 1,079 breast cancer patients, polymorphic variants of the MMP-7 gene associated with increased transcription were found to be significantly associated with poor prognosis [176]. In contrast to these tumor-promoting MMPs, strong immunohistochemical staining for MMP-26 in ductal carcinomas in situ was correlated with longer patient survival [177], indicating opposing effects of MMP-26 in breast cancers especially in early phase of tumorigenesis.

Inhibition of these proteinases might thus lead both to prevention of cancer development and to inhibition of dissemination. A series of synthetic low molecular weight MMP inhibitors has been produced [178]. Although several studies have shown that this class of drugs can significantly reduce the growth rate of both primary and secondary tumors and can block the process of metastasis [179], their use has so far been limited to patients with advanced disease.

Apoptosis

Several studies have indicated a role for apoptosis (programmed cell death) in a variety of human diseases and it has been found that suppression of apoptosis contributes to carcinogenesis by several mechanisms. This process involves an evolutionarily preserved multistep cascade and is regulated by proteins that promote or counteract apoptotic cell death [180]. **Survivin** is a novel member of inhibitors of the apoptosis (IAP) protein family implicated in the control of apoptosis and regulation of cell division [181]. Molecular mechanisms of regulation of survivin in cancer are not clearly understood but it appears to be overexpressed in histological samples of most common human cancers including breast carcinoma, being undetectable in normal differentiated adult tissue [182]. A recent meta-analysis was conducted to obtain a more precise estimation of the relationship between survivin expression and overall survival (OS) in breast cancer patients and results suggested that high survivin expression had an unfavorable prognostic role for patients with breast cancer [183]. Moreover survivin also appears to be involved in tumor resistance to some anticancer agents [184]. In particular the over expression of survivin is found to correlate with HER 2 and EGFR expression. Its presence has also been found to confer resistance to chemotherapy and radiation [183].

In prevention setting, data suggest that survivin could be detectable during the early phases of carcinogenesis and its inhibition with therapeutic intervention could be a new pathway of intervention in chemoprevention strategies. Several preclinical studies have shown that disrupting survivin expression or function in cancer cells decreases their proliferation and enhances apoptosis [185, 186]. However, Cazzaniga *et al.* have investigated survivin and Ki67 expression in breast epithelial cells obtained from a consecutive ductal lavage series in selected high risk women. They showed that survivin expression does not appear to be associated with cytological diagnosis, both in qualitative (presence/absence) or in quantitative evaluation (fraction of survivin-positive cells) either at a nuclear or a cytoplasmic level (AACR meeting abstract 2006).

A number of genetic abnormalities have been described in malignant breast tissue but the sequence of molecular events in breast carcinogenesis is poorly characterized. The tumor suppressor gene TP53 and its protein **p53** play a key role in many cellular pathways and its mutation is described in more than half of all of human cancers and in almost 20% of malignant breast tumors [187]. Recently mutation in p53 has been associated in the vast majority of triple negative breast cancers, and as such is a target of particular interest [188]. Its action plays a crucial role in response to various cellular stresses and stimuli, controlling cell proliferation, cell survival (apoptosis) and genomic integrity. Its disruption in fact promotes genomic instability, uncontrolled proliferation and inappropriate survival of damaged cells [189]. Loss of p53 function was reported to be related to worse prognosis and lower chemosensitivity [190], more aggressive tumors, early metastasis and decreased survival rates in breast cancer patients [191]. Several studies have also indicated that mutations in the p53 gene can occur in early phases of tumorigenesis, have been found in premalignant lesions [192, 193] and can be relevant for tumor progression [194]. In a recent case-control study of 4,888 women, Rohan *et al.* [195] suggest that p53 protein accumulation and polymorphic changes in p53 are associated with increased risk of progression to breast cancer in women to benign breast disease. Several interesting studies have also revealed a strong relationship between p53 and other breast cancer risk biomarkers. Tsuji *et al.* [196] showed that p53 mutation and loss of heterozygosity may up-regulate the survivin expression in breast cancer tissue. P53 antibodies (p53-abs) are associated with lack of estrogen receptor expression (ER) and also with antigen Ki67 but not with oncoprotein c-erbB2 [197]. A recent study demonstrated hormonal modulation of the p53 tumor suppression pathway with a specific endocrine stimulus necessary to activate p53 function and to mitigate the risk [198]. Despite this complex interplay (between hormones and heritable risk), the emerging pathways renew hope for interventions aimed at preventing breast cancer.

Several agents with potential activity against aberrant p53 signaling have been considered, (alone or in combination) as a novel approach to finding an effective targeted therapy for aggressive breast cancer subtype. PI3K/AKT/mTOR inhibitors (everolimus and temsirolimus) Chk1 inhibitors, HDAC inhibitors (vorinostat) and CDK inhibitors are the most important agent related by this pathway [199-204]. Their toxicity and the lack of evidence of their efficacy in early phases of the disease still limited their use in prevention setting.

Proliferation Antigens

Proliferative activity in breast tissue represents one of the biological processes that has been most thoroughly investigated for its association with tumor arises and progression. Several proliferation indices have provided independent information on breast carcinogenesis, prognosis and response to treatments in large retrospective studies. The absence of these molecules in quiescent cells and their expression in proliferating tissues [205] created great interest in their potential role as a proliferation marker and **Ki-67**, one of the most studied proliferative proteins, is frequently used as a static marker for proliferative activity over treatment efficacy. Thus although high Ki-67 is a variable predictor of poor prognosis in breast cancer evaluation, associated with a good chance of clinical response of chemotherapy [206], its role in precancerous lesions remains to be determined. Several studies have shown that in normal breast tissue or in benign diseases it is expressed at a very low level. Moreover it is interesting that only ER negative cells are proliferative in normal and benign breast while KI-67 is absent in ER positive cells in normal epithelium. This is lost in cancer tissue where Ki-67 is expressed in a higher percentage of cells and this seems to show a progressively changing pattern from normal to cancerous cells with an intermediated value in non-invasive precancerous lesions. An interesting work published in 2010 [207] authors have tried to understand if Ki67 expression could stratify risk in women with atypia and they examined Ki67 levels and 10-year and longer-term risk of breast cancer in a cohort of women with atypical hyperplasia. They interestingly found that the 30% of women with atypia had elevated expression of Ki67; these women had a fourfold increased risk of breast cancer within 10 years after their atypia biopsy. Conversely, those women with low Ki67 expression in their atypia tissue had an increased risk that was concentrated after 10 years of follow-up, compared to the general population. Thus authors concluded that Ki67 appears to be a time-varying biomarker that may help to better stratify risk in women with atypia. Previously these data, Cazzaniga *et al.* [208] showed that Ki-67 expression was associated with atypical cells and cell yield in a consecutive series of ductal lavage in high risk women. The authors suggest the use of Ki-67 as a surrogate biomarker in early-phase of chemoprevention trials. Another similar study [209], however, observed a good correlation of Ki-67 with total epithelial cell yield but no correlation was seen with cytological atypia. These controversial findings explain the necessity of further trials in order to clarify the real correlation between proliferation antigens and early phases of carcinogenesis. Moreover, pre-surgical model studies showed a change of Ki-67 expression after short-term exposure of patients to therapeutic agents [210, 211] and for this reason it is frequently used as a pharmacodynamic marker of efficacy in pre-surgical model. Actually Ki-67, is the biomarker preferentially used to select drugs in breast cancer because is accepted its prognostic value and its postulated role in predicting drug efficacy. These data could be used as a strong rationale for the choice of Ki-67 as a surrogate biomarker also in short-term phase II chemoprevention trials.

Epigenetic Modulation

Cancer is the result of multiple alterations in gene expression caused by genetic instability and epigenetics mechanisms. However, pathways which determine the malignant potential of premalignant breast lesions remains unclear. Epigenetics means the interaction between genes and environment in the development of particular phenotypical traits. In particular, epigenetic events are alterations in gene expression and these occur throughout all stages of carcinogenesis, early phases included, and they represent the major mechanism involved in silencing tumor suppressor genes. The role of aberrant epigenetic gene regulation has been proven in carcinogenesis of breast cancer. DNA Methylation, and in particular several tumor suppressor genes such as *RASSF1A, APC, H-cadherin, Rarβ2, Twist, HIN1* and *cyclin D2* are methylated more frequently in breast cancer than in adjacent benign tissue [212]. The possibility of using these epigenetic changes for early detection of breast cancer or to refine risk assessment is still under investigation. Recently, alterations in DNA methylation levels were monitored during benign, premalignant and malignant stages of ductal breast cancer development. Results have been very promising because seems that DNA hypermethylation of selected biomarkers - in particular (Methylated-IN-Tumour (MINT)17, MINT31, RAR*β*2 and RASSF1A) occurs early in breast cancer development, and may present a predictor of malignant potential [213].

This findings with the ability to reverse epigenetic changes using small molecules, makes them promising targets for cancer chemopreventive drugs development. Previous studies have reported methylation patterns of cellular DNA from NAF and DL fluid obtained from affected women compared with those with benign breast disease and healthy controls [214, 215]. Moreover in original study Locke [216] found levels of aberrant methylation in DL from breast of healthy BRCA mutation carriers compared with controls and suggested that methylation analysis may offer a useful surrogate marker of BRCA1/2 mutation status and or breast cancer risk. These data were confirmed in another similar study (ASCO meeting abstract 2007) and except *cyclin D2,* where methylation occurs almost exclusively in tumors (offering an excellent option for breast cancer detection), the presence of others methylated suppressor genes in benign breast epithelium could be associated with epidemiologic markers of increased breast cancer risk [217]. The significance of these findings in the context of breast cancer risk, prevention and treatment is highly promising but remains to be elucidated. The imperative to optimize assays and validate panels of DNA methylation markers in well-designed clinical studies in high risk and affected populations is fundamental.

Besides methylation, tumor suppressor genes could be involved in other epigenetic changes called post-translational modifications which could alter the structure of the chromatin (for example with acetylation) playing a role in regulating gene expression and concurring to the carcinogenesis process. Enzymes involved in these epigenetic events include **Histone deacetylases (HDAC)** and **histone acetyl transferases (HAT)** and there are data supporting altered HAT and/or HDAC activities in many cancers [218, 219]. Histone acetylation is controlled by a balance in activity between these two entities and in particular, the HDACs are critical in the regulation of expression of genes important for cell survival, proliferation, differentiation, and apoptosis [220]. High HDAC expression and histone hypoacetylation have been observed in breast cancer with associated transcriptional repression of genes, providing a rationale for the investigation of HDAC inhibitors in cancer therapeutics [221]. Several molecules have the ability to inhibit these enzymes inducing cancer cell growth arrest, apoptosis and differentiation [222] and a lot of these inhibitors are currently under investigation in clinical trials. Laboratory research conducted to date supports the investigation of HDAC inhibitors (Vorinostat, Entinostat) for the treatment of breast cancer. Vorinostat, for example, induces differentiation or arrests growth of a wide variety of human carcinoma cells including breast cancer cells [223, 224]. Recent experiments have provided the strong rationale for combining epigenetic modifiers with hormonal therapy in breast cancer clinical trials [225]. Interestingly, many of these studies also indicate that a strategy which combines HDAC and DNMT (DNA methyltransferase) inhibitors is more efficacious than either agent alone with respect to both re-expression of silenced genes and restoration of response to tamoxifen and aromatase inhibitors [226-228]. Accumulating evidence has demonstrated the effectiveness of HDAC inhibitors in combination with several other agents *in vitro* leading to new clinical trials in which HDAC inhibitors are combined with retinoids [229], antiHER2 strategies [230, 231], hypomethylating agents [232, 233], and many other novel agents.

Important questions remain regarding the optimal dose, schedule and combination of epigenetic modifiers in the breast cancer setting. In this era of personalized medicine, investigators continue to design preclinical experiments and clinical trials in order to answer these questions such that the right patients may benefit from these agents in the not too distant future.

Somatic loss of heterozygosity (**LOH**), is another frequent genetic event in the multistep process of breast cancer tumor development and progression [234]. Several studies have shown that in the presence of germ-line mutations in tumor suppressor genes (BRCA1-2) there is an elevated risk of LOH [235]. Not only but in sporadic breast cancer, although somatic mutations of these genes are rare, loss of heterozygosity (LOH) at BRCA1 and BRCA2 loci is common [236]. The presence of LOH reflects the insufficiency of different mechanisms of DNA repair and replication and finally in genetic instability. An interesting hypothesis is that the normal breast epithelium of high-risk women might contain occult genetic abnormalities and this could indicate a predisposition or vulnerability of this tissue to a neoplastic transformation. LOH has been reported both in normal tissue from women with and without breast cancer and in tissue adjacent to and distant from primary cancer [237]. However, the prevalence of LOH in normal breast epithelium of women at average risk is unknown and the relationship between LOH and increased risk for breast cancer is currently under investigation. Thus recurrent sites of LOH may identify pathways potentially important for the prevention and treatment of breast tumors. Interestingly, some investigators have evaluated the rates of LOH in ductal lavage specimens. Isaacs *et al.* [238] reported LOH in 58% of unaffected breast of BRCA1 mutation carriers with contralateral breast cancer. Locke *et al.* [239] reported LOH rates of 36-56% in BRCA1 and

45-61% in BRCA2 mutation carriers respectively. Moreover Yonekura [240] showed a rate of 74 to 93% in ductal lavage samples from breasts affected with cancer, 60 to 84% in contralateral unaffected breasts and almost 70% in women with benign breast disease. Although these data seem intriguing DNA quantity is highly variable between samples (probably due to contamination with non-epithelial cells in DL fluid) with low yields likely to detrimentally affect the interpretation of LOH.

Although almost 15% of breast cancer cases have some family history of the disease, only 7-10% can be explained by rare, highly penetrant mutation in genes such as BRCA 1-2. Since mutations that are recognized to increase breast cancer risk within families are quite rare, identification of variants known as SNPs is very important. Thus, other common, low-penetrance genetic variants which alter the predisposition to breast cancer may be present and it has been estimated that there are 7 million common SNPs in human genome often strongly correlated to one another. The research for other genetic markers of susceptibility to breast cancer and the recent technological advances has led to an increasing number of epidemiological studies regarding genetic general **polymorphisms** (low-penetrance mutation on several genes) and in particular the presence of **SNPs** (single-nucleotide polymorphisms) and the risk of breast cancer. Precise estimation of the risk associated with these and other as yet untested genes is actually unclear and more complex risks arising from gene-gene and gene-environment interactions are under investigation. In general, to address the association between variants and breast cancer, an increasing number of articles on genetic association studies, genome-wide association studies (GWASs), and related meta- and pooled analyses have been published. Results shown that about the total of genetic association studies 31.7% of the gene variant breast cancer associations were significant, and 21.7% of them were noteworthy. However, in GWASs, 80% of the significant associations were noteworthy [241]. There are also some polymorphisms strictly associated with the mammary field under investigation. For example Cytochrome P450 enzymes make up a multiple-gene "superfamily" that plays an important role in steroidogenesis and in modulation of some anticancer commonly used drugs. In fact some molecular studies seem to have found a relationship between breast cancer incidence (or therapy response) and some P450 cytochrome genotypes such as CYP1A1, CYP2D6 and CYP17 [242]. Moreover, a recent meta-analysis concluded and confirmed that CYP2D6 polymorphisms may influence tamoxifen treatment outcomes of DFS in BC patients [243].

Cellular Inducible Enzymes

Genetic instability and in particular chromosomal instability are other mechanisms which concur to alter the gene expression profile. These alterations appear early during breast carcinogenesis and are considered a major driving force in malignant transformation. **Telomeres** are terminal DNA-protein complexes with the function of stabilizing the chromosomes, playing thus a key role in the maintenance of chromosomal stability [244]. **Telomerase** is the enzyme responsible for maintenance of the telomeres. Cells with moderate telomere shortening enter an irreversible cell cycle arrest or initiate programmed cell death (apoptosis) while abrogation of this senescence checkpoint results in continued division and the initiation of chromosomal instability that, in turn, may foster carcinogenesis. Telomerase is stringently repressed in most normal somatic cells but is activated in a wide range of human cancers [245] including breast carcinoma where it is over-expressed in almost 90% of all cancers [246]. Moreover, while telomerase activity was found to be absent in fibrocystic changes, 45% of fibroadenomas showed low levels of these enzymes [247, 248]. This finding might explain the possible exponential activity of telomerase during carcinogenesis and makes it an attractive target for prevention. A recent systematic review and meta-analysis confirmed that telomerase activity was significantly present in breast cancer when compared with normal breast tissue or benign breast lesions [249]. Another multivariate analysis has revealed that telomerase activity is also strongly correlated with stage, nodal status [250] and lympho-vascular invasions [251]. Additionally, telomerase is also supposed to be associated with drug resistance. More than one hundred papers have been published on telomerase inhibitors but fewer of these agents have been tested in breast cancer cells. Zidovudine (AZT), which is currently used in the treatment of AIDS patients, has been shown to be effective in inhibiting breast cancer cell growth and telomerase activity at lower doses than in normal cells *in vitro* [252, 253]. Unfortunately, the antiproliferative effects of telomerase inhibition require extensive telomere shortening before they are fully present. Combining telomerase inhibition with common chemotherapeutic drugs can be used to reduce this lag phase and induce tumor cell death more effectively. For these reasons, standard chemopreventive agents have also been investigated for a possible role in telomerase inhibition and control of breast cancer. Retinoic acid and tamoxifen have already been shown to inhibit enzymatic activity in breast cancer cells, probably as a consequence of proliferation inhibition. Cells in which telomerase was suppressed were more sensitive to anticancer agents independently of their mechanism of action and this sensitization was dependent on the presence of shorter telomeres [254].

Finally, the expression of telomerase in various human cancers and its diminished expression in most normal cells suggest that the enzyme might serve as a good target for anticancer drugs. Due to telomerase inhibition, activity, or expression, these drugs might kill tumor cells but unfortunately most existing anticancer therapies disturb normal cells as well as malignant ones and often show some serious toxicity. Although these effects limit their use in prevention setting, several studies in this field are currently ongoing and Herbert *et al.* [255], have investigated the possibility of utilizing these agents or other specific telomerase inhibitors in breast cancer chemoprevention strategies and have shown that non-toxic doses of these agents significantly lowered the frequency of spontaneous immortalization.

Cell Cycle Regulators

The standard cell cycle is controlled by several mechanisms ensuring correct cell division. In particular cell cycle progression is controlled by sequential activation of **cyclin-dependent kinases** (CDKs) by **cyclins**, which are often deregulated in cancer [256, 257]. Consequently numerous pharmacological inhibitors of CDKs have been developed with the aim of treating cancers. The complexity of cell cycle regulation of is reflected in the different alterations, which can occur at different levels and lead to aberrant cell proliferation and development of cancer. CDK are different proteins, which regulate transition from one cell cycle phase to another, being activated during the cell cycle. In particular, while CDK levels remain stable during the cell cycle, the concentration of their activating proteins, the cyclins, rise and fall at specific stages throughout the cycle. Some cyclins have been identified but, like CDKs, not all of them are cell cycle and cancer related [258]. **Cyclin E** is the limiting factor G1 phase progression and S phase entry. Deregulation of this cyclin expression and/or high levels causes genomic instability and have been reported in a variety of tumors where is used as indicator of poor prognosis [259]. In breast cancer elevated levels of cyclin E were frequently found in ER-negative tumors [260] and it seems to be an independent prognostic factor for overall survival, but not to relapse-free survival [261]. As a predictive marker, high levels of cyclin E suggest resistance to tamoxifen adjuvant therapy [262]. Recently its overexpression has been associated with trastuzumab resistance in HER 2 positive breast cancer and this finding suggests that treatment with CDK inhibitors may be a valid strategy in patients with breast tumors with HER2 and cyclin E coamplification/overexpression [263] (Scalriti PNAS 2011).

D-type cyclins are other key regulator proteins in G1 phase progression. There are three cyclins in this family termed D1, D2 and D3, which have different effects in the development of the normal mammary gland and seem to play a key role in mediating mitogenic responses to steroids and growth factors. Aberrant expression of **Cyclin *D1*** has been reported in many human cancers [264] and it is over-expressed in almost 40% of invasive primary breast tumors. Moreover cyclin *D1* expression was detected at levels significantly greater than in normal breast epithelium in the early proliferative lesions and this level significantly increased during the progression to any form of cancer [265, 266]. Cyclin D1, in particular, is a central player both in the differentiation of mammary epithelium and breast cancer development. It appears to be closely involved in the regulation of mammary epithelial differentiation by C/EBPβ and PPARγ, as both a regulator and a target of these transcription factors. Cyclin D1 is also a conduit for the action of differentiation inducing therapeutics, including PPARγ agonists.. In the continuing study of differentiation pathways and therapeutics it will be relevant to observe the effect of expression of cell cycle proteins. This may allow a further understanding of the role of cell cycle proteins in differentiation, and also how they influence the progression of breast cancer. For these reasons targeting cell cycle and in particular the complex CDK-Cyclins presents a good opportunity for new drug discovery. The evidence in fact that CDK, their regulators (cyclins), the natural CDK-inhibitors (INK4 family as p15-16-18-19 proteins or Cip/Kip family as p21 and p27 proteins) and their substrates are targets of genetic alteration in different human cancers has stimulated the research of chemical inhibitors of these complexes. Several kinds of drugs have been tested against CDK (*i.e.*, purine analogues, pyrimidine analogues, flavonoids, indolinones and others) with some interesting results present in literature [267]. Several agents has also been tested against cyclins, especially cyclin *D1* in the breast cancer setting (*i.e.*, PPARγ activators, histone deacetylase inhibitors, all-trans retinoic acid, rosveratrol, lovastatin, aspirin, troglitazone and others) and it seems that PPARγ activators and HDAC inhibitors are able to induce cyclin *D1* degradation [268].

New Pathways and Biomarkers

Recent data indicate that primary dysfunction in the tumor **microenvironment**, in addition to epithelial dysfunction, can be crucial for carcinogenesis [269] and these findings make a compelling case for targeting the microenvironment for cancer chemoprevention [270]. It is now clear that stromal cells in the tumor microenvironment play an important role in cancer development. Molecular events through which reactive stromal cells affect cancer cells can be defined so that biomarkers and therapeutic targets can be identified and recognition of the important role of the stroma during the progression of breast cancers leads to the possibility of new targets for treatment of the initial breast cancer lesion as well as prevention of recurrence.

Molecular events through which reactive stromal cells affect cancer cells can be defined so that biomarkers and therapeutic targets can be identified. Cancer-associated fibroblasts (CAFs) make up the bulk of cancer stroma and affect the tumor microenvironment such that they promote cancer initiation, angiogenesis, invasion, and metastasis [271]. In breast cancer, CAFs not only promote tumor progression but also induce therapeutic resistance. Accordingly, targeting CAFs provides a novel way to control tumors with therapeutic resistance (anti-estrogen resistance in particular). It is increasingly clear that cells within the tumor stroma are communicating with other components of the tumor microenvironment (inflammatory cells, blood vessels and myofibroblasts, macrophages, other immune cells, adipocytes and endothelial cells, among others.) as well as with the tumor epithelial cells, thus, drug targets that can disrupt the tumor 'ecosystem' are highly sought after [272]. The most active avenues for drug development have been in targeting tumor-promoting inflammatory processes and tumor-associated angiogenesis. For example, the most clinically advanced of these are VEGF inhibitors that target tumor endothelial cells, such as anti-VEGF monoclonal antibodies bevacizimab and tyrosine kinase inhibitors [273, 274]. Moreover drugs already in wide clinical use for breast cancer such as tamoxifen and letrozole, while aimed at inhibiting the estrogen activity in breast tumor epithelial cells, have the dual benefit of acting on tumor-associated stroma as well. In conclusion recent efforts have been undertaken to identify and exploit potential drug targets associated specifically with CAFs and tumor-stroma paracrine signaling networks. And examining signaling interactions among the mammary epithelial cells and its associated stroma during normal development and tumorigenesis may provide critical insight to additional chemotherapeutic targets for future therapeutics.

While tumor-associated inflammatory cells were initially thought to represent the host response against tumors, evidence suggests that these cells may actually contribute to cancer development. **Macrophages** specifically play a key role in breast cancer, where they appear to be part of the pathogenesis of high-grade tumors. Tumor-associated macrophages (TAMs) produce factors that promote angiogenesis, remodel tissue and dampen the immune response to tumors. In detail, there are 2 types of macrophages named M1 and M2 and they are important because they express different features and function [275]. Given the tendency for TAMs to express the M2 phenotype [276] (which express relatively low IL-12 and high IL-10 levels) and contribute to tumor progression through the production of angiogenic factors, stromal breakdown factors and the suppression of adaptive immunity, targeting these cells could potentially have a significant therapeutic impact in breast cancer. TAMs are found in high-grade hormone receptor-negative breast cancers - aggressive tumor types for which new therapeutics are needed inhibiting their effects on angiogenesis and tissue remodeling, and interfering with their immunosuppressive properties by promoting a switch from the M2 to the M1 phenotype [277].

Metabolism

Metabolic activities in normal cells rely primarily on mitochondrial oxidative phosphorylation (OXPHOS) to generate ATP for energy. Unlike in normal cells, glycolysis is enhanced and OXPHOS capacity is reduced in various cancer cells [278]. It has long been believed that the glycolytic phenotype in cancer is due to a permanent impairment of mitochondrial OXPHOS, as proposed by Otto Warburg [279]. This view is challenged by recent investigations which find that the function of mitochondrial OXPHOS in most cancers is intact [280]. Aerobic glycolysis in many cancers is the combined result of various factors such as oncogenes, tumor suppressors, a hypoxic microenvironment, mtDNA mutations, genetic background and others. Understanding the features and complexity of the cancer energy metabolism will help to develop new approaches in early diagnosis and effectively target therapy of cancer. Cell proliferation as cancer cells, requires nutrients, energy, and biosynthetic activity to duplicate all macromolecular components during each passage through the cell cycle. It is therefore not surprising that metabolic activities in proliferating cells are fundamentally different from those in non-proliferating cells. Several pathways seems to be involved in supporting proliferation and tumorigenesis of diverse cell types including aerobic glycolysis, de novo lipid biosynthesis, the phosphatidylinositol 3-kinase (PI3K)/Akt/mTOR system and hypoxia-inducible factor 1 (HIF-1) [281] all of them considered interesting target for prevention and therapy. Moreover, recently observational studies have confirmed the evidence that impaired metabolism, obesity, hyperglycemia and hyperinsulinemia may have a role in cancer development, progression and prognosis, and actually diabetic and obese patients have increased cancer risk.

In detail, presence of overweight and/or the metabolic syndrome condition with visceral obesity, glucose intolerance, hyperinsulinemia and insulin resistance, have been strongly and repeatedly associated with BC recurrence and worse outcome after treatment [282]. This condition has become a worldwide health issue and it is now considered a central precursor for the development of most chronic diseases, including cardiovascular disease, diabetes and several types of common malignancies, including BC [283]. A meta-analysis of 43 studies found a HR of 1.33 (95% CI: 1.19-1.50) for BC-related mortality and a similar HR for all-cause mortality, when contrasting obese and non-obese patients with BC [284]. Hyperinsulinemia adversely affects prognosis in BC patients [285, 286] and is an independent risk factor for BC in healthy postmenopausal women, and can substantially explain the obesity-BC risk association [287]. Further, insulin can promote tumorigenesis *via* a direct effect on epithelial tissue, or indirectly by affecting the levels of other modulators, such as insulin-like growth factors, sex hormones and adipokines [288-290]. On the other hand, several studies found positive associations between high pretreatment insulin levels and poor prognosis. For example, in a recent study, those with high insulin levels had a two-fold worse distant disease-free survival (HR = 2.05; 95% CI: 1.16-3.62) and overall survival (HR = 2.57; 95% CI: 1.48-5.50) than other patients with BC [291]. Metformin an oral biguanide that inhibits hepatic gluconeogenesis and sensitizes insulin action at peripheral level has now been established as the drug of choice to reduce insulin resistance and improves glycemic control. Interest in this drug in the BC treatment setting reflects the recent convergence of several avenues of research. Exciting preclinical studies have demonstrated that metformin can inhibit the growth of BC cells [292-295]. More recently, a retrospective study [296] of patients who received neoadjuvant chemotherapy for BC showed that diabetic cancer patients receiving metformin during their neoadjuvant chemotherapy had a higher pathological complete response rate than diabetic patients not receiving metformin and non-diabetic patients (24% *vs* 8% *vs* 16%, respectively, p=0.02). Moreover, a recent pre-surgical, randomized, placebo-controlled, window of opportunity (WOP) clinical trial has shown the efficacy of metformin to reduce cell proliferation as measured by Ki-67 LI (now fully considered a standard surrogate biomarker to test the activity of candidate drugs) in BC cells particularly in metabolic unbalanced subjects treated before surgery [297.] This important study has shown that the effect of metformin on Ki-67 LI was modified by insulin resistance status (HOMA index), with a non-significant 10.5% decrease of BC proliferation in women with insulin resistance (HOMA>2.8). In additional analyses, similar modifications of metformin effects on Ki-67 LI by HOMA index were noted in women with luminal B tumors and in women who were overweight or obese, had abdominal obesity, had moderate alcohol intake, and had elevated CRP levels.

In conclusion increasing number of studies have associated with improved outcomes in cancer patients. These possible pleiotropic effects of metformin may establish metformin as a cancer prevention and treatment option.

Recently, the growing knowledge of the biologic heterogeneity of the disease has permitted to consider BC as a number of separate molecular pathological entities, to which therapy can be accordingly tailored. Furthermore, technological advances, particularly genomics and proteomics, have offered the possibility to improve treatment tailoring throughout the identification of novel targets for anticancer therapy. These molecules are implicated in several processes relevant to BC biology, such as signal transduction, cell cycle, apoptotic, pro-angiogenetic and metastatic pathways. In this field **miRNAs** are small, endogenous, non-coding RNAs that negatively regulate protein-coding mRNAs at the post-transcriptional level and in general it is estimated that in humans thousands of miRNAs are expressed and more than 700 miRNAs have been described to date. About 50% of annotated human miRNAs are detected in regions of fragile sites, which are associated with cancer. The available evidence has shown that miRNAs widely participate in the development or progression of many types of cancers, including breast cancer.

Researchers have recently shown that omics-based analyses of serum/plasma samples from high-risk individuals can accurately identify patients with early stage, asymptomatic disease [298, 299]. In particular, detection of extracellular microRNAs (EC-miRNAs) in body fluids is emerging as a promising approach for developing innovative, minimally invasive, cost-effective, diagnostic tests to be used as first-line screening procedures. miRNAs are short non-coding RNA molecules that are involved in the regulation of many cellular processes, including differentiation, proliferation and apoptosis [300, 301]. The expression of miRNAs is deregulated in tumors in a tissue and cancer-specific manner [302]. miRNAs have also been detected in body fluids due to their passive release from apoptotic cells or active release from cells in micro-vesicles or in complex with miRNA-binding proteins, which protect them from degradation [303-305]. Notably, fluctuations in ECmiRNAs have been associated with malignant and non-malignant diseases [306-308]. It is possible that tumor-associated EC-miRNA biomarkers are present in breast ductal fluid, which can be used to develop a sensitive and accurate molecular diagnostic test for breast cancer early detection. These fluids can be collected using non-invasive or mini-invasive procedures, such as ductal lavage and the Halo Breast Test that collects nipple aspirate fluid (NAF) [309]. Breast fluids offers advantages over serum as a source of breast cancer biomarkers as it is highly representative of the breast microenvironment and is likely to be enriched in biomarkers that signal subtle alterations in the breast during the very early phases of disease onset (*i.e.*, hyperplasia, atypical hyperplasia, ductal carcinoma *in situ*). Thus, ECmiRNAs could be excellent candidates for tumor markers that could be used in the diagnosis of early stage breast cancer.

USE OF BREAST BIOMARKERS IN RISK ASSESSMENT AND PREVENTION

The presence of biomarkers offers many opportunities in all aspects of risk assessment and chemoprevention of breast cancer. They can be used as a cancer risk marker for selecting cohorts for chemopreventive studies and their presence may predict response to mechanism-based intervention (surrogate endpoint biomarkers or SEBs). Moreover they may be molecular targets used for identifying new agents or optimizing lead agents. In addition, modulation of these biomarkers in early clinical studies is useful in determining the delivery of new drugs, biologically effective doses and their toxicity. Because many chemopreventive agents are likely to be used chronically in essentially healthy subjects, safety is critical. Thus biomarkers of potential toxicity could become very useful in evaluating candidate agents in preclinical development and in monitoring subjects in clinical trials (Fig. **3**).

At present these biomarkers are not yet used to monitor individual outcomes to prevention treatment but are commonly utilized in *Phase I prevention trials* for the purpose of dose findings and *Phase II trials* as preliminary evidence of the efficacy and toxicity profile. Eventual favorable modulation with acceptable side effect profile may then lead to a *Phase III trial* employing reduction in cancer incidence as the primary endpoint.

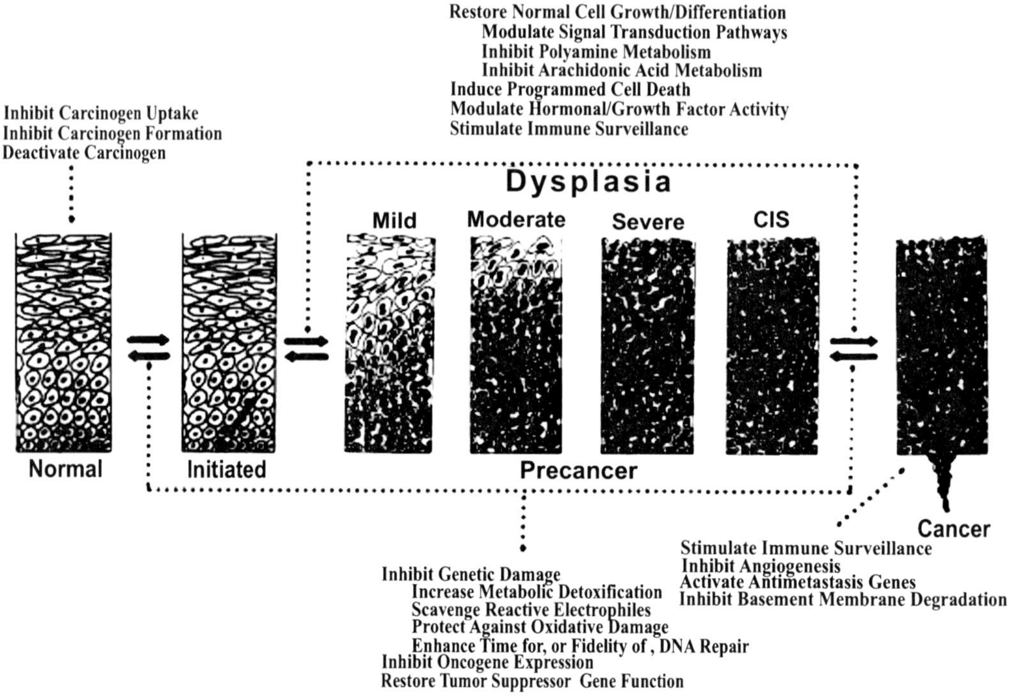

Fig. (3). Possible mechanisms of chemopreventive drugs.

Biomarkers for Risk Stratification

Biomarkers have the potential to further stratify risk prediction based on epidemiologic models and breast tissue morphology and could be used to improve discriminatory accuracy of ordinary risk prediction models. A number of biomarkers that are subject to modulation have been associated with breast cancer risk. For example, IEN and/or the presence of mammographic breast density are accepted at the moment as the two biomarkers with the highest reported relative risk. In an interesting prospective study performed by Fabian *et al.* [35] where immunocytochemical expression of ER, p53, EGFR and HER-2, obtained by RPFNA in high risk women was assessed, all the above-mentioned single markers were strongly predictive of cytologic atypia (and consequently improve the risk of cancer) and multiple marker expression of three of these biomarker set (HER-2 excluded) was strongly predictive of atypia in multivariable analysis. Moreover ER was the only single molecular marker predictive of cancer development. Cazzaniga *et al.* showed [208] that Ki-67 expression is associated with atypical cells and cell yield in a consecutive series of ductal lavage in high risk women suggesting the use of Ki-67 as a surrogate biomarker in early-phase of chemoprevention trials. Methylation-specific PCR to determine loss of expression of tumor suppressor genes is being utilized to help identify cancer in markedly atypical cytology specimens obtained by RPFNA or ductal lavage [213-216] and the possibility of determining whether it might identify proliferative disease likely to progress to cancer is under investigation.

Phase I Trial Models

The most popular phase I prevention model for dose findings is the *Pre-surgical model* where patients with a diagnostic core biopsy for intraductal neoplasia or a small invasive cancer are randomized to one of several doses of drug in the interval between the biopsy and surgical operation (generally 4-6 weeks). Remembering that the toxicity profile is generally well-known for most drugs being considered as potential prevention agents, it is necessary to bear in mind that even a minimal side effect might be unacceptable when a drug is administered to a healthy women for a long period. Thus the phase I prevention trials focus on establishing the lowest dose at which a drug modulates a risk and/or a mechanism of action biomarker. In detail, this type of trial could be considered separated into two independent phases with a first part (called Phase IA) (Fig. **4**) where the design is aimed at determining a dose effect on one or more bioactivity markers compared to a non randomized control and a second part (called Phase IB) where the dose selected in phase IA is tested for its reliability in modulating biomarkers over a 4-6 weeks interval compared to placebo (Fig. **4**).

Despite significant problems with these pre-surgical models (*i.e.*, difficulties of accrual, significant variations of biomarkers value in the different part of the lesion), these approaches showed good efficacy in affected women and could also be used as a first step to take advantage of the presence of these biomarkers in healthy high risk women (*i.e.*, when material recruited by NAF, ductal lavage or RPFNA expressing one of a combination of these biomarkers).

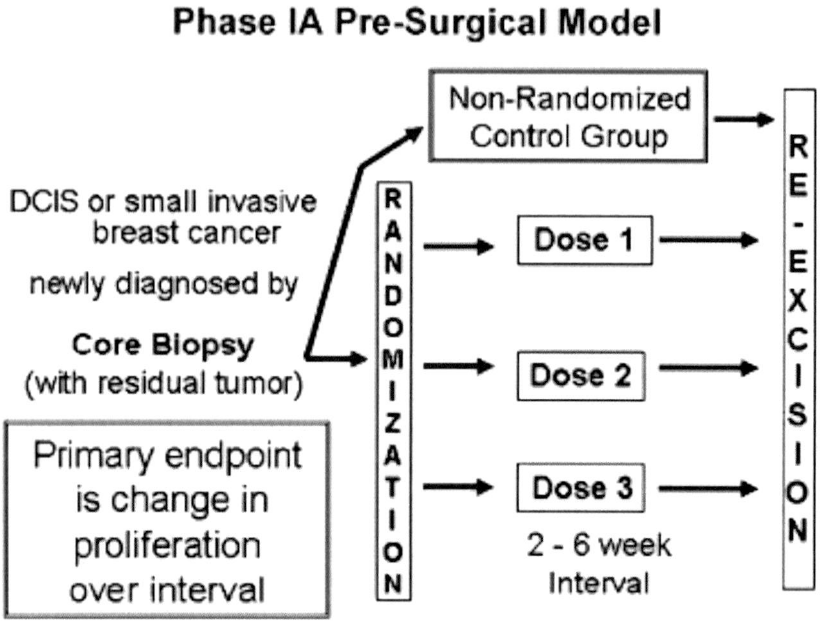

Fig. (4). Typical pre-surgical model phase IA biomarker chemoprevention trial. The dose selected in phase IA will be tested for its reliability in modulating biomarkers Phase IB trial over a 4-6 weeks interval compared to placebo. (Take from Fabian *et al.* Clin Cancer Res 2007).

Phase II Trial Models

Phase II trials are generally randomized, double blind, placebo-controlled studies in which high risk subjects are enrolled for 6-12 months where reversible risk biomarkers are sampled at baseline and at the conclusion of the trial period. Despite the placebo controlled, phase II trials are usually a single arm study because the effect of the agent on the primary endpoint biomarker is often uncertain or unknown. The kind of agent under investigation and the specific cohort of subjects used will dictate the choice of response biomarker. At present, breast intraepithelial neoplasia and their associated biomarkers (*i.e.*, ER and Ki67) are usually used as primary endpoints for these trials accompanied with serum biomarkers such as hormones and growth factors as a secondary endpoints. An example of phase II trial is explained in (Fig. **5**). Intervention showing favorable biomarker modulation with acceptable safety profile may then go on to a phase III trial employing cancer incidence as the primary endpoint.

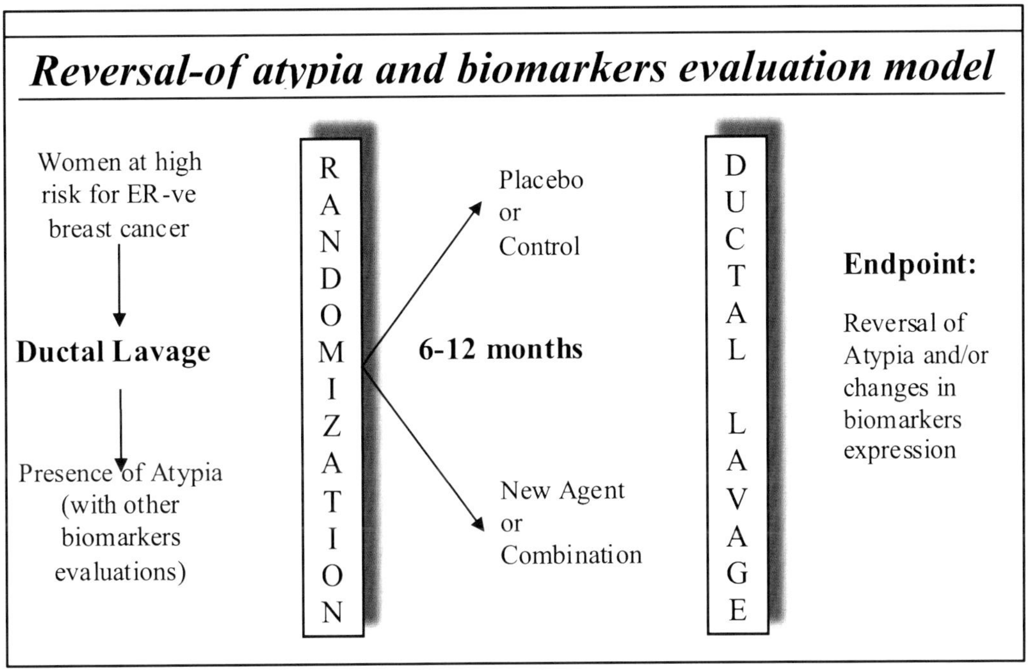

Fig. (5). Example of Phase II trial.

CONCLUSION

Breast cancer is a major cause of morbidity and mortality in women. Despite diagnostic and therapeutic innovation, there is still a lack of understanding about the natural history of the disease and its mechanisms which regulate the progression of carcinogenesis. The presence of several tumor-associated antigens called "biomarkers" that appear expressed during the different steps of this progression and the study of their characteristics, open up many opportunities to the refine risk profile (improving the accuracy of risk assessment usually confined, at present, to epidemiological models) in order to create a better and complete system of evaluation of the individual risk and improving our ability to harness this information for more targeted approaches to the prevention of breast disease.

Intraductal and transcutaneous approaches (NAF, ductal lavage, RPFNA and core biopsy) permit us to recruit adequate material from the mammary ductal system and contributes to a greater understanding of the tumor biology and the sophisticated mechanisms which regulate carcinogenesis.

Although some of these biomarkers, due to their role in the selection of patients likely to benefit for specific treatments and/or in prognosis, are ordinarily used in clinical practice (*i.e.*, ER, Ki67, Her-2), the importance of several others remains unknown and/or controversial and several of them are suggested for possible inclusion to ensure a high level of clinico-laboratory effectiveness. Novel findings, first of all a recognized biomarker of risk as the depurinating estrogen-DNA adducts, derived from gene expression analysis with genetic and epigenetic changes, will contribute to understanding the mechanisms that regulate the transformations which occur from the normal cell to cancer. Cancer chemoprevention, defined as treatment of carcinogenesis, is a prime field of intervention because these recent discoveries have provided us with a rich variety of potential targets for chemopreventive agents which might hopefully be able to reverse malignant tranformation. Ideally, one or a combination of chemopreventive agents should promote the differentiation of cells blocked in an undifferentiated state, inhibit cell replication and induce apoptosis but the first and essential requirement for a preventive method or agent is safety, as it is administered to healthy people who might never develop disease during their lifetime. Acceptability of adverse effects of preventive drugs is therefore lower than for therapeutic agents. The risk-benefits ratio of an agent with known adverse effects is optimized by the enrollment of individuals at high risk for the disease harnessing the presence of one or a combination of biomarkers. The time it takes to test new or usual chemopreventive agents could be shortened considerably if tools for morphological and molecular observation of breast cells were available for use in phase I and II prevention trials. Finally, the incorporation of tissue-based biomarkers, which reliably predict response, and their application to individuals who have been selected using better methods of risk assessment, could be an important tool for the short-term assessment of the benefits of chemoprevention strategies.

ACKNOWLEDGEMENTS

None declared.

CONFLICT OF INTEREST

The authors confirm that this chapter contents have no conflict of interest.

DISCLOSURE

The chapter submitted for the eBook Series entitled **"Advances in Cancer Drug Targets, Volume 2"** is an update of our article in **Current Cancer Drug Targets, Volume 9, Issue 4, 2009, pp. 482-499,** with additional text and references.

REFERENCES

[1] O'Shaughnessy JA. Kelloff GJ. Gordon GB, *et al.* Treatment and prevention of intraepithelial neoplasia: an important target for accelerated new agent development. Recommendations of the American Association of Cancer Research Task Force on the treatment and prevention of intraepithelial neoplasia. Clin Cancer Res 2002; 8; 314-346.

[2] Rockhill B, Spiegelman D, Byrne C, Hunter DJ, Colditz GA. Validation of the Gail model of breast cancer risk prediction and implications for chemoprevention. J Natl Cancer Inst 2001; 93; 358-366.

[3] Dua RS, Isacke CM, Gui GP. The intraductal approach to breast cancer biomarkers discovery. J Clin Oncol 2006; 24; 1209-1216.

[4] Locke I, Mitchell G, Eeles R. Ductal approaches to assessment and management of women at high risk for developing breast cancer. Breast Cancer Res 2004; 6; 75-81

[5] Janssens JP, Verlinden I, Gungor N, Raus J, Michiels L. Protein biomarkers for breast cancer prevention. Eur J Cancer Prev 2004; 13; 307-317.

[6] Wellings SR, Jensen HM, Marcum RG. An Atlas of subgross pathology of the human breast with special reference to possible precancerous lesions. J Natl Cancer Inst 1975; 55; 231-243.

[7] King EB, Chew KL, Petrakis NL, Ernster VL. Nipple aspirate cytology for the study of breast cancer precursor. J Natl Cancer Inst 1983; 71; 1115-1121.

[8] Fabian CJ, Kimler BF, Mayo MS, Khan SA. Breast-tissue sampling for risk assessment and prevention. Endocr Relat Cancer 2005; 12; 185-213.

[9] Proctor KA, Rowe LR, Bentz JS. Cytologic features of nipple aspirate fluid using an automated non-invasive collection device; a perspective observational study. BMC Womens Health 2005; 5; 10.

[10] Buehring GC, Letscher A, Mc Girr KM *et al.* Presence of epithelial cells in nipple aspirate fluid is associated with subsequent breast cancer: a 25-year prospective study. Breast Cancer Res Treat 2006; 98; 63-70.

[11] Dooley WC, Ljung BM, Veronesi U *et al.* Ductal lavage for detection of cellular atypia in women at high risk for breast cancer. J Natl Cancer Inst 2001; 93; 1624-1632.

[12] Khotari A, Beechey-Newman N, Kulkarni D. Breast duct-microendoscopy: a study of technique and a morphological classification of endo-luminal lesions. Breast 2006; 15; 363-369.

[13] Fabian CJ, Zalles C, Kamel S, Zeiger S, Simon C, Kimler BF. Breast cytology and biomarkers obtained by random fine needle aspiration: use in risk assessment and early chemoprevention trials. J Cell Biochem Suppl 1997; 28-29; 101-110.

[14] Kelloff GJ, Boone CW, Crowell JA *et al.* Risk biomarkers and current strategies for cancer chemoprevention. J Cell Biochem Suppl 1996; 25; 1-14.

[15] Renehan AG, Harvie M, Howell A. Insulin-like growth factor (IGF)-I, IGF binding protein-3, and breast cancer risk: eight years on. Endocr Relat Cancer 2006; 13; 273-278.
[16] Wu AH, Pike MC, Stram DO. Meta-analysis: dietary fat intake, serum estrogens levels and the risk of breast cancer. J Natl Cancer Inst 1999; 91; 529-534.
[17] Shaaban AM, Sloane JP, West CR, Foster CS. Breast cancer risk in usual ductal hyperplasia is defined by estrogen receptor α and Ki-67 expression. Am J Pathol 2002; 160; 597-604.
[18] Cavalieri E, Chakravarti D, Guttenplan J *et al.* Catechol estrogen quinones as initiators of breast and other human cancers: implications for biomarkers of susceptibility and cancer prevention. Biochim Biophys Acta 2006; 1766; 63-78.
[19] Endogenous Hormones and Breast Cancer Collaborative Group. Endogenous sex hormones and breast cancer in postmenopausal women: reanalysis of nine prospective studies. J Natl Cancer Inst 2002; 94; 606-616.
[20] Feigelson HS, Henderson BE. Estrogens and breast cancer. Carcinogenesis 1996; 17; 2279-2284.
[21] Mailander PC, Meza JL, Higginbotham S, Chakravarti D. Induction of A.T to G.C mutations by erroneous repair of depurinated DNA following estrogen treatment of the mammary gland of ACI rats. J Steroid Biochem Mol Biol 2006; 101; 204-215.
[22] Gaikwad NW, Yang L, Muti P *et al.* The molecular etiology of breast cancer: evidence from biomarkers of risk. Int J Cancer 2008; 122; 1949-1957.
[23] Tavassoli FA, Mammary intraepithelial neoplasia: a translational classification system for the intraductal epithelial proliferations. Breast 1997; 3; 48-58.
[24] Page DL, Dupont WD. Anatomic markers of human premalignancy and risk of breast cancer. Cancer 1990; 66; 1326-1335.
[25] Mitchell G, Antill YC, Murray W *et al.* Nipple aspiration and ductal lavage in women with germline BRCA1 or BRCA2 mutation. Breast Cancer Res 2005; 7; R1122-R1131.
[26] Dupont WD, Parl FF, Hartmann WH *et al.* Breast cancer risk associated with proliferative breast disease and atypical hyperplasia. Cancer 1993; 71; 1258-1265.
[27] Frykberg ER, Bland KI. Overview of the biology and management of ductal carcinoma in situ of the breast. Cancer 1994; 74; 350-361.
[28] Frykberg ER. Lobular carcinoma in situ of the breast. Breast J 1999; 5; 296-303.
[29] Degnim AC, Visscher DW, Berman HK *et al.* Stratification of breast cancer risk in women with atypia: a Mayo cohort study. J Clin Oncol 2007; 25; 2671-7.
[30] Tavassoli FA, Norris HJ. A comparison of the results of long-term follow-up for atypical intraductal hyperplasia and intraductal hyperplasia of the breast. Cancer 1990; 65; 518-529
[31] Hutchinson WB, Thomas DB, Hamlin WB, Roth GJ, Peterson AV, Williams B. Risk of breast cancer in women with benign breast disease. J Natl Cancer Inst 1980; 65; 13-20.
[32] Dupont WD, Page DL. Risk factors for breast cancer in women with breast proliferative disease. N Engl J Med 1985; 312; 146-151.
[33] Wrensch MR, Petrakis NL, King EB *et al.* Breast cancer incidence in women with abnormal cytology in nipple aspirates of breast fluid. Am J Epidemiol 1992; 135; 130-141.
[34] Wrensch MR, Petrakis NL, Miike R *et al.* Breast cancer risk in women with abnormal cytology in nipple aspirates of breast fluid. J Natl Cancer Inst 2001; 93; 1791-1798.
[35] Fabian CJ, Kimler BF, Zalles CM *et al.* Short-term breast cancer prediction by random periareolar fine-needle aspiration cytology and the Gail risk model. J Natl Cancer Inst 2000; 92; 1217-1227.

[36] Dupont WD, Page DL, Parl FF *et al.* Estrogen replacement therapy in women with a history of proliferative breast disease. Cancer 1999; 85; 1277-1283.

[37] Van Hoesel AQ, Sato Y, Elashoff DA *et al.* Assessment of DNA methylation status in early stages of breast cancer development. Br J Cancer 2013; 108; 2033-8.

[38] Agrawal A, Murphy RF, Agrawal DK. DNA methylation in breast and colorectal cancer. Mod Pathol 2007; 20; 711-721.

[39] Khan SA, Rogers MA, Khurana KK, Meguid MM, Numann PJ. Estrogen receptor expression in benign breast epithelium and breast cancer risk. J Natl Cancer Inst 1998; 90; 37-42.

[40] Lapidus RG, Ferguson AT, Ottaviano YL *et al.* Methylation of estrogen and progesterone receptor gene 5'CpG island correlates with lack of estrogen and progesterone receptor gene expression in breast tumor. Clin Cancer Res 1996; 2; 805-810.

[41] Kato S, Endoh H, Masuhiro Y *et al.* Activation of the estrogen receptor through phosphorylation by mitogen-activated protein kinase. Science 1995; 270; 1491-1494.

[42] Van Agthoven T, Timmermans M, Foekens JA, Dorssers LC, Henzen-Logmans SC. Differential expression of estrogen, progesterone and epidermal growth factors receptors in normal, benign and malignant human breast tissue using dual staining immunohistochemistry. Am J Pathol 1994; 144; 1238-1246.

[43] Stark A, Hulka BS, Joens S *et al.* HER-2/*neu* amplification in benign breast disease and the risk of subsequent breast cancer. J Clin Oncol 2000; 18; 267-274.

[44] Mommers EC, van Diest PJ, Leonhart AM, Meijer CJ, Baak JP. Expression of proliferation and apoptosis-related proteins in usual ductal hyperplasia of the breast. Hum. Pathol. 1998; 29; 1539-1545.

[45] Schimitt FC, Leal C, Lopes C. p53 protein expression and nuclear DNA content in breast intraductal proliferations. J Pathol 1995; 176; 233-241

[46] Rohan TE, Hartwick W, Miller AB, Kandel RA. Immunohistochemical detection of c-*erb*B-2 and p53 in benign breast disease and breast cancer risk. J Natl Cancer Inst 1998; 90; 1262-1269.

[47] O'Connell P, Pekkel V, Fukua SA, Osborne CK, Clark GM, Allred DC. Analysis of loss of heterozygosity in 399 premalignant breast lesions at 15 genetic loci. J Natl Cancer Inst 1998; 90; 697-703.

[48] Deroo BJ, Korach KS. Estrogen receptors and human disease. J Clin Invest 2006; 116; 561-570

[49] Soderqvist G. Effects of sex steroids on proliferation in normal mammary tissue. Ann Med 1998; 30; 511-524.

[50] Russo J, Russo IH. The role of estrogen in the initiation of breast cancer. J Steroid Biochem Mol Biol 2006; 102; 89-96

[51] Wilson CA, Slamon DJ. Evolving understanding of growth regulation in human breast cancer: interactions of the steroid and peptide growth regulatory pathways. J Natl Cancer Inst 2005; 97; 1238-1239.

[52] Cordera F, Jordan VC. Steroid receptors and their role in the biology and control of breast cancer growth. Semin Oncol 2006; 33; 631-641.

[53] Ricketts D, Turnbull L, Ryall G *et al.* Estrogen and progesterone receptors in the normal female breast. Cancer Res 1991; 51; 1817-1822.

[54] Shoker BS, Jarvis C, Clarke RB *et al.* Estrogen receptor-positive proliferating cells in the normal and precancerous breast. Am J Pathol 1999; 155; 1811-1815.

[55] Allred DC, Mohsin SK, Fuqua SA. Histological and biological evolution of human premalignant breast disease. Endocr Relat Cancer 2001; 8; 47-61.

[56] Barnes R, Masood S. Potential value of hormone receptor assay in carcinoma in situ of breast. Am J Clin Pathol 1990; 94; 533-537.

[57] Karayiannakis AJ, Bastounis EA, Chatzigianni EB *et al.* Immunohistochemical detection of oestrogen receptors in ductal carcinoma in situ of the breast. Eur J Surg Oncol 1996 ; 22 ; 578-582.

[58] Schmitt FC. Multistep progression from a oestrogen-dipendent growth towards an autonomous growth in breast carcinogenesis. Eur J Cancer 1995 ; 31 ; 2049-2052.

[59] Frasor J, Danes JM, Komm B *et al.* Profiling of estrogen up- and down-regulated gene expression in human breast cancer cells : insights into gene networks and pathways underlyng estrogenic control of proliferation and cell phenotype. Endocrinology 2003 ; 144 ; 4562-74

[60] Lin Y, Strom A, Vega VB *et al.* Discovery of estrogen receptor alpha target genes and response elements in breast tumor cells. Genome Biol 2004 ; 5 ; R66

[61] Alvarez-Baron CP, Jonsson P. Thomas C, Dryer SE, Williams C. The two-pore domain potassium channel KCNK5 : induction by estrogen receptor alpha and role in proliferation of breast cancer cells. Mol Endocrinol 2011 ; 25 ; 1326-36.

[62] Bhat-Nakshatri P, Wang G, Collins NR *et al.* Estradiol-regulated microRNAs control estradiol response in breast cancer cells. Nucleic Acid Res 2009 ; 37 ; 4850-61

[63] Blenkiron C, Goldstein LD, Thorne NP *et al.* MicroRNA expression profiling of human breast cancer identifies new marker of tumor phenotype. Genome Biol 2007 ; 8 ; R214

[64] Iorio MV, Ferracin M, Liu CG *et al.* MicroRNA gene expression deregulation in human breast cancer. Cancer Res 2005 ; 65 ; 7065-70

[65] Mattie MD, Benz CC, Bowers J *et al.* Optimized high-throughput microRNA expression profiling provides novel biomarker assessment of clinical prostate and breast cancer biopsies. Mol Cancer 2006 ; 5 ; 24.

[66] Katchy A, Edvardsson K, Aydogdu E, Williams C. Estradiol-activated estrogen receptor alpha does not regulate mature microRNA in T47D breast cancer cells. J Steroid Biochem Mol Biol 2012 ; 128 ; 145-53.

[67] Klinge GM. MiRNA and estrogen action. Trends Endocrinol Metab 2012; 23; 223-33.

[68] Yamagata K, Fujiyama S, Ito S *et al.* Maturation of microRNA is hormonally regulated by a nuclear receptor. Mol Cell 2009 ; 36 ; 340-7.

[69] Tontonoz P, Hu E, Spiegelman BM. Stimulation of adipogenesis in fibroblasts by PPARγ, a lipid-activated transcription factor. Cell 1994; 79; 1147-1156.

[70] Mueller E, Sarraf P, Tontonoz P *et al.* Terminal differentiation of human breast cancer through PPAR gamma. Mol Cell 1998; 1; 465-470.

[71] Crowe DL, Chandraratna RA. A retinoid X receptor (RXR)-selective retinoid reveals that RXR-α is potentially a therapeutic target in breast cancer cell lines, and that it potentiates antiproliferative and apoptotic responses to peroxisome proliferator-activated receptor ligands. Breast Cancer Res 2004; 6; R546-R555.

[72] Peters JM, Shah YM, Gonzales FJ. The role of peroxisome proliferator-activated receptors in carcinogenesis and chemoprevention. Nat Rev Cancer 2012; 12: 181-95.

[73] Elstner, E.; Muller, C.; Koshizuka, K.; Williamson, E. A.; Park, D.; Asou, H.; Shintaku, P.; Said, J. V.; Heber, D.; Koeffler, H. P. Ligand for PPAR gamma and retinoic acid receptor

inhibit growth and induce apoptosis of human breast cancer cells *in vitro* and in BNX mice. Proc. Natl. Acad. Sci. USA 1998, *95*, 8806-8811.

[74] Sertznig, P.; Seifert, M.; Tilgen, W.; Reichrath, J. Present concepts and future outlook: function of PPAR receptors for pathogenesis, progression, and therapy of cancer. J. Cell. Physiol. 2007, 212, 1-12.

[75] Suzuki T, Hayashi S, Miki Y *et al.* Peroxisome proliferator-activated receptor γ in human breast carcinoma: a modulator of estrogenic actions. Endocr Relat Cancer 2006; 13; 233-250.

[76] Fenner, M. H.; Elstner, E. PPAR gamma ligands for the treatments of breast cancer. Expert. Opin. Investig. Drugs 2005, 14, 557-568.

[77] Yee LD, Williams N, Wen P *et al.* Pilot study of rosiglitazone therapy in women with breast cancer: effects of short-term therapy on tumor tissue and serum markers. Clin Cancer Res 2007; 13; 246-252.

[78] Flageng MH, Moi LL, Dixon JM *et al.* Nuclear receptor co-activators and HER-2/neu are upregulated in breast cancer patients during neo-adjuvant treatment with aromatase inhibitors. Br J Cancer 2009; 101; 1253-60.

[79] Germain P, Chambon P, Eichele G *et al.* International Union of Pharmacology. LXIII. Retinoid X receptors. Pharmacol Rev 2006; 58; 760-772.

[80] Chambon P. A decade of molecular biology of retinoic acid receptors. FASEB J 1996; 10; 940-54.

[81] Simeone AM, Tari AM. How retinoids regulate breast cancer cell proliferation and apoptosis. Cell Mol Life Sci 2004; 61; 1475-84

[82] van der Leede BJ, Folkers GE, van den Brink CE, van der Saag PT, van der Burg B. Retinoic acid receptor α1 isoform is induced by estradiol and confers retinoic acid sensitivity in human breast cancer cells. Mol Cell Endocrinol 1995; 109; 77-86.

[83] Xu XC, Sneige N, Liu X *et al.* Progressive decrease in nuclear retinoic acid receptor β messenger RNA level during breast carcinogenesis. Cancer Res 1997; 57; 4992-4996.

[84] Veronesi U, De Palo G, Marubini E *et al.* Randomized trial of fenretinide to prevent second breast malignancy in women with early breast cancer. J Natl Cancer Inst 1999; 91; 1847-1856.

[85] Veronesi U, Mariani L, Decensi A *et al.* Fifteen-years results of a randomized phase III trial of fenretinide to prevent second breast cancer. Ann Oncol 2006; 17; 1065-1071.

[86] Decensi A, Bonanni B, Baglietto L *et al.* A two-by-two factorial trial comparing oral with transdermal estrogen therapy and fenretinide with placebo on breast cancer biomarkers. Clin Cancer Res 2004; 10; 4389-4397.

[87] Decensi A, Robertson C, Guerrieri-Gonzaga A *et al.* Randomized double-blind 2 x 2 trial of low-dose tamoxifen and fenretinide for breast cancer prevention in high-risk premenopausal women. J Clin Oncol 2009; 27; 3749-56

[88] Wu K, Zhang Y, Xu XC *et al.* The retinoid X receptor-selective retinoid, LGD1069, prevents the development of estrogen receptor-negative mammary tumors in transgenic mice. Cancer Res 2002; 62; 6376-80.

[89] Li Y, Zhang Y, Hill J *et al.* The rexinoid, bexarotene, prevents the development of premalignant lesions in MMTV-erbB2 mice. Br J Cancer 2008; 98; 1380-8

[90] Simpson ER, Mahendroo MS, Means GD *et al.* Aromatase cytochrome P450, the enzyme responsible for estrogen biosynthesis. Endocr Rev 1994; 15; 342-55

[91] Santen RJ, Brodie H, Simpson ER, Siiteri Pk, Brodie A. History of aromatase: saga of an important biological mediator and therapeutic target. Endocr Rev 2009; 30; 343-75

[92] Lu Q, Nakmura J, Savinov A *et al.* Expression of aromatase protein and messenger ribonucleic acid in tumor epithelial cells and evidence of functional significance of locally produced estrogen in human breast cancer. Endocrinol 1996; 137; 3061-3068.

[93] Mor G, Yue V, Santen RG *et al.* Macrofages, estrogens and the microinvironment of breast cancer. J Steroid Biochem Mol Biol 1998; 67; 403-411.

[94] Fisher B, Costantino JP, Wickerham DL *et al.* Tamoxifen for prevention of breast cancer: report of the National Surgical Adjuvant Breast and Bowel Project P-1 Study. J Natl Cancer Inst 1998; 90; 1371-1388.

[95] Cuzick, J. Aromatase inhibitors for breast cancer prevention. *J. Clin. Oncol.* 2005, *23*, 1636-1643.

[96] Mouridsen H, Sun Y, Gershanovich M *et al.* Superiority of letrozole to tamoxifen in the first-line treatment of advanced breast cancer: evidence from metastatic subgroups and a test of functional ability. Oncologist 2004; 9; 489-96

[97] Regan MM, Neven P, Giobbie-Hurder A *et al.* Assessment of letrozole and tamoxifen alone and in sequence for postmenopausal women with steroid hormone receptor-positive breast cancer: the BIG 1-98 randomised clinical trial at 8·1 years median follow-up. Lancet Oncol 2011; 12; 1101-8.

[98] Altundag, K.; Ibrahim, N. K. Aromatase inhibitors in breast cancer: An Overview. *Oncol.* 2006, *11*, 553-562.

[99] Autier, P.; Gandini, S. Vitamin D supplementation and total mortality: a meta-analysis of randomized controlled trials. *Arch. Intern. Med.* 2007, *167*, 1730-1737.

[100] Sperati F, Vici P, Maugeri-Sacca'M *et al.* Vitamin D supplementation and breast cancer prevention: a systematic review and meta-analysis of randomized clinical trials. PLoS One 2013; 8.

[101] Giovannucci E. The epidemiology of vitamin D and cancer incidence and mortality: a review. Cancer Causes Control 2005; 16; 83-95.

[102] Haussler MR, Whitfield GK, Haussler CA *et al.* The nuclear vitamin D receptor: biological and molecular regulatory properties revealed. J Bone Miner Res 1998; 13; 325-349.

[103] Friedrich M, Rafi L, Tilgen W, Schmidt W, Reichrath J. Expression of 1,25 dihydroxy vitamin D3 receptor in breast carcinoma. J Histochem Cytochem 1998; 46; 1335-1337.

[104] James SY, Mackay AG, Binderup L, Colston KW. Effects of a new synthetic vitamin D analogue, EB 1089, on the oestrogen-responsive growth of human breast cancer cells. J Endocrinol 1994; 141; 555-563.

[105] Dawson MI, Chao WR, Hobbs PD, Zhang XK. Effects of trans-retinoic acid, 9-cis retinoic acid, 1α,25-(dihydroxy)vitamin D3 and a novel apoptosis-inducing retinoid on breast cancer and endothelial cell growth. Cancer Lett 1998; 133; 1-8.

[106] Bouillon R, Eelen G, Verlinden L *et al.* Vitamin D and cancer. J Steroid Biochem Mol Biol 2006; 102; 156-162

[107] Colston KW, Hansen CM. Mechanisms implicated in the growth regulatory effects of vitamin D in breast cancer. Endocr Relat Cancer 2001; 9; 45-59.

[108] Mehta RG, Moriarty RM, Mehta RR *et al.* Prevention of preneoplastic mammary lesion development by a novel vitamin D analogue, 1 alpha-idroxyvitamin D5. J Natl Cancer Inst 1997; 89; 212-208.

[109] Welsh JE. Vitamin D and prevention of breast cancer. Acta Farmacol Sin 2007: 1373-1382.

[110] Freed-Pastor WA, Mizuno H, Zhao X *et al.* Mutant p53 disrupts mammary tissue architecture *via* the mevalonate pathway. Cell 2012; 148; 244-58.
[111] Chan KK, Oza AM, Siu LL. The statins as anticancer agents. Clin Cancer Res 2003; 9; 10-19.
[112] Coogan PF, Rosemberg L, Palmer JR *et al.* Statine use and the risk of breast and prostate cancer. Epidemiology 2002; 13; 262-267.
[113] Seeger H, Wallwiener D, Mueck AO. Statins can inhibit proliferation of human breast cancer cells *in vitro*. Exp Clin Endocrinol Diabetes 2003 ; 111 ; 47-48.
[114] Katz MS. Therapy insight: potential of statins for cancer chemoprevention and therapy. Nat Clin Pract Oncol 2005; 2; 82-89.
[115] Boudreau DM, Yu O, Miglioretti DL, Buist DS, Heckbert SR, Daling JR. Statin use and breast cancer risk in a large population-based setting. Cancer Epidemiol Biomarkers Prev 2007; 16; 416-421.
[116] Bonovas S, Filioussi K, Tsavaris N, Sitaras NM. Use of statins and breast cancer : A meta-analysis of seven randomized clinical trials and nine observational studies. J Clin Oncol 2005; 23; 8606-8612.
[117] Prowell TM, Stearns V, Trock B. Lipophilic statins merit additional study for breast cancer chemoprevention. J Clin Oncol 2006; 24; 2128-2129.
[118] Duncan RE, El-Sohemy A, Archer MC. Statins and cancer development. Cancer Epidemiol Biomarkers Prev 2005; 14; 1897-1898.
[119] Aaronson SA. Growth factors and cancer. Science 1991; 254; 1146-1153.
[120] Yarden Y. The EGFR family and its ligands in human cancer. Signalling mechanisms and therapeutic opportunities. Eur J Cancer 2001; 37(Suppl 4); S3-8.
[121] Knowlden JM, Hutcheson IR, Jones HE *et al.* Elevated levels of epidermal growth factor receptor/c-erbB2 heterodimers mediate an autocrine growth regulatory pathway in tamoxifen-resistant MCF-7 cells. Endocrinology 2003; 144; 1032-1044.
[122] Hudis CA. Trastuzumab—mechanism of action and use in clinical practice. N Engl J Med 2007; 357; 39-51.
[123] Harari PM, Allen GW, Bonner JA. Biology of interactions: antiepidermal growth factors receptors agents. J Clin Oncol 2007; 25; 4057-4065.
[124] Mendelsohn J, Beselga J. Status of epidermal growth factor receptor antagonists in the biology and treatment of cancer. J Clin Oncol 2003; 21; 2787-2799.
[125] Pavelic ZP, Pavelic L, Lower EE *et al.* C-myc, c-erbB2 and Ki-67 expression in normal breast tissue and in invasive and non invasive breast carcinoma. Cancer Res 1992; 52; 2597-2602.
[126] DiGiovanna, MP, Stern DF, Edgerton SM *et al.* Relationship of epidermal growth factor receptor expression to erbB-2 signaling activity and prognosis in breast cancer patients. J Clin Oncol 2005; 23; 1152-1160.
[127] Konecny G, Pauletti G, Pegram M *et al.* Quantitative association between HER-2/neu and steroid hormone receptors in hormone receptor-positive primary breast cancer. J Natl Cancer Inst 2003; 95; 142-153.
[128] Pritchard KI, Shepherd LE, O'Malley FP *et al.* HER-2 and responsiveness of breast cancer to adjuvant therapy. N Engl J Med 2006; 354; 2103-2111.
[129] Goldhirsh A, Ingle JN, Gelber RD *et al.* Thresholds for therapies: highlights of the St Gallen International Expert Consensus on the Primary Therapy of Early Breast Cancer Ann Oncol 2009; 20; 1319-1329.

[130] Vogel CL, Cobleigh MA, Tripathy D *et al.* Efficacy and safety of trastuzumab as a single agent in first-line treatment of HER2-overexpressing metastatic breast cancer. J Clin Oncol. 2002; 20(3): 719-726.

[131] Smith I, Procter M, Gelber RD *et al.* 2-year follow-up of trastuzumab after adjuvant chemotherapy in HER2-positive breast cancer: a randomised controlled trial. Lancet. 2007; 369(9555): 29-36.

[132] Decensi A, Puntoni M, Pruneri G *et al.* Lapatinib activity in premalignant lesions and HER-2-positive cancer of the breast in a randomized, placebo-controlled presurgical trial. Cancer Prev Res (Phila) 2011; 4; 1181-9,

[133] Sheen YY, Kim MJ, Park SA, Park SY, Nam JS. Targeting the Transforming Growth Factor-β Signaling in Cancer Therapy. Biomol Ther 2013; 21; 323-31.

[134] Wakefield LM, Piek E, Bottinger EP. TGF-beta signaling in mammary gland development and tumorigenesis. J Mammary Gland Biol Neoplasia 2001; 6; 67-82.

[135] Dumont L, Arteaga CL. Transforming growth factor-beta and breast cancer: tumor promoting effects of transforming growth factor-beta. Breast Cancer Res, 2000; 2; 125-132.

[136] Donovan J, Slingerland J. Transforming growth factor-beta and breast cancer: Cell cycle arrest by transforming growth factor-beta and its disruption in cancer. Breast Cancer Res 2000; 2; 116-124.

[137] Barcellos-Hoff MH, Ewan KB. Transforming growth factor-beta and breast cancer. Mammary gland development. Breast Cancer Res 2000; 2; 92-99.

[138] Ghellal A, LiC, Hayes M, Byrne M, Bundred N, Kumar S. Prognostic significance of TGF beta 1 and TGF beta 3 in human breast carcinoma. Anticancer Res 2000; 20; 4413-4418.

[139] Buck MB, Knabbe C. TGF-beta signaling and breast cancer. Ann N Y Acad Sci 2006; 1089; 119-126.

[140] Sachdev D, Yee D. The IGF system and breast cancer. Endocr. Relat. Cancer 2001; 8; 197-209.

[141] Schernhammer ES, Holly JM, Pollak MN, Hankinson SE. Circulating levels of insulin-like growth factors, their binding proteins and breast cancer risk. Cancer Epidemiol Biomarkers Prev 2005; 14; 699-704.

[142] Fletcher O, Gibson L, Johnson N *et al.* Polymorphisms and circulating level of insulin-like growth factor system and risk of breast cancer: a systematic review. Cancer Epidemiol Biomarkers Prev *2005*; 14; 2-19.

[143] Renehan AG, Egger M, Minder C, O'Dwyer ST, Shalet SM, Zwahlem M. IGF-I, IGF binding protein-3 and breast cancer risk: comparison of 3 meta-analyses. Int J Cancer 2005; 115; 1006-1007.

[144] Decensi A, Robertson C, Ballardini B *et al.* Effect of tamoxifen on lipoprotein(a) and insulin-like growth factor-I (IGF-I) in healthy women. Eur J Cancer 1999 : 35 ; 596-600.

[145] Bonanni B, Johansson H, Gandini S *et al.* Effect of low dose tamoxifen on the insulin-like growth factor system in healthy women. Breast Cancer Res Treat 2001; 69; 21-27.

[146] Eng-Wong J, Hursting SD, Venzon D, Perkins SN, Zujewski JA. Effect of raloxifene on insulin-like growth factor-I, insulin-like growth factor binding protein-3, and leptin in premenopausal women at high risk for developing breast cancer. Cancer Epidemiol. Biomarkers Prev 2003; 12; 1468-1473.

[147] Decensi A, Johansson H, Miceli R *et al.* Long-term effects of fenretinide, a retinoic acid derivative, on the insulin-like growth factor system in women with early breast cancer. Cancer Epidemiol Biomarkers Prev 2001; 10; 1047-1053.

[148] Jin M, Wang J, Buck E, Mulvihill MJ. Small-molecule ATP-competitive dual IGF-1R and insulin receptor inhibitors: structural insights, chemical diversity and molecular evolution. Fut Med Chem 2012; 4; 315-28

[149] Beevers CS, Li F, Liu L, Huang S. Curcumin inhibits the mammalian target of rapamycin-mediated signaling pathways in cancer cells. Int J Cancer 2006; 119; 757-764.

[150] Chen W, Wong MS. Genistein enhances insulin-like growth factor signaling pathway in human breast cancer (MCF-7) cells. J Clin Endocrinol Metab 2004; 89; 2351-2359.

[151] Khan N, Afaq F, Saleem M, Ahmad N, Mukhtar H. Targeting multiple signaling pathways by green tea polyphenol(-)-epigallocatechin-3-gallate. Cancer Res 2006; 66; 2500-2505.

[152] Vyas S, Asmerom Y, De Leon DD. Rosveratrol regulates insulin-like growth factor-II in breast cancer cells. Endocrinology 2005; 146; 4224-4233.

[153] Karas M, Amir H, Fishman D. Lycopene interferes with cell cycle progression and insulin-like growth factor I signaling in cancer cells. Nutr Cancer 2000; 36; 101-111.

[154] Shottenfeld D, Beebe-Donk J. Chronic inflammation: a common an important factor in the pathogenesis of neoplasia. CA Cancer J Clin 2006; 56; 69-83.

[155] Khuder SA, Mutgi AB. Breast cancer and NSAID use: a meta-analysis. Br J Cancer 2001; 84; 1188-92

[156] Sharpe CR, Collet JP, McNutt M, Belzile E, Boivin JF, Hanley JA. Nested case-control study of the effects of non-steroidal anti-inflammatory drugs on breast cancer risk and stage. Br J Cancer 2000; 83; 112-20.

[157] Hoellen F, Kelling K, Dittmer C, Diedrich K, Friedrich M, Thill M. Impact of cyclooxygenase-2 in breast cancer. Anticancer Res 2011; 31; 4359-67.

[158] Harris RE, Namboodiri KK, Farrar WB *et al.* Nonsteroidal antiinflammatory drugs and breast cancer. Epidemiology 1996; 7; 203-5.

[159] Harris RE, Beebe-Donk J, Alshafie GA. Reduction in the risk of human breast cancer by selective cyclooxygenase-2 (COX-2) inhibitors. BMC Cancer 2006; 6; 27-31.

[160] Half E, Tang XM, Gwyn K, Sahin A, Wathen K, Sinicrope FA. Cyclooxygenase-2 expression in human breast cancers and adjacent ductal carcinoma in situ. Cancer Res 2002; 62; 1676-81.

[161] Singh-Ranger G, Salhab M, Mokbel K *et al.* The role of cyclooxygenase-2 in breast cancer: review. Breast Cancer Res Treat 2008; 109; 189-98.

[162] Watanabe O, Shimizu T, Imamura H *et al.* Expression of cyclooxygenase-2 in malignant and benign breast tumors. Anticancer Res 2003; 23; 3215-21.

[163] Perrone G, Santini D, Vincenzi B *et al.* COX-2 expression in DCIS: correlation with VEGF, HER-2/neu, prognostic molecular markers and clinicopathological features. Hystopathology 2005; 46; 561-8.

[164] Glover JA Hughes CM, Cantwell MM, Murray LJ, A systematic review to establish the frequency of cyclooxygenase-2 expression in normal breast epithelium, ductal carcinoma in situ, microinvasive carcinoma of the breast and invasive breast cancer. Br J Cancer 2011; 105; 13-7.

[165] Brennan ME, Turner RM, Ciatto S *et al.* Ductal carcinoma in situ at core-needle biopsy: meta-analysis of underestimation and predictors of invasive breast cancer. Radiology 2011; 260; 119-28.

[166] Zhao YS, Zhu S, Li XW *et al.* Association between NSAIDs use and breast cancer risk: a systematic review and meta-analysis. Breast Cancer Res Treat 2009; 17; 141-50.

[167] Rothwell PM, Fowkes FG, Belch JF, Ogawa H, Warlow CP, Meade TW. Effect of daily aspirin on long-term risk of death due to cancer: analysis of individual patient data from randomised trials. Lancet 2011; 377; 31-41.

[168] Duffy MJ, Maguire TM, Hill A, McDermott E, O'Higgins N. Metalloproteinases: role in breast carcinogenesis, invasion and metastasis. Breast Cancer Res 2000; 252-257.

[169] Cheng CW, Yu JC, Wang HW *et al.* The clinical implications of MMP-11 and CK-20 expression in human breast cancer. Clin Chim Acta 2010; 411; 234-41

[170] Jiang WG, Davies G, Martin TA *et al.* Expression of membrane type-1 matrix metalloproteinase, MT1-MMP in human breast cancer and its impact on invasiveness of breast cancer cells. Int J Mol Med 2006; 17; 583-90.

[171] Kohrmann A, Kammerer U, Kapp M, Dietl J, Anacker J. Expression of matrix metalloproteinases (MMPs) in primary human breast cancer and breast cancer cell lines: New findings and review of the literature. BMC Cancer 2009; 9; 188

[172] Somiari SB, Somiari RI, Heckman CM *et al.* Circulating MMP2 and MMP9 in breast cancer -- potential role in classification of patients into low risk, high risk, benign disease and breast cancer categories. Int J Cancer 2006; 119; 1403-11.

[173] Stankovic S, Konjevic G, Gopcevic K, Jovic V, Inic M, Jurisic V. Activity of MMP-2 and MMP-9 in sera of breast cancer patients. Pathol Res Pract 2010; 206; 241-7

[174] Zhao YG, Xiao AZ, Ni J, Man YG, Sang QX. Expression of matrix metalloproteinase-26 in multiple human cancer tissues and smooth muscle cells. Ai Zheng 2009; 28; 1168-75.

[175] McGowan PM, Duffy MJ. Matrix metalloproteinase expression and outcome in patients with breast cancer: analysis of a published database. Ann Oncol 2008; 19; 1566-72.

[176] Beeghly-Fadiel A, Shu XO, Long J *et al.* Genetic polymorphisms in the MMP-7 gene and breast cancer survival. Int J Cancer 2009; 124; 208-14

[177] Savinov AY, Remacle AG, Golubkov VS *et al.* Matrix metalloproteinase 26 proteolysis of the NH2-terminal domain of the estrogen receptor beta correlates with the survival of breast cancer patients. Cancer Res 2006; 66; 2716-24.

[178] Brown PD. Matrix metalloproteinase inhibitors. Breast Cancer Res Treat 1998; 52; 125-136.

[179] Talbot DC, Brown PD. Experimental and clinical studies of the use of matrix metalloproteinase inhibitors for the treatment of cancer. Eur J Cancer 1996 ; 32 ; 2528-2533.

[180] Reed, JC. Dysregulation of apoptosis in cancer. J Clin Oncol 1999; 17; 2941-2953.

[181] Altieri DC. Survivin, versatile modulation of cell division and apoptosis. Oncogene 2003; 22; 8581-8589.

[182] Ambrosini G. Adida C. Altieri DC. A noble anti-apoptotic gene, survivin, is expressed in cancer and lymphoma. Nat. Med 1997; 3; 917-921.

[183] Song J, Su H, Zhou YY, Guo LL. Prognostic value of survivin expression in breast cancer patients: a meta-analysis. Tumour Biol 2013; 34; 2053-62.

[184] Hayes DF. Markers of increased risk for failure of adjuvant therapies. The Breast 2003; 12; 543-549.

[185] Blanc-Brude OP. Mesri M. Wall NR, Plescia J, Dohi T, Altieri DC. Therapeutic targeting of the survivin pathway in cancer: initiation of mithocondrial apoptosis and suppression of tumor-associated angiogenesis. Clin Cancer Res 2003; 9; 2683-2692.

[186] Wall NR, O'Connor DS, Plescia J, Pommier Y, Altieri DC. Suppression of survivin phosphorylation on Thr34 by flavopiridol enhances tumor cell apoptosis. Cancer Res 2003; 63; 230-235.

[187] Borresen-Dale AL. TP53 and breast cancer. Hum Mutat 2003; 21; 292-300.

[188] Turner N, Moretti E, Siclari O *et al.* Targeting triple negative breast cancer: is p53 the answer? Cancer Treat Rev 2013; 39; 541-50.

[189] Hartmann A, Blaszyk H, Kovach JS, Sommer SS. The molecular epidemiology of p53 gene mutation in human breast cancer. Trends Genet 1997; 13; 27-33.

[190] Elledge RM, Allred DC. Prognostic and predictive value of p53 and p21 in breast cancer. Breast Cancer Res Treat 1998; 52; 79-98.

[191] Pharoah P, Day NE, Caldas C. Somatic mutation in the p53 gene and prognosis in breast cancer. A meta-analysis. Br J Cancer 1999; 80; 968-973.

[192] Millikan R, Hulka B, Thor A *et al.* P53 mutations in benign breast tissue. J Clin Oncol 1995; 13; 2293-2300.

[193] O'Conell P, Pekkel V, Fuqua S, Osborne CK, Allred DC. Molecular genetic studies of early breast cancer evolution. Breast Cancer Res Treat 1994; 32; 5-12.

[194] Koutselini H, Malliri A, Field JK, Spandidos DA. P53 expression in cytologic specimens from benign and malignant breast lesions. Anticancer Res 1991; 11; 1415-1419.

[195] Rohan TE, Li SQ, Hartwick R, Kandel RA. P53 alterations and protein accumulation in benign breast tissue and breast cancer risk: A cohort study. Cancer Epidemiol Biomarkers Prev 2006; 15; 1316-1323.

[196] Tsuji N, Furuse K, Asanuma K *et al.* Mutations of p53 gene and loss of heterozygosity at chromosome 17p13.1 are associated with increased survivin expression in breast cancer. Breast Cancer Res Treat 2004; 87; 32-31.

[197] Sangrajrang S, Arpornwirat W, Cheirsilpa A *et al.* Serum p53 antibodies in correlation to other biological parameters of breast cancer. Cancer Detect Prev 2003; 27; 182-186.

[198] Sivaramen L, Conneely OM, Medina D, O'Malley BW. P53 is a potential mediator of pregnancy and hormone-induced resistence to mammary carcinogenesis. Proc Natl Acad Sci USA 2001; 98; 12379-12384.

[199] Courtney KD, Corcoran RB, Engelman JA. The PI3K pathway asdrug target in human cancer. J Clin Oncol 2010; 28; 1075-83.

[200] Baselga J, Campone M, Piccart M, *et al.* Everolimus inpostmenopausal hormone-receptor-positive advanced breast cancer. N Engl JMed 2012; 366; 520-9.

[201] Holm K, Hegardt C, Staaf J, *et al.* Molecular subtypes ofbreast cancer are associated with characteristic DNA methylation patterns. Breast Cancer Res 2010; 12; R36.

[202] Elsheikh SE, Green AR, Rakha EA, *et al.* Global histone modificationsinbreast cancer correlate with tumor phenotypes, prognostic factors, and patient outcome. Cancer Res 2009; 69; 3802-9.

[203] Fong PC, Boss DS, Yap TA, *et al.* Inhibition ofpoly(ADP-ribose)polymerase in tumors from BRCA mutation carriers. N Engl JMed 2009; 361; 123-34.

[204] Tutt A, Robson M, Garber J, *et al.* Phase IItrial ofthe oral PARP inhibitor olaparib (AZD2281) inBRCA-deficientadvanced breast cancer. J Clin Oncol 2009; 27. Abstr CRA501: 18s.

[205] Selim AG, El-Hayat G, Wells CA. Expression of c-erbB2, p53, Bcl-2, Bax, c-myc and Ki-67 in apocrine metaplasia and apocrine change with sclerosing adenosis of the breast. Virchows Arch 2002; 441; 449-455.

[206] De Azambuja E, Cardoso F, De Castro Jr G *et al.* Ki-67 as prognostic marker in early breast cancer: a meta-analysis of published studies involving 12155 patients. Br J Cancer 2007; 96; 1504-1513.

[207] Santisteban M, Reynolds C, Barr Fritcher EG *et al.* Ki67: a time-varying biomarker of risk of breast cancer in atypical hyperplasia. Breast Cancer Res Treat 2010; 121; 431-7

[208] Cazzaniga M, Severi G, Casadio C, Chiapparini C, Veronesi U, Decensi A. Atypia and Ki-67 expression from ductal lavage in women at different risk for breast cancer. Cancer Epidemiol Biomarkers Prev 2006; 15; 1311-1315.

[209] Bhandare D, Bryk M, Nayar N. Effect of tamoxifen on estrogen-related biomarkers in ductal lavage samples. A study on follow-up lavages. Breast Cancer Res Treat 2004; 88; S158.

[210] Dowsett M, Smith IE, Ebbs SR *et al.* IMPACT Trialist. Short-term changes in Ki-67 during neoadjuvant therapy of primary breast cancer with anastrazole or tamoxifen alone or combine correlated with recurrence-free survival. Clin Cancer Res 2005; 11; 951 s-8s.

[211] Decensi A, Robertson C, Viale G *et al.* A randomized trial of low-dose tamoxifen on breast cancer proliferation and blood estrogenic biomarkers. J Natl Cancer Inst 2003; 95; 779-790.

[212] Widschwendter M, Jones PA. DNA methylation and breast carcinogenesis. Oncogene 2002; 21; 5462-5482.

[213] Euhus DM, Bu D, Milchgrub S *et al.* DNA methylation in benign breast epithelium in relation to age and breast cancer risk. Cancer Epidemol Biomarkers Prev 2008; 17: 1051-9

[214] Evron E, Dooley WC, Umbricht CB *et al.* Detection of breast cancer cells in ductal lavage fluid by methylation-specific PCR. Lancet 2001; 357; 1335-1336.

[215] Krassenstein R, Sauter E, Dulaimi E, *et al.* Detection of breast cancer in nipple aspirate fluid by CpG island hypermethylation. Clin. Cancer Res 2004; 10; 28-32.

[216] Locke I, Kote-Jarai Z, Fackler MJ *et al.* Gene promoter hypermethylation in ductal lavage fluid from healthy BRCA gene mutation carriers and mutation-negative controls. Breast Cancer Res 2007; 9; R20.

[217] Lewis CM, Cler LR, Bu DW *et al.* Promoter hypermethylation in benign breast epithelium in relation to predicted breast cancer risk. Clin Cancer Res 2005; 11; 166-172.

[218] Timmermann S, Lehrmann H, Polesskaya A, Harel-Bellan A. Histone acetylation and disease. Cell Mol Life Sci 2001; 58; 728-736.

[219] Wang C, Fu M, Mani S, Wadler S, Senderowicz AM, Pestell RG. Histone acetylation and the cell-cycle in cancer. Front Biosci 2001; 6; 610-629.

[220] Jones PA, Baylin SB. The fundamental role of epigenetic events in cancer. Nat Rev Genet 2002; 3; 415-28.

[221] Prince HM, Bishton MJ, Harrison SJ. Clinical studies of histone deacetylase inhibitors. Clin Cancer Res. 2009; 15; 3958-69.

[222] Marks PA, Richon VM, Miller T, Kelly WK. Histone deacetylase inhibitors. Adv Cancer Res 2004; 91; 137-168.

[223] Said TK, Moraes RC, Sinha R, Medina D. Mechanisms of suberoylanilide hydroxamic acid inhibition of mammary cell growth. Breast Cancer Res. 2001; 3; 122-33.

[224] Munster PN, Troso-Sandoval T, Rosen N, Rifkind R, Marks PA, Richon VM. The histone deacetylase inhibitor suberoylanilide hydroxamic acid induces differentiation of human breast cancer cells. Cancer Res 2001; 61; 8492-7.

[225] Sabnis GJ, Goloubeva O, Chumsri S, Nguyen N, Sukumar S, Brodie AM. Functional activation of the estrogen receptor-alpha and aromatase by the HDAC inhibitor entinostat sensitizes ER-negative tumors to letrozole. Cancer Res 2011; 71; 1893-903.

[226] Keen JC, Yan L, Mack KM, *et al.* A novel histone deacetylase inhibitor, scriptaid, enhances expression of functional estrogen receptor alpha (ER) in ER negative human breast cancer cells in combination with 5-aza 2′-deoxycytidine. Breast Cancer Res Treat. 2003; 81; 177-86.

[227] Yang X, Phillips DL, Ferguson AT, Nelson WG, Herman JG, Davidson NE. Synergistic activation of functional estrogen receptor (ER)-alpha by DNA methyltransferase and histone deacetylase inhibition in human ER-alpha-negative breast cancer cells. Cancer Res. 2001; 61; 7025-9.

[228] Fan J, Yin WJ, Lu JS, *et al.* ER alpha negative breast cancer cells restore response to endocrine therapy by combination treatment with both HDAC inhibitor and DNMT inhibitor. J Cancer Res Clin Oncol. 2008; 134; 883-90.

[229] Raffoux E, Cras A, Recher C, *et al.* Phase 2 clinical trial of 5-azacitidine, valproic acid, and all-trans retinoic acid in patients with high-risk acute myeloid leukemia or myelodysplastic syndrome. Oncotarget. 2010; 1; 34-42.

[230] http://clinicaltrials.gov/ct2/show/NCT00258349term=swaby&rank=2 [Acccessed on: February13th, 2012].

[231] http://clinicaltrials.gov/ct2/show/NCT01118975term=vorinostat+and+breast+cancer&rank=2 [Acccessed on: February13th, 2012].

[232] Gore SD, Baylin S, Sugar E, *et al.* Combined DNA methyltransferase and histone deacetylase inhibition in the treatment of myeloid neoplasms. Cancer Res. 2006; 66; 6361-9.

[233] Juergens RA, Wrangle J, Vendetti FP, *et al.* Combination epigenetic therapy has efficacy in patients with refractory advanced non-small cell lung cancer. Cancer Discovery. 2011; 1(7); 598-607.

[234] Miller BJ, Wang D, Krahe R, Wright FA. Pooled analysis of loss of heterozygosity in breast cancer: a genome scan provides comparative evidence for multiple tumor suppressors and identifies novel candidated regions. Am J Hum Genet 2003; 73; 748-767.

[235] Hedenfalk I, Duggan D, Chen Y, *et al.* Gene-expression profiles in hereditary breast cancer. N Engl J Med 344; 539-548.

[236] Okada S, Tokunaga E, Kitao H *et al.* Loss of heterozygosity at BRCA1 locus is significantly associated with aggressiveness and poor prognosis in breast cancer. Ann Sur Oncol 2012; 19; 1499-507.

[237] Cavalli LR, Singh B, Isaacs C, Dickson RB, Haddad BR. Loss of heterozygosity in normal breast epithelial tissue and benign breast lesions in BRCA1-2 carriers in breast cancer. Cancer Genet Cytogenet 2004; 149; 38-43.

[238] Isaacs C, Cavalli LR, Cohen Y *et al.* Detection of LOH and mitochondrial DNA alterations in ductal lavage and nipple aspirate fluids from high-risk patients. Breast Cancer Res Treat 2004; 84; 99-105.

[239] Locke I, Kote-Jarai Z, Bancroft E, *et al.* Loss of heterozygosity at the BRCA1 and BRCA2 loci detected in ductal lavage fluid from BRCA gene mutation carriers and controls. Cancer Epidemiol Biomarkers Prev 2006; 15; 1399-1402.

[240] Yonekura Y, Yamamoto D, Okugawa H, Tanaka K, Kamiyama Y. Loss of heterozygosity in ductal lavage for breast tumor and the contalateral breast. Oncol Rep 2005; 13; 739-743.

[241] Peng S, Lü B, Ruan W, Zhu Y, Sheng H, Lai M. Genetic polymorphisms and breast cancer risk: evidence from meta-analyses, pooled analyses, and genome-wide association studies. Breast Cancer Res Treat 2011; 127; 309-24
[242] Coughlin, S. S.; Piper, M. Genetic polymorphisms and risk of breast cancer. *Cancer Epidemiol. Biomarkers Prev.* 1999, *8*, 1023-1032.
[243] Zeng Z, Liu Y, Liu Z *et al.* CYP2D6 polymorphisms influence tamoxifen treatment outcomes in breast cancer patients: a meta-analysis. Cancer Chemother Pharmacol 2013; 72; 287-303.
[244] Krupp G, Klapper W, Parwaresch R. Cell proliferation, carcinogenesis and diverse mechanisms of telomerase regulation. Cell Mol Life Sci 2000; 57; 464-486.
[245] Shay JW. Meeting report: the role of telomeres and telomerase in cancer. Cancer Res 2005; 65; 3513-3517.
[246] Poremba C, Bocker W, Willenbring H *et al.* Telomerase activity in human proliferative breast lesions. Int J Oncol 1998; 12; 641-648.
[247] Hiyama E, Gollahon L, Kataoka T, *et al.* Telomerase activity inhuman breast tumors. J Natl Cancer Inst 1996; 88; 116-122.
[248] Meeker MA, Argani, P. Telomere shortening occurs early during breast tumorigenesis: a cause of chromosome destabilization underlying malignant transformation. J Mammary Gland Biol Neoplasia 200; 9; 285-296.
[249] Winnikow EP, Medeiros LR, Edelweiss MI *et al.* Accuracy of telomerase in estimating breast cancer risk: a systematic review and meta-analysis. Breast 2012; 21; 1-7.
[250] Rha SY, Park KH, Kim TS *et al.* Changes of telomerase and telomere lengths in paired normal and cancer tissues of breast. Int J Oncol 1999; 15; 839-845.
[251] Mokbel K. The role of telomerase in breast cancer. Eur J Surg Oncol 2000; 26; 509-514.
[252] Melana SM, Holland JF, Pogo BG. Inhibition of cell growth and telomerase activity of breast cancer cells *in vitro* by 3'-azido-3'-deoxythymidine. Clin Cancer Res 1998; 4; 693-696.
[253] White LK, Wright WE, Shay JW. Telomerase inhibitors. Trends Biotechnol 2001; 19; 114-120.
[254] Cerone MA, Londoño-Vallejo JA, Autexier C. Telomerase inhibition enhances the response to anticancer drug treatment in human breast cancer cells. Mol Cancer Ther 2006; 5; 1669-75.
[255] Herbert BS, Wright AC, Passons CM *et al.* Effects of chemopreventive and antitelomerase agents on the spontaneous immortalization of breast epithelial cells. J Natl Cancer Inst 2001; 93; 39-45.
[256] Malumbres M, Harlow E, Hunt T *et al.* Cyclin-dependent kinases: a family portrait. Nat Cell Biol 2009; 11; 1275-1276.
[257] Lim S, Kaldis P: Cdks, cyclins and CKIs: roles beyond cell cycle regulation. Development 2013; 140; 3079-3093.
[258] Grana X, Reddy EP. Cell cycle control in mammalian cells: role of cyclins, cyclins dependent kinases (CDKs), growth suppressor genes and cyclins-dependent kinase inhibitors (CDIs). Oncogene 1995; 11; 211-219.
[259] Nielsen NH, Arnelov C, Emdin SO, Landberg G. Cyclin E overexpression, a negative prognostic factor in breast cancer with strong correlation to oestrogen receptor status. Br J Cancer 1996; 74; 874-880.

[260] Sutherland RL, Musgrove EA. Cyclins and breast cancer. J Mammary Gland Biol Neoplasia 2004; 9; 95-104.

[261] Wang L, Shao ZM. Cyclin E expression and prognosis in breast cancer patients: a meta-analysis of published studies. Cancer Invest 2006; 24; 581-587.

[262] Span PN, Tjan-Heijnen VC, Manders P, Beex LV, Sweep CG. Cyclin-E is a strong predictor of endocrine therapy failure in human breast cancer. Oncogene 2003; 22; 4898-4904.

[263] Scaltriti M, Eichhorn PJ, Cortés J *et al.* Cyclin E amplification/overexpression is a mechanism of trastuzumab resistance in HER2+ breast cancer patients. Proc Natl Acad Sci USA 2011; 108; 3761-6.

[264] Alao JP. The regulation of cyclin D1 degradation: role in cancer development and the potential for therapeutic intervention. Mol Cancer 2007; 2; 6-24.

[265] Alle KM, Henshall SM, Field AS, Sutherland RL. Cyclin D1 protein is overexpressed in hyperplasia and intraductal carcinoma of the breast. Clin Cancer Res 1998; 4; 847-854.

[266] Umekita Y, Yoshida H. Cyclin D1 expression in ductal carcinoma in situ, atypical ductal hyperplasia: an immunohistochemical study. Pathol Int 2000; 50; 527-530.

[267] Fisher PM, Gianella-Borradori A. Recent progress in the discovery and development of cyclin-dependent kinase inhibitors. Expert Opin Investig Drugs 2005; 14; 457-477.

[268] Fu M, Rao M, Bouras T *et al.* Cyclin D1 inhibits peroxisome proliferator-activated receptor gamma-mediated adipogenesis throught histone deacetylase recruitment. J Biol Chem 2005; 280; 16934-16941.

[269] Mbeunkui F, Johann DJ Jr. Cancer and the tumor microenvironment: a review of an essential relationship. Cancer Chemother Pharmacol 2009; 63; 571-82.

[270] Albini A, Sporn MB. The tumour microenvironment as a target for chemoprevention. Nat Rev Cancer 2007; 7; 139-47.

[271] Aboussekhra A. Role of cancer-associated fibroblasts in breast cancer development and prognosis. Int J Dev Biol 2011; 55; 841-9.

[272] Togo S, Polanska UM, Horimoto Y, Orimo A. Carcinoma-associated fibroblasts are a promising therapeutic target. Cancers (Basel). 2013; 5: 149-69.

[273] Mueller MM, Fusenig NE. Friends or foes - bipolar effects of the tumour stroma in cancer. Nat Rev Cancer. 2004; 4: 839-49.

[274] Ellis LM, Hicklin DJ. VEGF-targeted therapy: mechanisms of anti-tumour activity. Nat Rev Cancer. 2008; 8: 579-91.

[275] Mukhtar RA, Nseyo O, Campbell MJ, Esserman LJ. Tumor-associated macrophages in breast cancer as potential biomarkers for new treatments and diagnostics. Expert Rev Mol Diagn. 2011; 11: 91-100.

[276] Siveen KS, Kuttan G. Role of macrophages in tumour progression. Immunol Lett 2009; 123: 97-102.

[277] Allavena P, Sica A, Solinas G, Porta C, Mantovani A. The inflammatory micro-environment in tumor progression: the role of tumor-associated macrophages. Crit Rev Oncol Hematol. 2008; 66: 1-9

[278] Yadava N, Schneider SS, Jerry DJ, Kim C. Impaired mitochondrial metabolism and mammary carcinogenesis. J Mammary Gland Biol Neoplasia. 2013; 18: 75-87

[279] Warburg, O. On the origin of cancer cells. Science. 1956; 123: 309-314.

[280] Kroemer G and Pouyssegur J: Tumor cell metabolism: cancer's Achilles' heel. Cancer Cell 2008; 13: 472-482.

[281] Ward PS, Thompson CB. Metabolic reprogramming: a cancer hallmark even warburg did not anticipate. Cancer Cell. 2012; 21: 297-308.

[282] RH. Eckel, SM. Grundy and PZ. Zimmet. The metabolic syndrome. The Lancet 2005; 365(9468): 1415-28.

[283] F. Xue, KB Michels. Diabetes, metabolic syndrome and breast cancer: a review of the current evidence. Am J Clin Nutr. 2007; 86(3): 823-35.

[284] Protani M, Coory M, Martin JH. Effect of obesity on survival of women with breast cancer: Systematic review and meta-analysis. Breast Cancer Res Treat. 2010; 123: 627-635.

[285] PJ. Goodwin, M. Ennis, KI. Pritchard, *et al.* Fasting insulin and outcome in early stage breast cancer: results of a prospective cohort study. J Clin Oncol 2002; 20: 42-51.

[286] P. Pasanisi, F. Berrino, M. De Petris, *et al.* Metabolic syndrome as a prognostic factor for breast cancer recurrences. Int J Cancer. 2006; 119: 236-38.

[287] Gunter MJ, Hoover DR, Yu H, *et al.* Insulin, insulin-like growth factor-I, and risk of breast cancer in postmenopausal women. J Natl Cancer Inst 2009; 101(1): 48-60.

[288] I. Wolf, S. Sadetzki, R. Catane, *et al.* Diabetes mellitus and breast cancer. Lancet Oncol 2005; 6: 103-11.

[289] EE. Calle, R. Kaaks. Overweight, obesity and cancer: epidemiological evidence and proposed mechanisms. Nat Rev Cancer 2004; 4: 579-91.

[290] MN. Pollak, ES. Schernhammer, SE. Hankinson. Insulin-like growth factors and neoplasia. Nat Rev Cancer 2004; 4: 505-18.

[291] PJ. Goodwin, M. Ennis, KI. Pritchard, *et al*: Insulin- and obesity-related variables in early-stage breast cancer: Correlations and time course of prognostic associations. J Clin Oncol.30: 164-171.

[292] IN. Alimova, B. Liu, Z. Fan, *et al.* Metformin inhibits breast cancer cell growth, colony formation and induces cell cycle arrest *in vitro*. Cell Cycle 2009; 8: 910-5.

[293] M. Zakikhani, R. Dowling, IG. Fantus, *et al.* Metformin is an AMP kinase-dependent growth inhibitor for breast cancer cells. Cancer Res 2006; 66: 10269-73.

[294] RJ. Dowling, M. Zakikhani, IG. Fantus, *et al.* Metformin inhibits mammalian target of rapamycin dependent translation initiation in breast cancer cells. Cancer Res 2007; 67: 10804-12.

[295] I. Ben Sahra, K. Laurent, A. Loubat, *et al.* The antidiabetic drug metformin exerts an antitumoral effect *in vitro* and *in vivo* through a decrease of cyclin D1 level. Oncogene 2008; 27: 3576-86.

[296] S. Jiralerspong, SL. Palla, SH. Giordano, *et al*: Metformin and pathologic complete responses to neoadjuvant chemotherapy in diabetic patients with breast cancer. J Clin Oncol 2009; 27: 3297-3302.

[297] B. Bonanni, M. Puntoni, M. Cazzaniga, *et al.* Dual effect of metformin on breast cancer proliferation in a randomized pre surgical trial. J Clin Oncol 2012; 30: 2593-2600.

[298] Bianchi F, Nicassio F, Marzi *et al.* A serum circulating miRNA diagnostic test to identify asymptomatic high-risk individuals with early stage lung cancer. EMBO Mol Med. 2011; 3: 495-503.

[299] Boeri M, Verri C, Conte D, Roz L, Modena P, Facchinetti F, *et al.* MicroRNA signatures in tissues and plasma predict development and prognosis of computed tomography detected lung cancer. Proc Natl Acad Sci USA 2011; 108: 3713-8.

[300] Yendamuri S, Kratzke R. MicroRNA biomarkers in lung cancer: MiRacle or quagMiRe? Transl Res. 2011; 157: 209- 15.

[301] Krol J, Loedige I, Filipowicz W. The widespread regulation of microRNA biogenesis, function and decay. Nat Rev Genet. 2010; 11: 597-610.

[302] Volinia S, Calin GA, Liu CG, Ambs S, Cimmino A, Petrocca F, *et al.* A microRNA expression signature of human solid tumors defines cancer gene targets. Proc Natl Acad Sci U S A. 2006; 103: 2257-61.

[303] Hunter MP, Ismail N, Zhang X, Aguda BD, Lee EJ, Yu L, *et al.* Detection of microRNA expression in human peripheral blood microvesicles. PLoS One. 2008; 3.

[304] Turchinovich A, Weiz L, Langheinz A, Burwinkel B. Characterization of extracellular circulating microRNA. Nucleic Acids Res. 2011; 39: 7223-33.

[305] Wang K, Zhang S, Weber J, Baxter D, Galas DJ. Export of microRNAs and microRNA-protective protein by mammalian cells. Nucleic Acids Res. 2010; 38: 7248-59.

[306] Chen X, Ba Y, Ma L, Cai X, Yin Y, Wang K, *et al.* Characterization of microRNAs in serum: a novel class of biomarkers for diagnosis of cancer and other diseases. Cell Res. 2008; 18: 997-1006.

[307] Shen J, Todd NW, Zhang H, Yu L, Lingxiao X, Mei Y, *et al.* Plasma microRNAs as potential biomarkers for nonsmall- cell lung cancer. Lab Invest. 2011; 91: 579-87.

[308] Hu Z, Chen X, Zhao Y, Tian T, Jin G, Shu Y, *et al.* Serum microRNA signatures identified in a genome-wide serum microRNA expression profiling predict survival of non-small-cell lung cancer. J Clin Oncol. 2010; 28: 1721-6.

[309] Sauter ER, Ross E, Daly M, Klein-Szanto A, Engstrom PF, Sorling A, *et al.* Nipple aspirate fluid: a promising noninvasive method to identify cellular markers of breast cancer risk. Br J Cancer. 1997; 76: 494-501.

CHAPTER 7

Modulation of the Myostatin/Follistatin Axis by Deacetylase Inhibitors: Improvement of TNFα-Induced Myotube Atrophy But Not of Experimental Cancer Cachexia

Andrea Bonetto[1], Fabio Penna[2,3], Gabriella Bonelli[2], Francesco M. Baccino[2] and Paola Costelli[*,2,3]

Department of Surgery, Indiana University School of Medicine, IUPUI, Indianapolis, IN, USA; [2]Department of Clinical and Biological Sciences, University of Turin, Italy; [3]Interuniversitary Institute of Myology, Italy

Abstract: Myostatin, a negative regulator of skeletal muscle mass, is increased in several conditions characterized by muscle wasting, among which cancer cachexia. Physiological inhibitors, such as follistatin, negatively regulate myostatin bioactivity.

Histone deacetylase inhibitors have been shown to improve muscle wasting and function in dystrophic *mdx* mice, mainly by modulating the myostatin/follistatin axis.

The present study was aimed at investigating the efficacy of two histone deacetylase inhibitors, namely valproic acid and trichostatin A, in preventing muscle atrophy in C26 tumor-bearing mice and in C2C12 myotubes exposed to TNFα.

The progressive muscle depletion that occurs in the C26 hosts was associated with increased expression of myostatin and muscle-specific ubiquitin ligases. Administration of valproic acid, but not trichostatin A, resulted in decreased muscle myostatin expression and increased follistatin levels. Neither agent, however, was able to effectively counteract muscle atrophy or ubiquitin ligase hyperexpression. By contrast, morphological analysis suggested that both valproic acid and trichostatin A are protective against TNFα-induced myotube atrophy.

Altogether, these results suggest that modulation of the myostatin/follistatin axis can prevent TNFα-associated myofiber atrophy, although it is not sufficient to correct muscle atrophy in cancer cachexia.

Keywords: Cancer cachexia, deacetylase inhibitors, follistatin, myostatin, TNFα.

INTRODUCTION

The maintenance of skeletal muscle mass is a finely tuned process that depends on several factors. Among these, myostatin, a member of the transforming growth

***Corresponding Author Paola Costelli:** Department of Clinical and Biological Sciences, Corso Raffaello, 30, 10125 Torino, Italy; Tel: +39-0116707062; Fax: +39-0116707753; E-mail: paola.costelli@unito.it

factor-β (TGF-β) superfamily [1], is known to negatively regulate skeletal muscle mass. Indeed, the lack of intact myostatin-dependent signaling results in marked muscle hypertrophy [1], while increased myostatin expression has been reported in situations characterized by depletion of muscle mass, such as sarcopenia of aging, denervation-induced atrophy, cancer-related muscle wasting [3-6].

Myostatin circulates in the blood in a latent form, complexed with physiological inhibitors such as myostatin propeptide and follistatin [7]. Active myostatin binds the activin type IIB receptor (ActRIIB) and, after recruitment and phosphorylation of ALK (Activin-Like Kinase)-4 or ALK-5 [2,8], leads to phosphorylation of Smads 2 and 3, and to their interaction with the co-Smad 4. The resulting complex translocates to the nucleus, where it regulates the transcription of myostatin target genes [9], among which those coding for the muscle-specific ubiquitin ligases atrogin-1 and MuRF1 [10], MyoD and other myogenic regulatory factors [11]. Myostatin has been reported to signal independently from Smads as well, activating either the ERK/MAPK [12] or the JNK-dependent [13] pathways.

Histone deacetylase inhibitors (DIs) such as valproic acid (VPA), trichostatin A (TSA), or sodium butyrate have been reported to increase follistatin expression in the skeletal muscle, inhibiting myostatin activity and favoring myoblast recruitment and differentiation [14,15]. TSA, in particular, has been reported to improve the dystrophic muscle phenotype in *mdx* mice [16]. Quite recently histone deacetylase (HDAC)-I has been involved in the activation of FoxOs, a family of transcription factors required for the expression of atrophy-related genes such as atrogin-1 and MuRF1. In this regard, HDAC-1 inhibition by TSA has been shown to prevent disuse-induced muscle atrophy [17].

In order to test if DIs administration could improve cancer-induced muscle wasting, mice bearing the C26 colon adenocarcinoma, a well characterized experimental model of cancer cachexia, have been treated with VPA or TSA. The results obtained clearly demonstrate that, despite being able to restore physiologic myostatin and follistatin expression, DIs are not protective against C26-induced muscle wasting. Cancer cachexia is a complex multifactorial syndrome that results from the interplay of several factors, among which malnutrition, dysmetabolism and systemic inflammation. This latter, in particular, plays a crucial role. Indeed, proinflammatory cytokines, such as TNFα, IL-6, IL-1β, have been shown to be associated with the pathogenesis of cancer-related muscle atrophy [reviewed in 18]. In order to determine whether DIs can modulate the atrophic stimulus induced by proinflammatory cytokines, C2C12 cells were exposed to TNFα, whose effects in terms of muscle atrophy and protein hypercatabolism are well known [19]. The results obtained suggest that VPA improves myotube atrophy and restores the myostatin/follistatin axis in C2C12 cells exposed to TNFα.

MATERIALS AND METHODS

Animals and Experimental Design

Balb-c mice weighing about 20 g were purchased from Charles River Laboratories (Calco, LC, Italy). They were maintained on a regular dark-light cycle (light: 08:00-20:00), with free access to food (Piccioni, Brescia, Italy) and water, and cared for in compliance with the Italian Ministry of Health Guidelines (n° 86609 EEC) and the *Policy on Humane Care and Use of Laboratory Animals* (NIH 1996). The experimental protocol was approved by the Bioethical Committee of the University of Torino.

The C26 adenocarcinoma cells were seeded in plastic culture flasks (TPP, St. Louis, MO, USA) in DMEM medium supplemented with 10% fetal bovine serum (GIBCO Laboratories, Grand Island, NY, USA), 100 U/ml penicillin, 100 mg/ml streptomycin, 100 mg/ml sodium pyruvate, 2 mM L-glutamine and grown to subconfluency in humidified atmosphere containing 5% CO_2. C26 cells were trypsinized and resuspended in sterile saline [5×10^6 cells/ml] for *in vivo* transplantation.

Mice were randomized and divided into four groups, namely controls (C; n=6), untreated (C26; n=8), VPA- (C26+VPA; n=8) and TSA-treated tumor bearers (C26+TSA; n=8). Tumor hosts were inoculated *s.c.* dorsally with $5x10^5$ C26 cells (100 μl of the initial cell suspension). In another set of experiments, a group of healthy animals (C+VPA; n = 6) was treated with VPA for 13 days and compared with untreated controls (C; n = 6). Treated groups received daily *s.c.* injections of either VPA (100 mg/kg) or TSA (0.6 mg/kg; Sigma, St. Louis, MO, USA; 17).

These doses were chosen in view of the results obtained in dose-response experiments. Starting point was the dose commonly used in the rat, about 300 mg/kg, that resulted in greater toxicity in the mouse. Mice were weighed every day, while fore- and hindlimb grip strength was measured in all the animals at days 8 and 13 after tumor transplantation by means of a grip strength meter (Columbus Instruments, Columbus, OH, USA; see 25). At days 11 (beginning of significant body weight loss) or 13 (terminal point) after tumor transplantation the animals were sacrificed under anesthesia.

Gastrocnemius, tibialis anterior, and heart were rapidly excised, weighed, frozen in liquid nitrogen, and stored at -80°C. Further analysis was performed on the gastrocnemius muscle only.

Cell Cultures

Murine C2C12 skeletal myoblasts (ATCC, Manassas, VA, USA) were grown in high glucose Dulbecco's Modified Eagle's Medium (DMEM) supplemented with 10% FBS, 100 U/ml penicillin, 100 mg/ml streptomycin, 100 mg/ml sodium pyruvate, 2 mM L-glutamine, and maintained at 37°C in a humidified atmosphere of 5% CO_2 in air. Cultures were regularly checked for mycoplasma contamination by staining with the DNA specific fluorochrome 4'-6-diamidine-2-phenylindole dihydrochloride (DAPI; Boehringer, Mannheim, Germany). For the experiments, cells were seeded at 35000/cm^2 to obtain full confluence 24 h later. C2C12 myoblasts were exposed to either valproic acid (VPA, 5 mM; 14) or trichostatin-A (TSA, 50 nM; 15) for 24 and 18 h, respectively. Subsequently, cells were induced to differentiate by shifting confluent cultures to DMEM supplemented with 2% horse serum. The medium was replaced every other day, and within 5 days most of the cells in control cultures were fused to form myotubes. On day 6, the cultures were exposed to 100 ng/ml TNFα (Immunological Sciences, Rome, Italy), and cells collected after 24-48 h. Both TNFα-treated and untreated cultures were photographed under phase contrast microscopy. Cells were collected and stored at -80°C for further analysis.

Histology

Tibialis anterior muscles were excised, weighed, mounted in OCT (VWR, Milan, Italy) and frozen in melting isopentane cooled in liquid nitrogen. Ten-micrometer thick cross sections from the midbelly region were cut on a cryostat and later stained with hematoxylin and eosin (H&E). The tibialis anterior CSA was determined by the Image J software [20].

Reverse Transcription-PCR

Total RNA was obtained using the TriPure reagent (Roche, Indianapolis, IN, USA) following the instructions provided by the manufacturer. RNA concentration was determined spectrophotometrically (SmartSpec 3000, Bio-Rad, Hercules, CA, USA) and its purity ensured by evaluating the 260/280 nm ratio. RNA integrity was checked by electrophoresis on 1.2% agarose gel, containing morpholino propane-sulfonic acid (MOPS) 0.02 M and 18% formaldehyde.

Follistatin, atrogin-1 and MuRF-1 mRNA levels were determined by semiquantitative reverse-transcription polymerase chain reaction using the kit 'Ready-to-Go RT-PCR Beads' (Amersham Biosciences, Milano, Italy). Following manufacturer's protocol, 0.5 μg total RNA and 400 nM mixture of each couple of primers were added to a RT-PCR reaction mixture containing ~2.0 units *Taq* DNA-polymerase, 10 mM Tris-HCl pH 9.0, 60 mM KCl, 1.5 mM $MgCl_2$, 200 μM dNTP, Moloney Murine Leukemia Virus (M-MuLV) Reverse Transcriptase, ribonuclease inhibitor and stabilizers to reach a final volume of 50 μl in each reaction tube. Table **1** shows primers sequences and accession numbers for glyceraldehyde-3-phosphate dehydrogenase (GAPDH), follistatin, atrogin-1 and MuRF-1, obtained according to published sequences (Invitrogen, Milano, Italy).

Retrotranscription was performed at 42°C for 30 min; before entering the cycling protocol the samples were denatured (2 min, 95°C). Amplification conditions for atrogin-1 and MuRF-1 consisted of 1 min denaturation (95°C), 1 min annealing (60°C), 2 min polymerization (72°C) for 30 or 35 cycles respectively, followed by extension (72°C, 7 min). As for follistatin, 35 cycles consisting in 1 min denaturation (95°C), 1 min annealing (55°C), 1 min polymerization (72°C) were followed by extension at 72°C for 7 min. Both positive and negative controls were performed. PCR products were electrophoresed on 2% agarose gels and visualized with ethidium bromide. A 100 bp-standard DNA ladder (Fermentas, Burlington, ON, Canada) was used to estimate the length of each PCR product (follistatin:

345 bp; atrogin-1: 75 bp; MuRF-1: 58 bp). Quantification was performed by densitometric analysis. The results were normalized according to GAPDH expression (177 bp), amplified under the following conditions: denaturation (95°C, 1 min), annealing (60°C, 1 min), polymerization (72°C, 1 min), for 20 cycles, extension (72°C, 7 min). Comparisons among groups were made in the linear phase of amplification.

Table 1: List of Oligonucleotides Used as PCR Primers

	Primer Sequence
Follistatin *(NM_008046)*	5'-CTCTTCAAGTGGATGATTTTC-3' 5'-ACAGTAGGCATTATTGGTCTG-3'
Atrogin-1 *(NM_026346)*	5'-CCATCAGGAGAAGTGGATCTATGTT-3' 5'-GCTTCCCCCAAAGTGCAGTA-3'
MuRF-1 *(AF_294790)*	5'-TGTCTGGAGGTCGTTTCCG-3' 5'-ATGCCGGTCCATGATCACTT-3'
GAPDH *(AF_106860)*	5'- TGCACCACCAACTGCTTA-3' 5'- GGATGCAGGGATGATGTTC -3'

Western Blotting

Both gastrocnemius muscle (100 mg) and C2C12 myotubes (~1.5x10^6 cells) were homogenized in 80 mM TRIS-HCl, pH 6.8 (containing 100 mM DTT, 70 mM SDS, and 1 mM glycerol), kept on ice for 30 min, centrifuged at 15000 x g for 10 min at 4°C, and the supernatant collected. Protein concentration was assayed according to Lowry *et al.* [21] using BSA as working standard. Equal amounts of protein (30 μg) were heat-denaturated in sample-loading buffer (50 mM TRIS-HCl, pH 6.8, 100 mM DTT, 2% SDS, 0.1% bromophenol blue, 10% glycerol), resolved on a SDS-PAGE (12% polyacrilamide, 0.1% SDS) and transferred for 2 h to nitrocellulose membranes (Bio-Rad, Hercules, CA, USA). Protein transfer was checked by Ponceau S staining. The filters were then blocked with Tris buffered saline (TBS) containing 0.05% Tween and 5% non-fat dry milk and incubated overnight with either a polyclonal anti-myostatin antibody (1:1000; Società Italiana Chimici, Roma, Italy) or a polyclonal antibody against phospho-GSK-3β (Ser 9, 1:1000; Cell Signaling Technology, Danvers, MA, USA). The latter binds the ~46 kDa phosphorylated form of the kinase, while the former, specific for the ~30 kDa processed myostatin, was raised against a synthetic peptide (aa 133-148) representing a portion of human GDF-8 encoded within exon 3 (LocusLink ID 2660). Goat anti-rabbit peroxidase-conjugated IgG (Bio-Rad, Hercules, CA, USA) was used as secondary antibody. The filters were then stripped by incubation in 62.5 mM Tris-HCl, pH 6.7, containing 100 mM 2-mercaptoethanol and 2% SDS for 30 min at 50° C, and reprobed with a mouse polyclonal antibody directed against tubulin (~50 kDa; Sigma, St. Louis, MO, USA) to normalize sample loading. The membrane-bound immune complexes were detected by enhanced chemiluminescence (Santa Cruz Biotechnology, USA) on a photon-sensitive film (Hyperfilm ECL; Amersham Biosciences, Milano, Italy). Band quantification was performed by densitometric analysis with a specific software (TotalLab, NonLinear Dynamics, Newcastle upon Tyne, UK).

Data Analysis and Presentation

All results were expressed as means ± SD. Significance of the differences was evaluated by analysis of variance (ANOVA) followed by Tukey's test.

RESULTS

Mice bearing the C26 tumor experienced a marked and progressive body weight loss, reaching 75% of control values at the end of the experimental period (day 13; Fig. **1**). Body weight loss was paralleled by a significant decrease in the size of the fast-twitch muscles gastrocnemius and tibialis anterior (77% and 68% of controls, respectively; Fig. **1A**), as well as of the heart, although the reduction in this tissue was less pronounced (Fig. **1A**). Daily administration of VPA or TSA to the C26 hosts did not exert any positive effect on cancer-induced muscle and body wasting (Fig. **1**). Interestingly, the kinetic of body weight loss was quite different between VPA-treated and untreated C26 hosts (Fig. **1B**). Indeed, body weight appeared reduced soon after tumor implantation in the former group, while remained unchanged until day 10 after transplantation in the latter.

The lack of effect in the VPA-treated group also extended to muscle function: the significant reduction of grip strength that occurs in the C26 hosts was not modified by 12-days VPA treatment (Fig. **2**). Similarly, forelimb grip strength in healthy animals was not significantly affected by VPA (Fig. **2**).

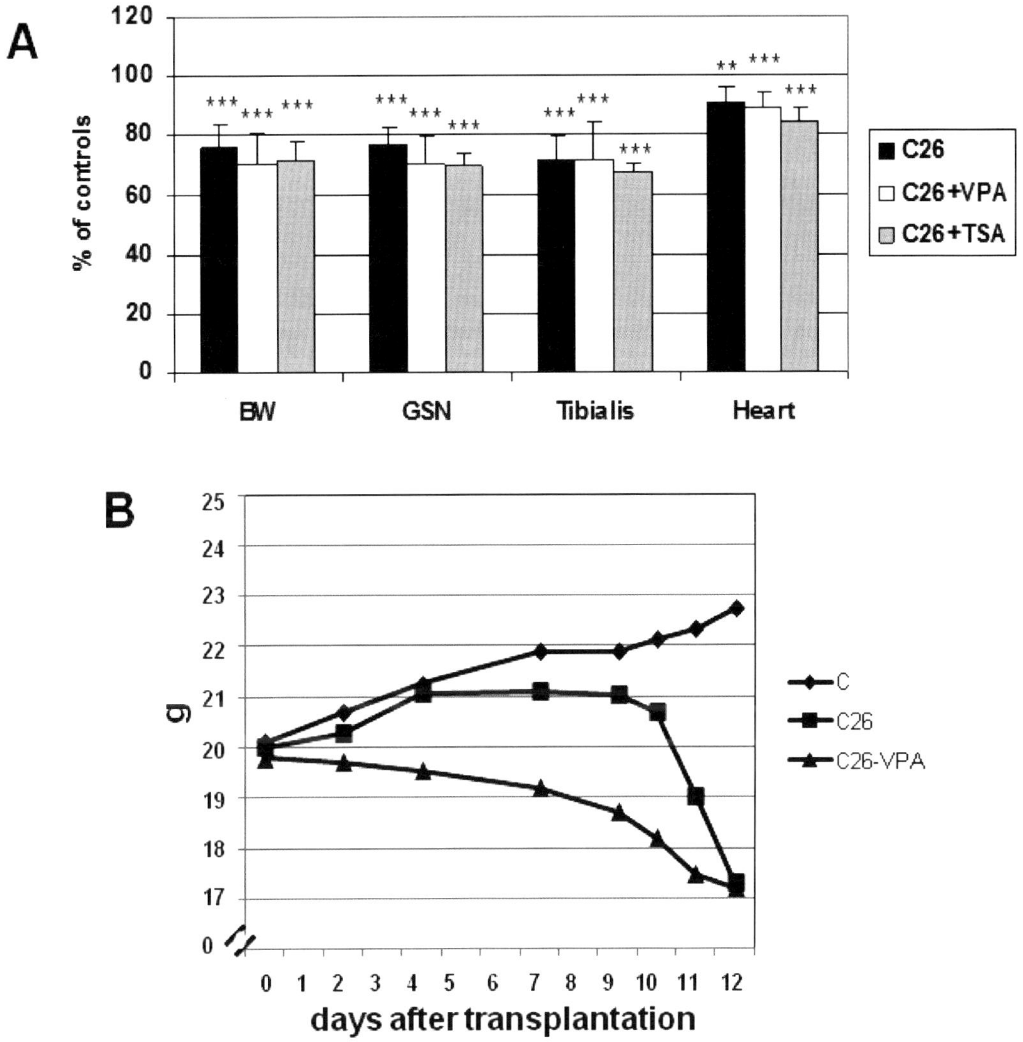

Fig. (1): (**A**) Body and muscle weight in untreated, VPA- or TSA-treated C26- bearing mice. All the tumor-bearing mice (n=8) were sacrificed at day 13 after C26 transplantation. Data (means ± SD) are expressed as percentage of controls (day 13, n=6); BW = body weight, GSN = gastrocnemius. Significance of the differences *vs* controls: $^{**}p<0.01$, $^{***}p<0.001$; (**B**) Kinetic of body weight loss in mice bearing the C26 tumor, treated or not with VPA.

Growth of the C26 tumor also resulted in a significant decrease of cumulative food intake (C = 35±0.3 g; C26 = 24±0.8 g, $p<0.001$ *vs* C); such a reduction was not improved by treatment with VPA or TSA (C26+VPA = 25±0.9 g; C26+TSA = 23±1.1 g, $p<0.01$ *vs* C).

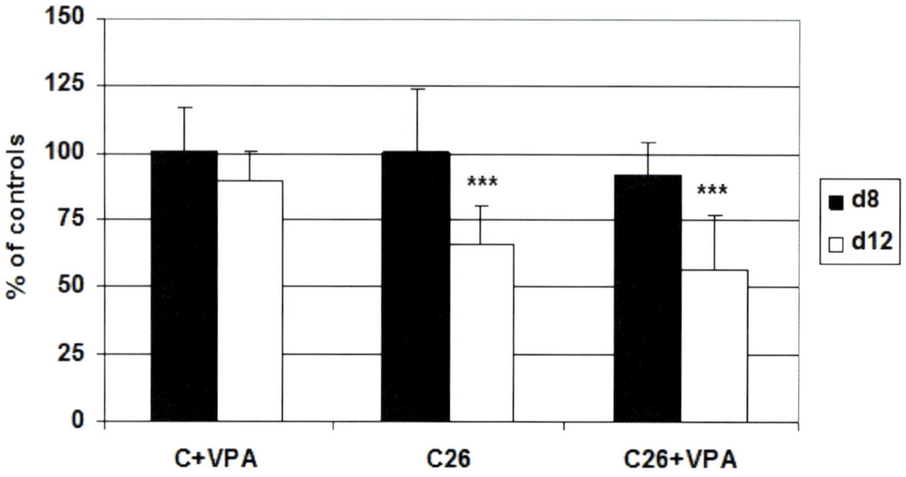

Fig. (2): Fore and hindlimbs grip strength. Measurement performed in VPA-treated controls (n=6), untreated (n=8) and VPA-treated (n=8) tumor bearers 8 and 12 days after C26 transplantation. Each force measurement consists of two separate trials. Data (means ± SD) are expressed as percentage of untreated controls at the same time points (n=6). Significance of the differences *vs* untreated controls: ***p<0.001.

Consistently with the lack of effect on skeletal muscle mass, myofiber CSA in the tibialis anterior was not modified by VPA administration in both controls (C = 5261±881 a.u., C + VPA = 5233±654 a.u.; Fig. **3**) and C26 hosts (C26 = 3971±648 a.u., C26 + VPA = 4048±152 a.u.; Fig. **3**).

In the C26-bearing mice myostatin protein levels progressively increased with respect to controls at days 11 and 13 after tumor transplantation (C d11 = 1.64±0.45 a.u., C26 d11 = 2.89±0.97 a.u., $p < 0.05$ *vs* C; C d13 = 0.8±0.2, C26 d13 = 1.70±0.7, $p < 0.05$ *vs* C), while follistatin mRNA expression is not modified (Fig. **4**). By contrast, VPA markedly increased follistatin mRNA levels in both controls and tumor bearers (Fig. **4**). Interestingly, TSA did not affect myostatin levels in C26-bearing animals (Fig. **4**).

TSA treatment was unable to restore the myostatin levels in the C26 hosts, while VPA resulted in a marked reduction (about 49%; Fig. **5**). Of note, VPA did not modify myostatin levels in control mice (Fig. **5**).

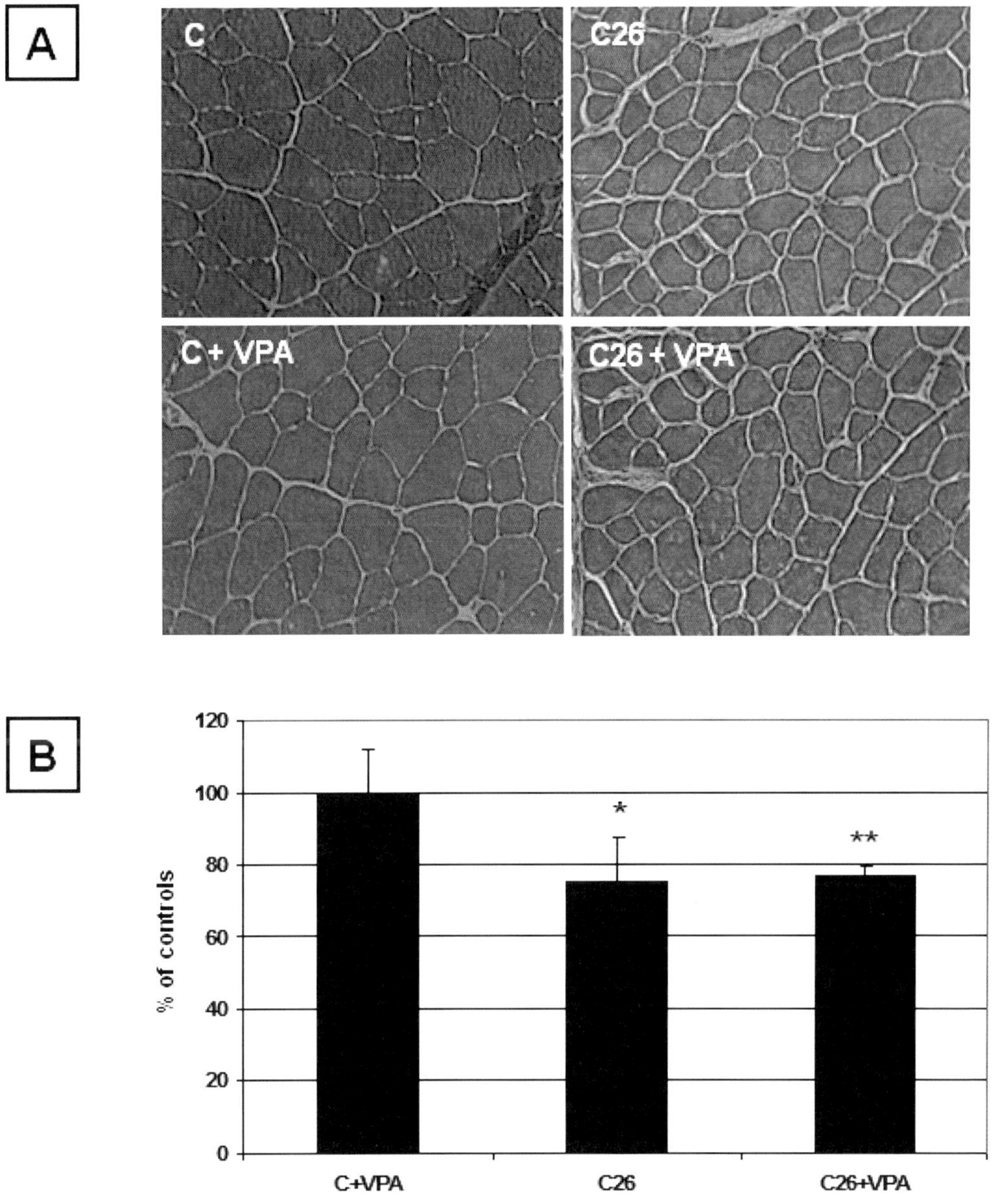

Fig. (3): Tibialis anterior myofiber cross-sectional area (CSA). Panel **A**: H&E staining of tibialis anterior transverse sections. Panel **B**: Tibialis anterior myofiber CSA. Both treated (n=8) and untreated (n=8) tumor-bearing mice were sacrificed at day 13 after C26 transplantation. Treated controls received VPA for 13 days before sacrifice (n=6). Data (means ± SD) are expressed as percentage of untreated controls. Significance of the differences: *p<0.05, **p<0.01 *vs* untreated controls.

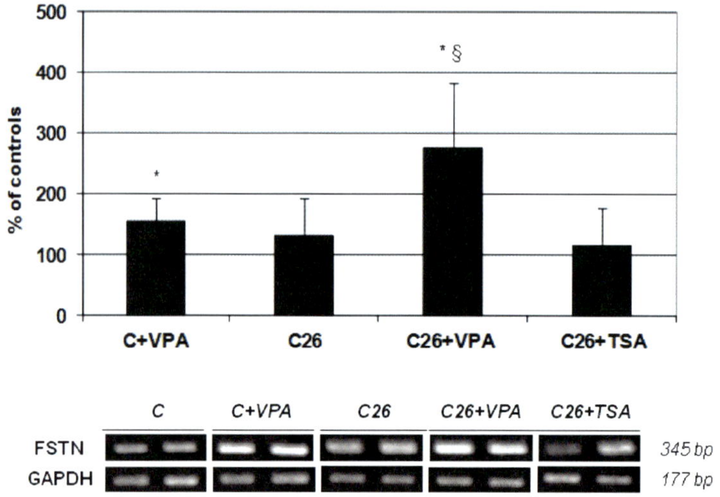

Fig. (4): Follistatin (FSTN) mRNA expression in treated and untreated C26 hosts. Representative RT-PCR pattern of FSTN mRNA expression in the gastrocnemius muscle. Both treated (n=8) and untreated (n=8) tumor-bearing mice were sacrificed at day 13 after C26 transplantation. Treated controls received VPA for 13 days before sacrifice (n=6). Data (means ± SD) are expressed as percentage of untreated controls at the same time point (n=6). Significance of the differences: *p<0.05 *vs* untreated controls, §p<0.05 *vs* C26.

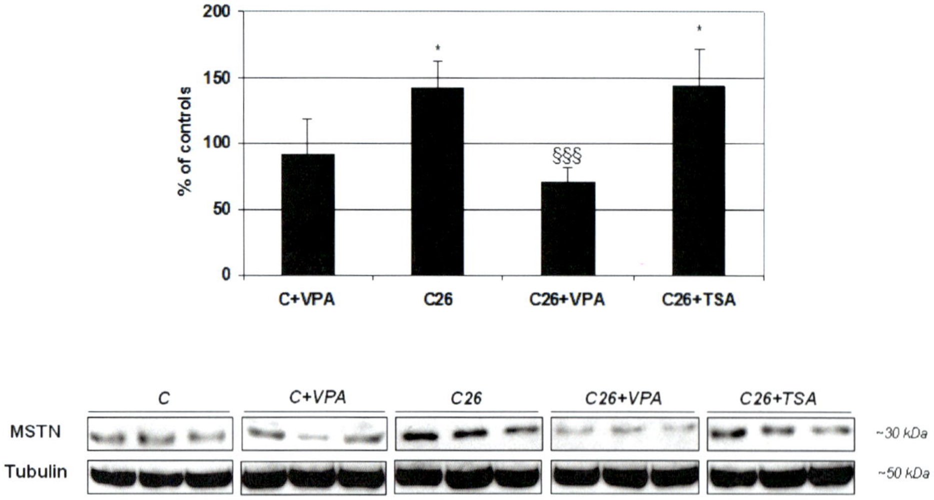

Fig. (5): Myostatin (MSTN) protein levels in in treated and untreated C26 hosts. Representative western blotting of myostatin expression in the gastrocnemius muscle. Treated controls received VPA for 13 days before sacrifice (n=6). All the tumor-bearing mice were sacrificed at day 13 (n=8) after C26 transplantation. Data (means ± SD) are expressed as percentage of untreated controls at the same time point (n=6). Significance of the differences: *p<0.05 *vs* untreated controls, §§§p<0.001 *vs* C26.

Since VPA has been shown to inhibit glycogen synthase kinase (GSK)-3β [22, 23], the state of activation of this kinase was also evaluated in the gastrocnemius muscle of both controls and C26 hosts treated with VPA. The results showed that phosphorylated (inactive) GSK-3β is more abundant in VPA-treated than in untreated tumor-bearing mice, while no differences could be observed in control mice (Fig. **6**).

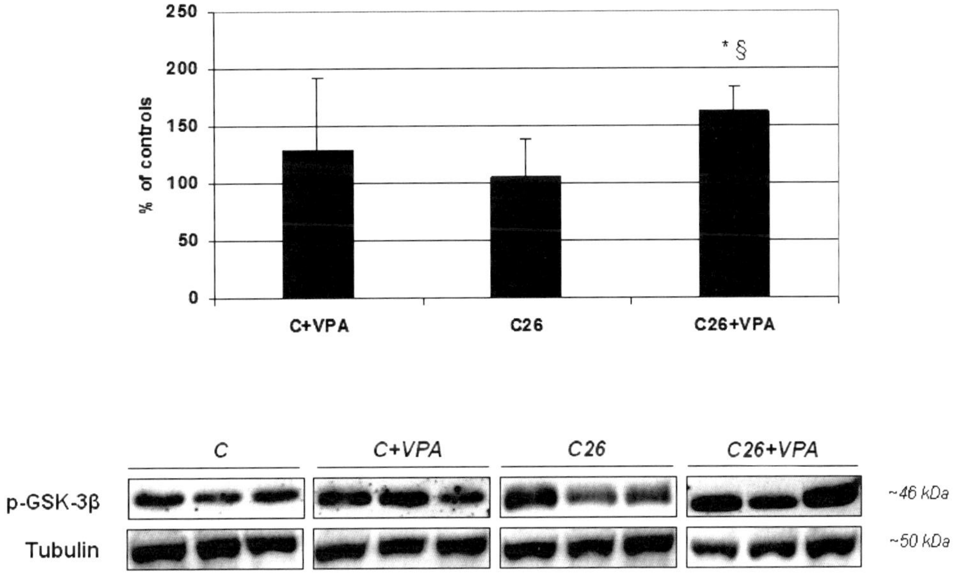

Fig. (6): Levels of phosphorylated GSK-3β (p-GSK-3β) in the gastrocnemius. Treated controls received VPA for 13 days before sacrifice (n=6). Treated (n=8) and untreated (n=8) tumor-bearing mice were sacrificed at day 13 after C26 transplantation. Data (means ± SD) are expressed as percentage of controls at the same time point (n=6). Significance of the differences: *$p<0.05$ *vs* controls, $^{\S}p<0.05$ *vs* C26.

The mRNA levels of atrogin-1 and MuRF-1, two ubiquitin ligases that are generally overexpressed in pathological conditions associated with muscle atrophy [24-26], were evaluated after DIs treatment. The expression levels of these ubiquitin ligases remained significantly elevated in tumor hosts *vs* controls, both in the presence and in the absence of VPA or TSA treatment (Fig. **7**).

Finally, DIs were tested for their capacity of counteracting cytokine-induced myotube atrophy. As reported above, pro-inflammatory cytokines play a central role in the pathogenesis of cancer-induced muscle wasting [reviewed in 18]. In this regard, previous studies reported that C2C12 myotubes exposed to TNFα show a marked reduction in size, associated with decreased expression of fast-type myosin heavy-chain [19,27], increased atrogin-1 expression and activation of the Ca^{2+}-dependent proteolytic system [19]. TNFα exposure also affects the myostatin/follistatin axis, with increased myostatin abundance and SMAD DNA-binding activity [19].

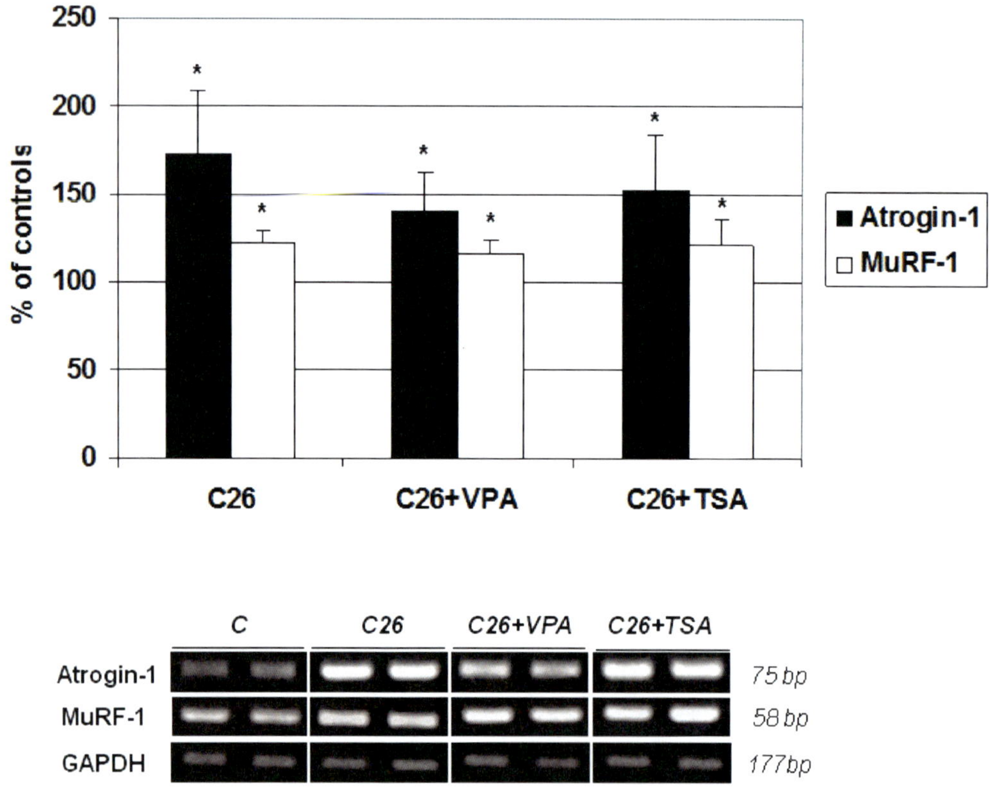

Fig. (7): Atrogin-1 and MuRF-1 mRNA levels in the gastrocnemius of untreated or treated C26-bearing mice. Representative RT-PCR pattern of ubiquitin ligases expression. Both treated (n=8) and untreated (n=8) tumor-bearing mice were sacrificed at day 13 after C26 transplantation. Data (means ± SD) are expressed as percentage of untreated controls (day 13, n=6). Significance of the differences *vs* untreated controls: *p<0.05.

The data reported in Fig. (**8**) showed that myotubes obtained by C2C12 myoblast differentiated in the presence of either VPA or TSA and subsequently exposed to TNFα display a hypertrophic phenotype when compared to cultures differentiated in the absence of DIs.

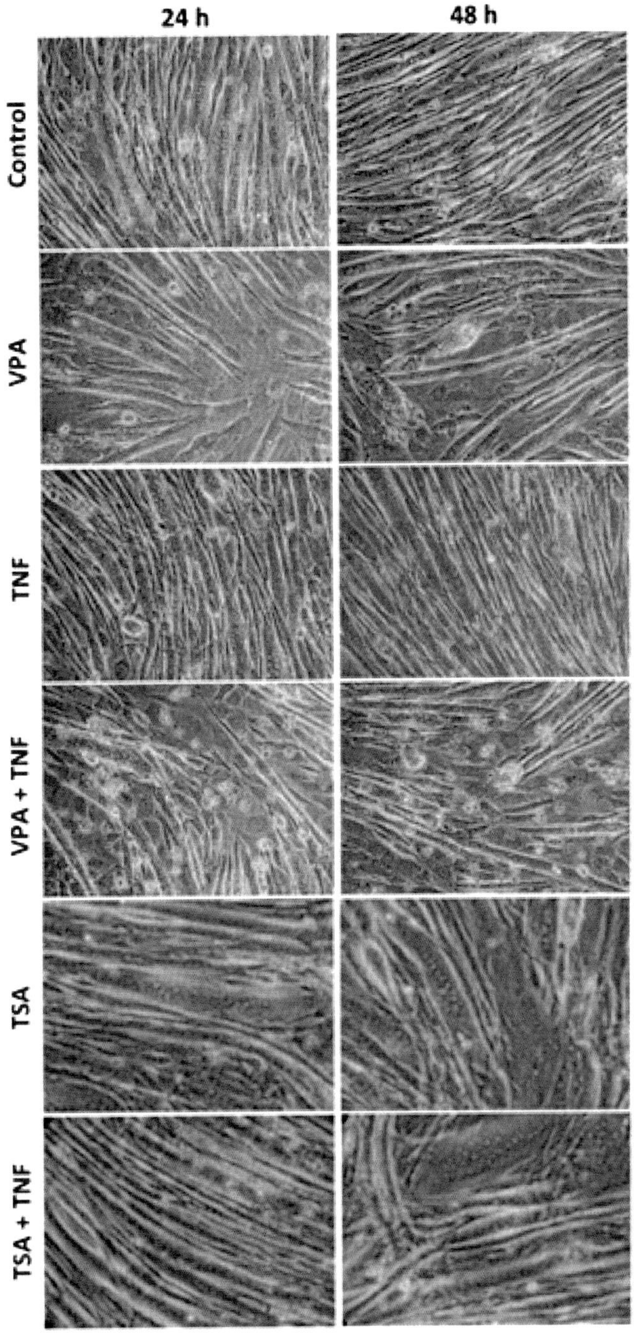

Fig. (8): Effect of DIs on TNFα-treated C2C12 myotubes. Phase contrast images of myotube cultures differentiated in the presence or in the absence of VPA (5 mM) or TSA (50 nM), treated for 24 or 48 hours with TNFα (100 ng/ml).

The effects exerted by VPA were associated with enhancement of both follistatin mRNA and protein expression in both control and TNFα-treated myotubes (Fig. **9B**, **D**). Consistently with previous results [19], no differences with respect to controls could be observed in cells differentiated in VPA-free medium and then exposed to TNFα (Fig. **9**). As for myostatin (Fig. **9A**, **C**), both protein and mRNA levels were comparable to controls (or even reduced) in the presence of the combined treatment (TNF+VPA), while VPA or TNFα alone resulted in increased expression.

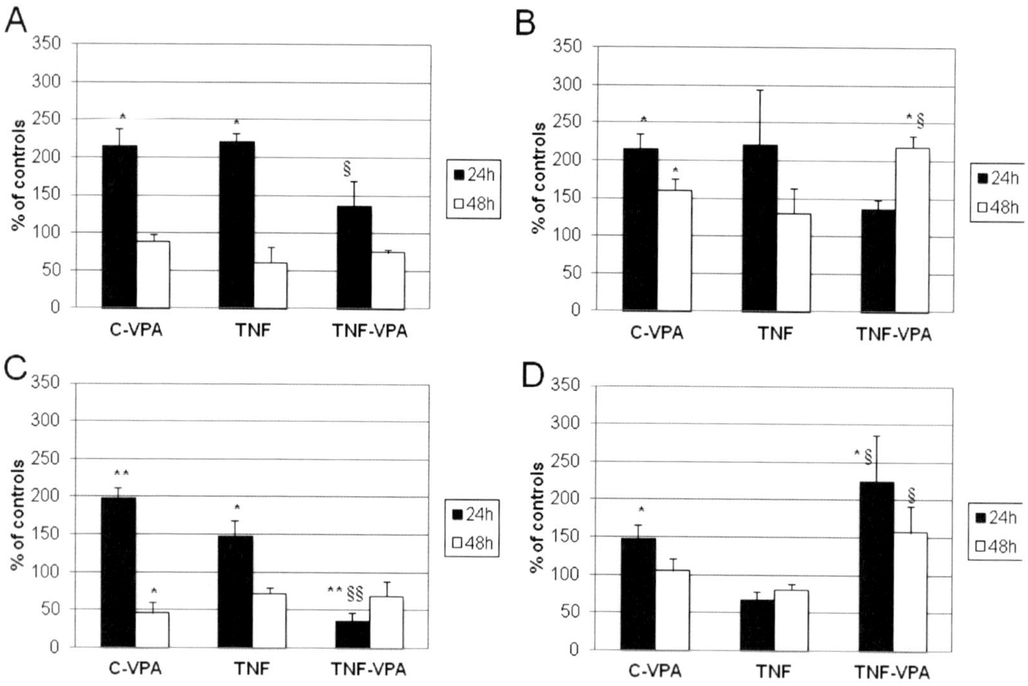

Fig. (9): Effect of DIs on myostatin and follistatin expression in TNFα-treated C2C12 myotubes differentiated in medium containing or not VPA (5 mM). Myostatin (**A**) and follistatin (**B**) mRNA levels, myostatin (**C**) and follistatin (**D**) protein expression. Data (means ± SD n = 3, from 3 independent experiments) are expressed as percentage of untreated controls. Significance of the differences: $^{*}p<0.05$, $^{**}p<0.01$ *vs* C; $^{\S}p<0.05$ *vs* TNFα.

By contrast, myostatin protein levels in myotubes differentiated in the presence of TSA and subsequently exposed to TNFα seemed to increase with respect to cultures treated with TNFα alone, though not significantly (Fig. **10**). A similar increase could also be detected in TSA-diffrentiated myotubes in the absence of TNFα (Fig. **10**).

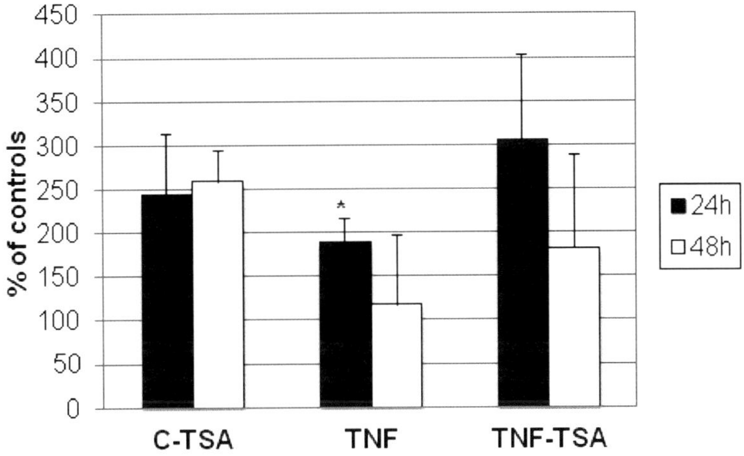

Fig. (10): Effect of DIs on myostatin expression in TNFα-treated C2C12 myotubes differentiated in medium containing or not TSA (50 nM). Data are means ± SD (n = 3, from 3 independent experiments), expressed as percentage of untreated controls. Significance of the differences: $^{*}p<0.05$ *vs* C.

DISCUSSION

The connection between increased myostatin expression and muscle wasting has been suggested by a number of studies [reviewed in 28]. However, conflicting findings have been reported. In this regard, muscle atrophy induced by hindlimb suspension seems to affect myostatin-deficient mice more than wild-type animals [29]. In addition, the occurrence of a correlation between myostatin mRNA levels and muscle atrophy is not a general finding. Indeed, this is lacking, for example, in muscle wasting due to disuse [30,31].

Previous results have shown that myostatin expression and signaling are altered in cancer-induced muscle wasting. Indeed, myostatin protein and mRNA levels were increased in the skeletal muscle of both rats bearing the AH-130 Yoshida hepatoma and mice transplanted with the C26 tumor [32-34; present study], while they were unchanged in mice bearing the Lewis lung carcinoma [35]. Consistently, myostatin inhibition by antisense mRNA has been shown to improve muscle wasting in mice bearing the S-180 tumor [36]. In addition, treatments protective against cancer cachexia also proved effective in restoring normal myostatin expression levels [32,34].

The present study has been aimed at investigating whether modulations of the myostatin signaling by means of DIs could also result in protection against cancer-induced muscle wasting. For this reason mice implanted with the C26 tumor have been administered VPA or TSA. In comparison to untreated C26-bearing mice, the former drug lead to increased follistatin and reduced myostatin levels. Increased follistatin expression after DIs administration has been previously reported also in the skeletal muscle of dystrophic *mdx* mice, leading to improved muscle phenotype [15,16,37]. Similarly, TSA strongly induced follistatin expression in porcine satellite cells [38]. Myostatin has been proposed to negatively regulate skeletal muscle mass through antagonism of hypertrophy-inducing signals, mainly driven by down-regulation of the Akt-FoxO pathways [10]. In this regard, VPA has been shown to inhibit GSK-3β [22,23], an essential kinase acting both as a downstream target and as a negative regulator of the PI3K/Akt pathway [39]. Indeed, in the present study VPA administration to the C26 hosts results in markedly increased phosphorylated (inactive) GSK-3β. Such inhibition does not affect skeletal muscle mass in tumor bearers. This observation is not surprising, since previous studies have shown that the PI3K/Akt pathway is not down-regulated in C26-induced cachexia [24,40].

Skeletal muscle wasting in chronic pathologies, cancer included, mainly reflects the onset of a protein hypercatabolic state due to increased activity of different intracellular proteolytic systems [41]. Among these, the degradative pathway dependent on ubiquitin and proteasome is considered to play a crucial role, although the signals that precisely lead to its hyperactivation are still unclear. In this regard, myostatin has been shown to mediate the increased transcription of atrogin-1 and MuRF1, likely by inhibiting the IGF-1/PI-3K/Akt axis [10]. Consistently, myostatin-deficient mice exposed to glucocorticoids are not able to up-regulate muscle-specific ubiquitin ligase expression [42]. In the present study the increased levels of both atrogin-1 and MuRF1 observed in the muscle of the C26 hosts are not down-regulated by VPA administration, despite treated animals display a restoration of the physiological myostatin/follistatin ratio. In this regard,

DIs have been shown to activate rather than inhibit protein breakdown in myotube cultures exposed to glucocorticoids [43]. These results have been confirmed by a study showing that muscle protein breakdown rates and atrogin-1 expression increase in rats treated with TSA [44]. On this line, ubiquitin ligase hyperexpression in the C26 hosts treated with VPA could result from DIs-dependent activation of the ubiquitin-proteasome pathway [45], possibly counterbalacing the effect exerted by myostatin normalization on skeletal muscle mass. Not only, VPA has also been shown to activate lysosomal-autophagic proteolysis in glioma cell lines [46]. While VPA effect of autophagy in the skeletal muscle has not been described, recent data show that this proteolytic pathway is activated in C26-induced cancer cachexia [47], suggesting that induction of autophagy might contribute to mask VPA effectiveness in tumor-bearing mice.

The lack of effect of DIs on C26-induced muscle wasting is in contrast with the TSA-dependent improvement of muscle phenotype in *mdx* mice [16]. However, the marked differences existing among the experimental models used, in terms of inflammatory response, regenerative stimuli and treatment schedule, likely account for such a discrepancy. The impairment of myogenesis that has been reported in the C26 hosts [48] could well be responsible for the absence of effect of VPA in correcting muscle wasting. Indeed, DIs appear to up-regulate myogenesis only in the presence of a regenerative stimulus [15], such as that occurring in the *mdx* mice [16].

Another important factor that possibly modulates the response to DIs in tumor-bearing animals is the inflammatory response. To clarify this point DIs have been tested for their ability to prevent TNFα-induced myotube atrophy. The results obtained demonstrate that myotubes deriving from myoblast differentiation in the presence of both VPA and TSA are resistant to TNFα in terms of myotube size. VPA is also effective in increasing and decreasing follistatin and myostatin expression, respectively. These results demonstrate that VPA affects the myostatin/follistatin axis also in C2C12 cultures. However, while modulations of the myostatin system result in protection against TNFα-induced myotube atrophy, they are unable to modify cancer-induced muscle wasting. These results suggest that VPA affects the inflammatory component of C26-induced muscle wasting; such efficacy however, is likely masked by other pathways that are not inhibited by the drug, or that might be even enhanced (see the effects on protein degradation cited above).

In contrast to VPA, myoblast differentiation in the presence of TSA appears to stimulate myostatin expression. This is even more evident when when myotubes are exposed to TNFα. These observations are consistent with those reported by Han *et al.* [49], showing that myostatin expression is increased in TSA-treated C2C12 myotubes, while follistatin levels remain comparable to controls. However, myotubes differentiated in the presence of TSA are resistant to TNFα-induced myotube atrophy, suggesting that this drug likely modulates pathways different from the myostatin-dependent one, at least in an *in vitro* model system.

In conclusion the results shown in the present paper demonstrate that treatment of C26-bearing mice with VPA effectively modifies the myostatin/follistatin axis in the skeletal muscle. However, such modulation does not result in improvement of cachexia. By contrast, VPA-differentiated myotubes are resistant to TNFα effects in terms of both myotube size and myostatin/follistatin ratio. One possible explanation of the different DIs effects reported in the present studies could be that cachexia induced by the C26 tumor is mainly dependent on IL-6 [50]. A more general view, however, would suggest that, the multifactorial pathogenesis of cancer cachexia might be responsible for the absence of effects associated with VPA treatment in C26-induced muscle wasting.

ACKNOWLEDGEMENTS

Work supported by 'Ministero per l'Università e la Ricerca' (MIUR, Roma; PRIN projects 2001 and 2003), University of Torino (ex-60% funds), Regione Piemonte, Italian Association for Cancer Research (AIRC), Milan, Italy.

CONFLICT OF INTEREST

The authors confirm that this chapter contents have no conflict of interest.

DISCLOSURE

The chapter submitted for the eBook Series entitled **"Advances in Cancer Drug Targets, Volume 2"** is an update of our article in **Current Cancer Drug Targets, Volume 9, Issue 5, 2009, pp. 608-616,** with additional text and references.

REFERENCES

[1] McPherron AC, Lee SJ. Double muscling in cattle due to mutations in the myostatin gene. Proc Natl Acad Sci USA 1997; 94: 12457-61.

[2] Lee SJ, McPherron AC. Regulation of myostatin activity and muscle growth. Proc Natl Acad Sci USA 2001; 98: 9306-11.

[3] Baumann AP, Ibebunjo C, Grasser WA, Paralkar VM. Myostatin expression in age and denervation-induced skeletal muscle atrophy. J Musculoskelet Neuronal Interact 2003; 3: 8-16.

[4] Ma K, Mallidis C, Bhasin S, *et al.* Glucocorticoid-induced skeletal muscle atrophy is associated with upregulation of myostatin gene expression. Am J Physiol Endocrinol Metab 2003; 285: E363-E371.

[5] Holzbaur ELF, Howland DS, Weber N, *et al.* Myostatin inhibition slows muscle strophy in rodent models of amyotrophic lateral sclerosis. Neurobiol Dis 2006; 23: 697-707.

[6] Gonzalez-Cadavid NF, Taylor WE, Yarasheski K, *et al.* Organization of the human myostatin gene and expression in healthy men and HIV-infected men with muscle wasting. Proc Natl Acad Sci USA 1998; 95: 14938-43.

[7] Hill JJ, Davies MV, Pearson AA, *et al.* The myostatin propeptide and the follistatin-related gene are inhibitory binding proteins of myostatin in normal serum. J Biol Chem 2002; 277: 40735-41.

[8] Rebbapragada A, Benchabane H, Wrana JL, Celeste AJ, Attisano, L. Myostatin signals through a transforming growth factor beta-like signaling pathway to block adipogenesis. Mol Cell Biol 2003; 23: 7230-42.

[9] Zhu X, Topouzis S, Liang LF, Stotish RL. Myostatin signaling through Smad2, Smad3 and Smad4 is regulated by the inhibitory Smad7 by a negative feedback mechanism. Cytokine 2004; 26: 262-72.

[10] McFarlane C, Plummer E, Thomas M, *et al.* Myostatin induces cachexia by activating the ubiquitin proteolytic system through an NF-kappaB-independent, FoxO1-dependent mechanism. J Cell Physiol 2006; 209: 501-14.

[11] Rodino-Klapac LR, Haidet AM, Kota J, Handy C, Kaspar BK, Mendell JR. Inhibition of myostatin with emphasis on follistatin as a therapy for muscle disease. Muscle Nerve 2009; 39: 283-96.

[12] Yang W, Chen Y, Zhang Y, Wang X, Yang N, Zhu D. Extracellular signal-regulated kinase 1/2 mitogen-activated protein kinase pathway is involved in myostatin-regulated differentiation repression. Cancer Res 2006; 66: 1320-6.

[13] Huang Z, Chen D, Zhang K, Yu B, Chen X, Meng J. Regulation of myostatin signaling by c-Jun N-Terminal kinase in C2C12 cells. Cell Signal 2007; 19: 2286-95.

[14] Iezzi S, Cossu G, Nervi C, Sartorelli V, Puri PL. Stage-specific modulation of skeletal myogenesis by inhibitors of nuclear deacetylases. Proc Natl Acad Sci USA 2002; 99: 7757-62.

[15] Iezzi S, Di Padova M, Serra C, *et al.* Deacetylase inhibitors increase muscle cell size by promoting myoblast recruitment and fusion through induction of follistatin. Develop Cell 2004; 6: 673-84.

[16] Minetti GC, Colussi C, Adami R, *et al.* Functional and morphological recovery of dystrophic muscles in mice treated with deacetylase inhibitors. Nat Med 2006; 12: 1147-50.

[17] Beharry AW, Sandesara PB, Roberts BM, Ferreira LF, Senf SM, Judge AR. HDAC1 activates FoxO and is both sufficient and required for skeletal muscle atrophy. J Cell Sci 2014; doi: 10.1242/jcs.136390.

[18] Penna F, Bonelli G, Baccino FM, Costelli P. Mechanism-based therapeutic approaches to cachexia. Vitam Horm 2013; 92: 271-99.

[19] Bonetto A, Penna F, Minero VG, *et al.* Glutamine prevents myostatin hyperexpression and protein hypercatabolism induced in C2C12 myotubes by tumor necrosis factor-α. Amino Acids 2011; 40: 585-94.

[20] Rasband WS. ImageJ. US National Institutes of Health, Bethesda, Maryland, USA. http://rsb.info.nih.gov/ij/. 1997-2007.

[21] Lowry OH, Rosebrough NJ, Farr AL, Randall RJ. Protein measurement with the Folin phenol reagent. J Biol Chem 1951; 193: 265-275.

[22] Kim AJ, Shi Y, Austin RC, Werstck GH. Valproate protects from ER stress-induced lipid accumulation and apoptosis by inhibiting glycogen synthase kinase-3. J Cell Sci 2005; 118: 89-99.

[23] Kozlovsky N, Belmaker RH, Agam G. Low GSK-3 activity in frontal cortex of schizophrenic patients. Schizophr Res 2001; 52: 101-5.

[24] Acharyya S, Butcbach MER, Sahenk Z, *et al.* Dystrophin glycoprotein complex dysfunction: A regulatory link between muscular dystrophy and cancer cachexia. Cancer Cell 2005; 8: 421-31.

[25] Lecker SH, Jagoe RT, Gilbert A, *et al.* Multiple types of skeletal muscle atrophy involve a common program of changes in gene expression. FASEB J 2004; 18: 39-51.

[26] Acharyya S, Ladner KJ, Nelsen LLN, *et al.* Cancer cachexia is regulated by selective targeting of skeletal muscle gene products. J Clin Invest 2004; 114: 370-8.

[27] Li YP, Reid MB. NF-kappaB mediates the protein loss induced by TNF-alpha in differentiated skeletal muscle myotubes. Am J Physiol Regul Integr Comp Physiol 2000; 279: R1165-70.

[28] Argilés JM, Orpí M, Busquets S, López-Soriano FJ. Myostatin: more than just a regulator of muscle mass. Drug Discov Today 2012; 17: 702-9.

[29] McMahon CD, Popovic L, Oldham JM, *et al.* Myostatin-deficient mice lose more skeletal muscle mass than wild-type controls during hindlimb suspension. Am J Physiol Endocrinol Metab 2003; 285: E82-7.

[30] Carnac G, Ricaud S, Verms B, Bonnieu A. Myostatin: biology and clinical relevance. Mini Rev Med Chem 2006; 6: 765-70.

[31] Carlson CJ, Booth FW, Gordon SE. Skeletal muscle myostatin mRNA expression is fiber-type specific and increases during hindlimb unloading. Am J Physiol Regul Integr Comp Physiol 1999; 277: R601-6.

[32] Costelli P, Muscaritoli M, Bonetto A, *et al.* Muscle myostatin signaling is enhanced in experimental cancer cachexia. Eur J Clin Invest 2008; 38: 531-8.

[33] Bonetto A, Penna F, Minero VG, *et al.* Deacetylase inhibitors modulate the myostatin/follistatin axis without improving cachexia in tumor-bearing mice. Curr Cancer Drug Targets 2009; 9: 608-16.

[34] Busquets S, Toledo M, Marmonti E, *et al.* Formoterol treatment downregulates the myostatin_system in skeletal muscle of cachectic tumour-bearing rats. Oncol Lett 2012; 3: 185-9.

[35] Busquets S, Toledo M, Orpí M, *et al.* Myostatin_blockage using actRIIB antagonism in mice bearing the Lewis lung carcinoma results in the improvement of muscle wasting and physical performance. J Cachexia Sarcopenia Muscle 2012; 3: 37-43.

[36] Liu, C-M, Yang Z, Liu C-W *et al.* Myostatin antisense RNA-mediated muscle growth in normal and cancer cachexia mice. Gene Ther 2008; 15: 155-60.

[37] Berdaux R, Goebel N, Banaszynski L, *et al.* SIK1 is a class II HDAC kinase that promotes survival of skeletal myocytes. Nat Med 2007; 13: 597-603.

[38] Fan H, Zhang R, Tesfaye D, *et al.* Sulforaphane causes a major epigenetic repression of myostatin_in porcine satellite cells. Epigenetics 2012; 7: 1379-90.

[39] Hanada M, Feng J, Hemmings BA. Structure, regulation and function of PKB/AKT - a major therapeutin target. Biochim Byophis Acta 2004; 1697: 3-16.

[40] Penna F, Bonetto A, Muscaritoli M, *et al.* Muscle atrophy in experimental cancer cachexia: is the IGF-1 signaling pathway involved? Int J Cancer 2010; 127: 1706-17.

[41] Costelli P, Baccino FM. Mechanisms of skeletal muscle depletion in wasting syndromes: role of the ATP-ubiquitin-dependent proteolysis. Curr Opin Clin Nutr Metab Care 2003; 6: 407-12.

[42] Gilson H, Schakman O, Combaret L, *et al.* Myostatin gene deletion prevents glucocorticoid-induces muscle atrophy. Endocrinology 2007; 148: 452-60.

[43] Yang H, Wei W, Menconi M, Hasselgren PO. Dexamethasone-induced protein degradation in cultured myotubes is p300/HAT dependent. Am J Physiol Regul Integr Comp Physiol 2007; 292: R337-44.

[44] Alamdari N, Smith IJ, Aversa Z, Hasselgren PO. Sepsis and glucocorticoids upregulate p300 and downregulate HDAC6 expression and activity in skeletal muscle. Am J Physiol Regul Integr Comp Physiol 2010; 299: R509-20.

[45] Krämer OH, Baus D, Knauer SK, *et al.* Acetylation of Stat1 modulates NF-kappaB activity. Genes Dev 2006; 20: 473-85.

[46] Fu J, Shao CJ, Chen FR, Ng HK, Chen ZP. Autophagy induced by_valproic_acid is associated with oxidative stress in glioma cell lines. Neuro Oncol 2010; 12: 328-40.

[47] Penna F, Costamagna D, Pin F, *et al.* Autophagic degradation contributes to muscle wasting in cancer cachexia. Am J Pathol 2013; 182: 1367-78.

[48] Penna F, Costamagna D, Fanzani, Bonelli G, Baccino FM, Costelli P. Muscle wasting and impaired myogenesis in tumor bearing mice are prevented by ERK inhibition. PLoS One 2010; 5: e13604.

[49] Han DS, Huang HP, Wang TG, *et al.* Transcription activation of myostatin by trichostatin A in differentiated C2C12 myocytes *via* ASK1-MKK3/4/6-JNK and p38 mitogen-activated protein kinase pathways. J Cell Biochem 2010; 111: 564-73.

[50] Bonetto A, Aydogdu T, Jin X, *et al.* JAK/STAT3 pathway inhibition blocks skeletal muscle wasting downstream of IL-6 and in experimental cancer cachexia. Am J Physiol Endocrinol Metab 2012; 303: E410-21.

CHAPTER 8

Indoleamine 2,3-Dioxygenase, An Emerging Target for Anti-Cancer Therapy

Xiangdong Liu*, Robert C. Newton, Steven M. Friedman and Peggy A. Scherle

Incyte Corporation, Wilmington, DE 19880, USA

Abstract: The inability of the host immune system to control tumor growth appears to result from dominant mechanisms of immune suppression that prevent the immune system from effectively responding in a way that consistently results in tumor rejection. Among the many possible mediators of tumoral immune escape, the immunoregulatory enzyme, indoleamine 2,3-dioxygenase (IDO), has recently gained considerable attention. IDO is a heme-containing, monomeric oxidoreductase that catalyzes the first and rate-limiting step in the degradation of the essential amino acid tryptophan to N-formyl-kynurenine. Tryptophan depletion as well as the accumulation of its metabolites results in a strongly inhibitory effect on the development of immune responses by blocking T cell activation, inducing T cell apoptosis and promoting the differentiation of naïve T cells into cells with a regulatory phenotype (T_{regs}). Recent data obtained from preclinical tumor models demonstrate that IDO inhibition can significantly enhance the antitumor activity of various chemotherapeutic and immunotherapeutic agents. These results, coupled with data showing that increased IDO expression is an independent prognostic variable for reduced overall survival in cancer patients, suggest that IDO inhibition may represent an effective strategy to treat malignancies, either alone or in combination with chemotherapeutics or other immune based therapies. This review will focus on the role of IDO as a mediator of peripheral immune tolerance, evidence that IDO becomes dysregulated in human cancers, and the latest progress on the development of IDO inhibitors as a novel anti-cancer therapy.

Keywords: Cancer and anti-cancer, dendritic cells, immune suppression or tolerance, indoleamine 2,3-dioxygenase, L-tryptophan, kynurenine, T cells.

INTRODUCTION

Tryptophan is the least abundant essential amino acid, comprising only 1% of total proteins [1]. The tryptophan that is not utilized in protein synthesis is catabolized by two pathways: the first pathway is through tryptophan hydroxylase (TPH) which is expressed in certain cell types in the central nervous system

***Corresponding Author Xiangdong Liu:** Incyte Corporation, Wilmington, DE 19880, USA; Tel: 302-498-6815; Fax: 302-425-2760 E-mail: xliu@incyte.com

Atta-ur-Rahman (Ed)

(CNS) and is the first step in the synthesis of serotonin [2]; and the second pathway, by which 99% of tryptophan catabolism occurs, is the salvage pathway for nicotinamide adenine dinucleotide (NAD^+) synthesis that is active when niacin is limiting in the diet [3]. The first and rate-limiting step in the second pathway is the conversion of tryptophan to kynurenine. This is catalyzed by two enzymes – tryptophan dioxygenase (TDO) and indoleamine 2,3-dioxygenase (IDO) in an oxidative reaction that requires superoxide. As shown in Fig. (**1**), TDO and IDO catabolize tryptophan to yield N-formylkynurenine [4]. Kynurenine is further catabolized leading to a number of biologically active metabolites, including the excitoxin quinolinic acid, the N-methyl D-aspartate (NMDA) receptor antagonist kynurenic acid and ultimately, the production of NAD^+ [3].

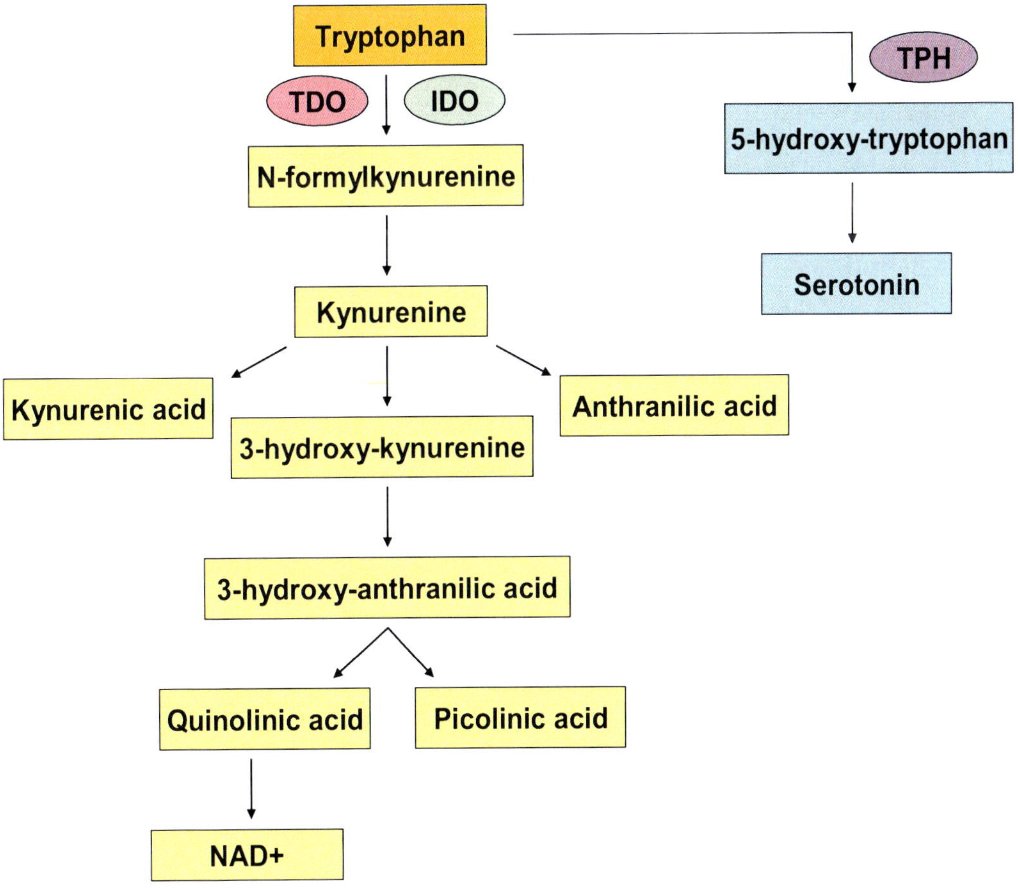

Fig. (1): The tryptophan catabolic pathways.

Although TDO and IDO are both heme-containing enzymes and catalyze the same reaction, they have very low sequence homology (11% identity, 26% similarity) and exhibit a number of other striking differences [3, 5]. For example, tryptophan is the only substrate for TDO whereas IDO recognizes a spectrum of indoleamine derivatives, including L-tryptophan, D-tryptophan, melatonin, tryptamine and serotonin. TDO is functionally active as a homotetramer and is only found in the liver where it is solely responsible for maintaining homeostatic levels of tryptophan in response to dietary uptake. IDO, on the other hand, is active as a monomer and is expressed in a variety of tissues, with particularly high levels observed within the epididymis, the placenta of pregnant females, and across large mucosal surfaces such as the gut and lung epithelium [6]. It was recognized early on that IDO activity is induced at sites of inflammation [7] and that interferon gamma (IFN-γ), a type II interferon, is a particularly potent inducer of systemic IDO activity [5].

Prior to 1998, the prevailing view had been that IDO functions to suppress microbial infections by reducing tryptophan availability in infected tissues [8]. This hypothesis was supported by studies demonstrating that the replication of certain parasites was reduced by IFN-γ and that this effect could be reversed by the addition of exogenous tryptophan to the media. However, in 1998, the biological relevance of IDO-mediated tryptophan catabolism to peripheral immune tolerance was first established by Munn *et al.* when they showed that treating female mice with a small molecule inhibitor of IDO, 1-methyl-tryptophan (1-MT), could break the toleragenic state that protects allogeneic concepti from the maternal immune system [9]. Subsequent studies have led to the hypothesis that the IDO pathway is a key regulatory element responsible for induction and maintenance of peripheral immune tolerance in normal physiological situations as well as in pathological conditions including autoimmunity, neuropathology, infection and cancer. This review will focus on the structure, expression and regulation of IDO, studies supporting the role of IDO as a mediator of immune tolerance, evidence that IDO becomes dysregulated in human cancers, and the latest progress on the development of IDO inhibitors as a novel anti-cancer therapy.

IDO BIOLOGY

Structure and Biochemical Activity

IDO is a 41 kDa, heme-containing monomeric oxidoreductase that is encoded by the *IDO1* gene which, in humans, is comprised of 10 exons spanning approximately 15 kb and is mapped to chromosome 8p12-p11 [10, 11]. Based on X-ray crystallography, the tertiary structure of IDO was shown to contain two helical domains with the heme positioned between them [12]. The smaller domain contains nine alpha-helices and two beta sheets while the larger domain consists of fifteen helices as well as the catalytic domain. Access to the catalytic site is governed by a flexible loop that runs parallel to the heme plane. While the unbound enzyme favors an open conformation of the loop, the substrate bound complex promotes closure of this region, thereby stabilizing the substrate within the catalytic site [13].

In the inactive form of IDO, the heme contains the iron in its ferric state (IDO-Fe^{3+}). Catalytic activation of IDO first requires the reduction of the ferric state to the ferrous state (IDO-Fe^{2+}) which then allows binding of L-tryptophan and oxygen to form a ternary complex [14, 15]. Once activated, IDO can bind L-tryptophan with high affinity ($K_m = 20$ μM) and catalyze the oxidative cleavage of the 2,3 double bond in the indole moiety of L-tryptophan [16], resulting in the production of N-formylkynurenine. N-formylkynurenine is then catabolized to formic acid and kynurenine, which can be further metabolized to the additional biologically active products as described above (Fig. **1**).

Another enzyme, named IDO2, was recently discovered [17, 18]. The gene encoding IDO2 is adjacent and structurally similar (43% identity) to the *IDO1* gene, suggesting that it might have arisen *via* gene duplication. The IDO2 protein is expressed in the murine kidney, liver, male and female reproductive systems and like IDO, the IDO2 enzyme appears to catalyze the oxidative cleavage of a broad range of indole-containing substrates. More detailed information of the IDO1/IDO2 gene structures and expression has been reviewed by Ball *et al.* [18]. A recent study indicated that IDO2 is the preferred enzyme target for the D isomer of 1-MT (D-1-MT) [19]. The study further demonstrated that D-1-MT has little activity against IDO – a finding that has been corroborated by the data obtained independently by other groups [20, 21]. In addition, it should be noted that IDO2 is significantly weaker than IDO in an *in vitro* assay measuring tryptophan to kynurenine conversion. Furthermore, inactivating IDO2 polymorphisms frequently occur in human populations. Another study revealed that although IDO2 is expressed in human tumors, tryptophan degradation in tumor cells is entirely mediated by IDO [22]. Together, these data raise a question about the exact biological role of IDO2, especially in humans. More studies will be required to address this question.

Regulation of Expression

IDO is expressed in various tissues throughout the body, but predominately in cells within the immune system where it is specifically induced at the transcriptional level in dendritic cells (DCs) and macrophages by cytokines at sites of inflammation. IFN-γ is one particularly potent and well-characterized inducer of IDO activity [5]. The IDO promoter contains multiple transcriptional elements, including interferon regulatory factor 1 (IRF-1) and signal transducer and activator of transcription 1 (STAT1) binding elements, that confer responsiveness to IFN-γ. Because IDO appears to be integrated within the complex milieu of regulatory factors that promote immune tolerance, a number of other immune modulators impact its expression and activity as well and have been described in greater detail in other reviews [6, 23]. Immunomodulatory agents such as Toll receptor agonists including LPS and CpGs, type I interferons and transforming growth factor beta (TGF-β) have been shown to induce IDO expression in the $CD11c^{+}$ $CD19^{+}$ subpopulation of plasmacytoid DCs, and in $CD8^{+}$ and $CD8^{-}$ DCs [24, 25]. The prostaglandin E2 (PGE2) has also been shown to dramatically increase IDO expression although tumor necrosis factor alpha (TNF-α) was additionally required to elicit enzymatic activity [26]. In contrast, interleukin 4 (IL-4) [27], interleukin 10 (IL-10) [28], inducible nitric oxide synthase (iNOS) [29] and tryptophan [30] have all been reported to antagonize IFN-γ mediated induction of IDO expression.

In addition to pro-inflammatory cytokines, signals from T cells can also influence IDO expression. For example, the immunoregulatory molecules CTLA-4 (cytotoxic T lymphocyte-associated antigen 4), CD40 (TNF receptor superfamily member 5) and 4-1BB (TNF superfamily member 9 or CD137) have all been shown to increase IDO expression [31-33]. $CD4^+CD25^+$ T_{regs} (regulatory T cells) that constitutively express CTLA-4 on their surface can promote IDO activity in DCs through a CTLA-4 dependent mechanism [34]. CD28-Ig (cluster of differentiation 28 and immunoglobulin fusion protein) binds the B7 T cell costimulatory molecule like CTLA-4-Ig, but has the opposite effect on IDO expression [35]. DCs treated with CD28-Ig exhibited rapid and sustained production of interleukin 6 (IL-6) that was shown to upregulate suppressor of cytokine signaling 3 (SOCS3) and inhibit the STAT-dependent IFN-γ signaling required for IDO induction.

IDO can also be regulated post-translationally in addition to its regulation at the transcriptional level [36]. Changes in intracellular redox status may contribute to this regulation [37] as well as the actions of certain cytokines [6, 26]. The precise mechanisms involved are unclear although gene expression profiling in $CD8\alpha^+$ DCs led to the identification of the *Tyrobp*-encoded DAP12 (DNAX-activating protein of molecular mass 12 kilodaltons or TYRO protein tyrosine kinase binding protein) as involved in post-translational suppression of IDO activity [38]. In addition, it was recently shown that SOCS3 can bind to IDO and target it for ubiquitination and proteosomal degradation [39], thus suggesting that proteolysis can also contribute to the complexity of IDO regulation.

Biological Function as a Mediator of Immune Tolerance

The importance of IDO as a regulator of T cell function has been demonstrated in both rodent and human model systems and has been covered extensively in other reviews [6]. The first indications of a mechanistic involvement of IDO in the suppression of T cell activation were obtained in a study using human macrophages exposed to colony stimulating factor 1 (CSF-1) *in vitro*, which promoted the induction of IDO activity in these cells in the context of the mixed lymphocyte reaction (MLR) and led to a block of T cell activation by inducing G1 arrest [40]. Most recent attention has focused on the expression of IDO in DCs and has come from investigating the toleragenic mechanism elicited by $CD11c^+CD8\alpha^+$ DCs in the context of challenge with tumor/self antigens. For example, in an *in vivo* rodent delayed type hypersensitivity (DTH) skin test model, fractionated CD8α⁻ myeloid DCs presented with tumor/self peptide were actively immunogenic but could be effectively inhibited by reintroduction of a minority population of $CD8\alpha^+$ lymphoid DCs which were shown to express IDO. This effect was reversed by the addition of the IDO inhibitor, 1-MT [41]. Of particular note has been the seminal finding that IDO activity in DCs can act as an important downstream effector for the immunoregulatory molecule CTLA-4. Murine $CD8\alpha^-$ DCs treated with CTLA-4-Ig displayed IDO activity and were rendered toleragenic both *in vitro* and *in vivo* [42, 43]. Again, the effect of CTLA-4-Ig was abrogated by 1-MT treatment or by using IDO-null mice as hosts [44].

How IDO-mediated tryptophan catabolism can elicit immune tolerance has not yet been fully elucidated as there is evidence for different but not mutually exclusive mechanisms of action. Some studies have indicated that induction of IDO activity may only be necessary for the acquisition of a suppressor phenotype [41, 45, 46]. Most attention, however, has focused on the direct suppression of T cells by IDO-mediated tryptophan catabolism, which involves both the degradation of growth-essential tryptophan and the production of pro-apoptotic tryptophan catabolites [47-50]. The finding that T cells from *Gcn2*-null mice are no longer responsive to IDO-expressing DCs also suggests that IDO-mediated induction of proliferative arrest and energy is signaled through the GCN2 kinase pathway in response to environmental tryptophan depletion [51].

In addition to the effects on T cell proliferation, several studies have shown that IDO expressed in DCs results in the generation of T_{regs} by promoting the conversion of naïve $CD4^+$ T cells into $Foxp3^+$ T cells with a regulatory phenotype [52, 53]. It has also been shown that IDO expression in DCs contributes to DC maturation and T_{regs} expansion [54]. Finally, a recent study has demonstrated that IDO can activate T_{regs} through the GCN2 pathway and that the IDO-activated T_{regs} mediate their suppression through the PD-1/PD-L (programmed cell death 1/programmed cell death ligands) pathway [55]. IDO-mediated tryptophan catabolism has also been shown to have a number of additional effects on immune cells including downmodulation of T cell receptor zeta chain expression in $CD8^+$ cells, inhibition of NK cell proliferation, and impaired generation of memory $CD8^+$ cells [23]. Together, the data suggest that IDO-mediated suppression of T cell responses occurs through multiple mechanisms, including decreased T cell proliferation, increased T cell apoptosis and induction of T_{regs}, that together lead to impairment of the cellular immune response (Fig. **2**).

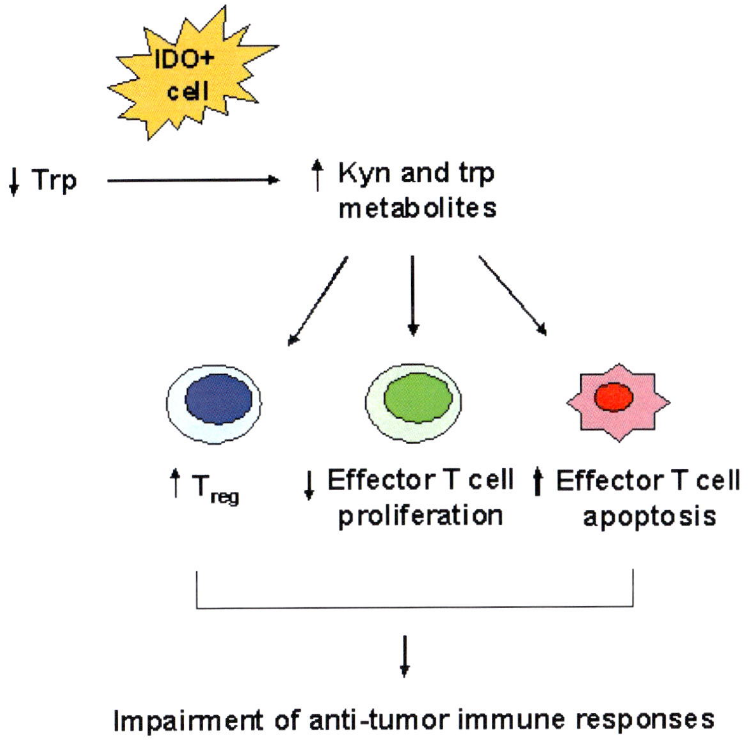

Fig. (2): IDO-mediated immune suppression.

IDO DYSREGULATION IN HUMAN CANCERS

Aberrant IDO activity has been associated with a wide variety of non-oncologic human pathological conditions, including but not limited to autoimmune diseases, infectious diseases, depression, obesity, organ and bone marrow transplantation, and atherosclerosis. Direct evidence for this has been obtained by studying patients as well as relevant animal models [6, 56-61] and together, the data suggest that IDO agonists and antagonists could have utility in treating these conditions. Since most of these topics have previously been reviewed or described by others [6, 56-61], the remainder of this review will focus on the dysregulation of IDO in human cancers.

Several lines of evidence suggest that the IDO pathway plays a key role in regulating immune evasion by tumors. This includes data showing that: 1) IDO is overexpressed by a wide variety of human tumors, tumor infiltrating lymphocytes (TILs) and DCs that localize to the tumor draining lymph nodes (TDLNs); 2) IDO activation in patients correlates with disease progression and reduced overall survival, as well as drug resistance; and 3) IDO inhibition significantly reduces tumor growth and increases the antitumor activities of various chemotherapeutic and immunotherapeutic agents in relevant animal models. These findings are detailed in the sections below.

Numerous studies have shown that elevated IDO expression or activity can be found in patients with various cancers, and in some cases it is associated with poor clinical outcome and drug resistance (Table **1**). For example, upon examining a series of tumor tissues of various origins, Uyttenhove *et al.* found that most human tumor types expressed IDO [62]. Strikingly, all tested tumor samples of prostatic, colorectal, pancreatic and cervical carcinomas, as well as many samples of other tumor types were IDO positive. Another study of prostate cancer patients confirmed that higher IDO levels were more frequently detected in prostate cancer tissues than in benign prostatic hyperplasia [63]. Because tryptophan (trp) degradation and kynurenine (kyn) production are indicative of IDO activity in cancer patients, this study also revealed that higher IDO levels in the tumor tissues correlated with a higher kyn/trp ratio in patients' sera. IDO expression was also detected in tumor tissues of breast cancer patients [64], and tryptophan degradation was detected in patients with gynecological cancer [65].

In addition to its expression in tumor cells, IDO has also been found in tumor infiltrating cells or cells from the stroma and lymph nodes. In a study of uterine cervical cancer, IDO expression in tumor cells as well as T_{regs} was found in cervical intraepithelial neoplasia CIN-3 of the uterine cervix [66]. Interestingly, IDO^+ T_{regs} and cancer cells co-localized and were found predominantly at the invasive border of the tumor. Another study of small cell lung cancer revealed that IDO was expressed in the tumor-infiltrating eosinophils and the level of IDO^+ eosinophil infiltrate was further associated with shortened overall survival [67].

Table 1: IDO Dysregulation in Human Cancers

Cancer Type	Comments	Refs.
Acute monocyte leukemia	High IDO (in cancer cells)	[80]
Acute lymphocyte leukemia	High IDO (in cancer cells)	[80]
Acute myeloid leukemia	High IDO (in cancer cells); higher kyn/trp ratio (in blood) linked to poor survival	[81, 82]
T cell leukemia/lymphoma	High IDO (in cancer cells); higher kyn levels & kyn/trp ratio (in blood) inversely linked to chemotherapy	[62, 83]
Bladder	Various IDO levels (in cancer cells)	[62]
Breast	High IDO (in tumor tissue)	[62, 64]
Cervical	IDO detection (in cancer cells and T_{regs}), not linked to prognosis	[62, 66]
Colorectal	High IDO (in cancer cells) and reduced $CD3^+$ infiltrating T cells, linked to liver metastasis and poor survival	[62, 70, 71]
Endometrial	High IDO (in cancer cells) and reduced infiltrating lymphocytes and NK cells, linked to impaired progression-free survival	[62, 68, 69]
Gastric	High IDO (in cancer cells)	[62]
Glioblastoma	High IDO (in cancer cells)	[62]
Gynecological	Higher kyn levels and kyn/trp ratio and lower trp (in blood)	[65]
Head and neck	IDO detection (in cancer cells)	[62]
Pediatric Hodgkin's lymphoma	High IDO (in cancer cells) and higher kyn/trp ratio (in blood)	FN #2
Liver	Conflicting data regarding IDO involvement	[62, 85, 86]
Lung	IDO detection (in tumor tissues and non-malignant lung tissues), not linked to prognosis	[84]
Non-small cell lung	IDO detection (in cancer cells)	[62]
Small cell lung	IDO detection (in infiltrating eosinophils), linked to poor overall survival	[62, 67]
Melanoma	High IDO (in cancer cells and DCs of TDLNs) and higher kyn/trp ratio and neopterin (in blood), increased T_{regs}, linked to metastasis and poor survival	[62, 75-77, 79]
Mesothelioma	IDO detection (in cancer cells)	[62]
Oral squamous cell	High IDO (in cancer cells), linked to metastasis, chemoresistance and prognosis	FN #1
Ovary	High IDO (in cancer cells), linked to poor survival and paclitaxel resistance in serous type	[62, 73, 74]
Pancreatic ductal adenocarcinoma	IDO upregulation (in cancer cells) and increased T_{regs}	[62, 72]
Prostate	High IDO (in cancer cells) and higher kyn/trp ratio (in blood)	[62, 63]
Renal cell carcinoma (clear cell)	High IDO (in endothelial cells of newly formed blood vessels), inversely correlated with tumor cell growth	[62, 87]

Several studies have attempted to link IDO expression/activity with its proposed mechanism of action, demonstrating that IDO expression/activation is associated with reduced intratumoral T cell infiltration, disease progression, as well as overall survival. For example, in a study of endometrial cancer patients, high IDO expression in tumor cells was found in 32 of 65 cases and was positively correlated with myometrial invasion, nodal metastasis, and lymph-vascular space involvement [68]. There was also a significant correlation between high IDO expression and reduced numbers of $CD3^+$ and $CD8^+$ lymphocytes and $CD57^+$ natural killer (NK) cells infiltrating into both the tumor epithelium and stroma. Significantly shortened progression-free survival (PFS) was observed in patients with high IDO levels, a low number of stromal $CD3^+$ cells, and low intraepithelial $CD8^+$ or low stromal $CD8^+$ lymphocytes. In fact, IDO expression and the number of stromal $CD3^+$ lymphocytes were shown to be independent prognostic factors for impaired PFS [68, 69]. These results suggest that tumoral IDO expression correlates with a reduced number of TILs and NK cells in endometrial cancer, possibly contributing to disease progression and poor clinical outcome.

A survival trend was also observed when the role of IDO was investigated in colorectal cancer (CRC) patients (n = 143) [70]. In this study, high IDO expression was associated with a significant reduction of infiltrating $CD3^+$ T cells compared to patients with low IDO. Further, high IDO staining significantly correlated with the frequency of liver metastases. Fifty percent of patients with high IDO primary tumors had metastases while metastases were detected in only 29% of patients with low IDO. Again, high IDO expression was shown to be an independent prognostic variable. Separately, decreased serum tryptophan also correlated with decreased immune activation and impaired quality of life in colorectal cancer patients [71].

Another interesting study of metastatic pancreatic ductal adenocarcinoma (PDA) showed that IDO upregulation in metastatic PDA cells was associated with an increased number of T_{reg} cells [72]. Although IDO protein was present in all tumors (primary and metastatic) from patients with lymph node metastases, intensity of staining was stronger in the corresponding metastatic foci when compared with the primary tumor. Three nonmetastatic PDAs were negative or only focally positive for IDO. Strikingly, forkhead box p3 (Foxp3) positive T_{reg}

cells were increased in lymph nodes containing IDO^+ metastatic tumor cells. The data indicate that metastatic PDA cells may be selected for IDO overexpression to evade immunologic detection. A study of oral squamous cell cancer patients revealed that IDO was overexpressed in 39/88 (44.3%) tumor specimens and high IDO immunoreactivity significantly correlated with the frequency of metastases (Kronberger IE *et al.*[1]). By multivariate Cox's analysis high IDO expression emerged as independent prognostic variable.

IDO may also be involved in mechanism(s) leading to chemoresistance in cancer patients. In a study of ovarian cancer patients (n = 122), IDO staining was positive in 57.5% of serous adenocarcinomas (SA), 49.2% of clear cell adenocarcinomas (CCA), and 73.3% of endometrioid adenocarcinomas (EA), respectively [73]. The Kaplan-Meier analysis showed a clear relationship between IDO staining score and overall survival in patients (n = 33) with advanced (stages III and IV) SA who underwent optimal surgery and paclitaxel-carboplatin (TC) chemotherapy as a first-line regimen. In addition, a positive correlation between IDO expression and paclitaxel resistance was reported by the same group in a separate study of patients with serous type ovarian cancer [74].

Several studies have addressed the role of IDO in melanoma – a tumor type in which many immunotherapeutic agents have been evaluated. In addition to the fact that tumor cells from melanoma patients often express IDO [62, 75], IDO stained positively in DCs from the TDLNs of many patients, which was also correlated with poor prognosis [76]. Furthermore, the presence of IDO^+ DCs in the sentinel nodes was frequently noted prior to overt metastasis. When archival cutaneous melanoma tumors (n = 14) and regional lymph nodes (n = 328) were examined [77], an abnormal accumulation of IDO^+ cells with a monocytoid or plasmacytoid morphology was identified in the perisinusoidal regions of draining lymph nodes in 45% of the nodes studied. It was thus hypothesized that these IDO^+ antigen-presenting cells (APCs) may be recruited and contribute to the acquired tolerance to tumor antigens. In another study of a DC-based vaccine, IDO mRNA was detected in a series of human DCs prior to vaccination of

---

[1]Kronberger, I. E., Laimer, K., Perathoner, A.; Fuchs, D.; Margreiter, R.; Amberger, A.; Brandacher, G. Increased expression of indoleamine 2,3-dioxygenase contributes to response to adjuvant therapy and overall survival in patients with oral squamous cell carcinoma. *The 98th AACR Annual Meeting*. **2007**, Abstract # 172.

advanced melanoma patients [78]. In biopsies obtained 24 hour after vaccination, a prominent infiltrate of IDO^+ cells was observed. Moreover, the cell infiltrate of these sites stained positive for Foxp3, indicating an IDO-associated accumulation of T_{reg} cells. Further, all analyzed patients receiving the DC-based vaccine exhibited rapid disease progression with a short overall survival, suggesting a potential immune suppressive role of IDO in DC-based vaccines *via* the attraction of T_{reg} cells. In a separate study, lower trp levels were reported in a group of patients ($n = 87$) with malignant melanoma compared to healthy volunteers ($n = 49$) [79]. This was especially true for the subgroup of patients with distant metastases ($p = 0.01$). There existed a positive correlation between kyn/trp ratio and neopterin (an immune activation marker) levels ($p < 0.001$). In patients who died due to tumor dissemination, median trp levels were significantly decreased ($p = 0.006$), and the kyn/trp ratio ($p = 0.03$) and neopterin levels ($p = 0.002$) were higher compared to survivors. In addition, lower trp levels as well as higher kyn/trp ratio and neopterin levels predicted a shorter survival. Thus, decreased serum trp levels and elevated serum neopterin levels may be useful as predictive markers for the future course in melanoma patients. The data are also consistent with the notion that higher IDO activity may contribute to tumor progression.

In addition to solid tumors, aberrant IDO expression has also been reported in hematological malignancies. A study showed high IDO levels in 29.4 % of acute monocyte leukemia patients and 24.7% of acute lymphocyte leukemia (ALL) patients [80]. IDO was also detected in primary cancer cells from 40 out of 76 (52%) acute myeloid leukemia (AML) patients [81]. In addition, a higher serum kyn/trp ratio was detected in AML patients and was further shown to be associated with reduced survival [82]. Similar findings were reported in pediatric Hodgkin's disease where tumor tissues from 17 out of 20 patients were stained positively for IDO and an increased serum kyn/trp ratio was observed (Shahlaee AH *et al*[2]). Hoshi *et al.* found that serum kyn levels, kyn/trp ratio, IDO mRNA/protein levels in T cell leukemia/lymphoma (ATLL) cells were all significantly increased in ATLL patients compared to healthy individuals, while trp levels were significantly decreased in the same group of the patients.

---

[2]Shahlaee, A. H.; Al-Quran, S, Z.; Hou, W.; Schwartz, C.; Munn, D. H. Aberrant indoleamine 2,3 dioxygenase (IDO) expression is present in pediatric patients with Hodgkin's lymphoma. *Journal of Clinical Oncology, 2007 ASCO Annual Meeting Proceedings*. **2007**, 25 (18S), 9531.

Interestingly, upon receiving chemotherapy, serum kyn levels as well as soluble IL-2 receptor levels were significantly reduced while trp levels were significantly increased, suggestive of IDO pathway activation [83].

There are also studies in which a correlation between IDO expression and poor clinical outcome could not be established or conflicting data were reported. For example, the study of uterine cervical cancer by Nakamura *et al.* [66] did not reveal significant correlation between IDO expression in tumor cells and/or T_{regs} and patient prognosis, despite the significant increase of these cells in metastatic lymph nodes compared with non-metastatic lymph nodes. Another study of lung cancer showed that IDO mRNA was detected in most patients' tumor samples and non-malignant lung tissues, and no significant correlations between IDO expression and clinicopathological parameters were found [84]. Conflicting data were reported in patients with hepatocellular carcinoma (HCC). One study of primary HCC clinical surgical specimens (n = 138) revealed that IDO was overexpressed in 35.5% of tumor resection samples, whereas 64.5% of cases showed weak staining. IDO overexpression was significantly correlated with high metastasis rates ($p = 0.049$) and was further associated with significantly poor prognosis ($p = 0.017$). Multivariate Cox's analysis suggested that IDO expression was an independent prognostic factor for overall survival of HCC patients ($p = 0.010$) [85]. However, another study of HCC patients found that IDO mRNA was only detected in tumor infiltrating cells but not in tumor cells, and the recurrence-free survival rate of IDO^+ HCC patients was significantly higher than that of IDO^- patients [86]. Finally, a study examined IDO expression in tumor cell and microvessel endothelial cells of clear cell renal cell carcinoma (RCC, 55 primary and 52 metastatic, along with 32 normal kidneys) [87]. Over 75% of the patient samples had elevated IDO levels compared to normal kidneys. Low IDO mRNA levels in primary tumors represented an unfavorable independent prognostic factor ($p = 0.016$). Unexpectedly, IHC analyses revealed that IDO was nearly exclusively expressed in endothelial cells of newly formed blood vessels and was virtually absent from tumor cells. A highly significant inverse correlation between the density of IDO^+ microvessels and the content of proliferating K_i67^+ tumor cells in primary and metastatic patients was found ($p = 0.004$). The authors proposed that IDO in endothelial cells might limit the influx of tryptophan from the blood to the tumor or generate tumor-toxic metabolites, thus restricting tumor growth and contributing to patient survival.

In summary, although the results of a few studies are contradictory and if confirmed may point to different roles of IDO in different cancer types, the vast majority of the data support the involvement of IDO in promoting tumor progression by suppressing local tumor immunity. Therefore, IDO represents an attractive target for therapeutic intervention.

THERAPEUTIC POTENTIAL OF IDO INHIBITION

Abnormal tryptophan metabolism and kynurenine accumulation in the urine of cancer patients were first reported over a half century ago [88-91]. The early belief was that IDO activation imposes an inhibitory effect on human tumors by depleting tryptophan essential for tumor cell survival [92]. However, the direct evidence supporting the involvement of IDO in controlling tumor growth came from a series of recent experiments, demonstrating that ectopic expression of *IDO1* promoted tumor growth in immuno-competent mice and that this effect could be reversed by the specific suppression of IDO enzymatic activity or expression [62]. Significantly, a novel mechanism of local immune suppression was proposed a few years ago as the potential mechanism of action [6], namely that IDO available from various sources in the tumor microenvironment helps tumor cells to evade local immune destruction by suppressing tumor-reactive lymphocytes. Since then, this proposed mechanism has been corroborated by numerous subsequent studies.

For example, it was shown in an animal model that mononuclear cells that invaded tumors and TDLNs expressed IDO [93]. In this study, Lewis lung carcinoma (LLC) cells promoted a more effective allogeneic T cell response *in vitro* in the presence of 1-MT. Moreover, when administered *in vivo,* 1-MT resulted in the inhibition of LLC tumor growth in syngeneic mice. The data suggest that tumors evade immune rejection at least in part through IDO and that inhibiting IDO led to an antitumor effect. The seminal work conducted by Uyttenhove *et al.* [62] further showed that ectopic expression of IDO by immunogenic mouse tumor cells prevented their rejection by preimmunized mice.

This effect was accompanied by the lack of accumulation of specific T cells at the tumor site and could be partly reversed by the systemic treatment of mice with 1-MT. Additionally, using an engineered leukemia mouse model, it was shown that 1-MT inhibited tumor growth and offered significant survival benefit compared to control mice [80]. These data suggest that IDO is involved in the suppression of local immune activity that could otherwise prevent or slow tumor growth *in vivo,* and that an IDO inhibitor may have therapeutic utility.

Several studies of multiple tumor types indicate that an IDO-mediated immunosuppressive mechanism may be involved in attenuating the antitumor efficacy of both chemotherapeutic agents and vaccines. One such study utilized the IDO expressing AMEC human endometrial carcinoma cell and showed that IDO expression markedly enhanced tumor growth in IDO^+ AMEC xenografted mice when compared with control mice. Interestingly, the numbers of splenic NK cells in IDO^+ AMEC xenografted mice were significantly decreased. Further, oral administration of D-1-MT in combination with paclitaxel in IDO^+ AMEC xenografted mice strongly potentiated the antitumor effect of paclitaxel, resulting in significantly prolonged survival [94]. Another group showed that 1-MT prevented tryptophan depletion and further enhanced the inhibitory effects of chemotherapeutic agents such as temozolomide, bischloroethylnitrosourea, etoposide and cisplatin in glioma cells [95]. A similar observation was made in a study utilizing the spontaneous mammary tumors that develop in the MMTV-*Neu* transgenic mouse model, where IDO inhibition alone was less effective than when it was deployed in combination with various chemotherapeutic agents [96]. Moreover, the antitumor activity of IDO inhibition appeared to be mediated by T cells as the effect was abolished by the depletion of either $CD4^+$ or $CD8^+$ T cells prior to treatment.

In another assessment of efficacy of a DC/Lewis lung carcinoma (LLC) fusion vaccine in a LLC-derived mouse model [97], it was noted that IDO^+ cells accumulated in TDLNs. Further, vaccination with fusion DC/LLC cells alone caused significant upregulation of IDO in spleens, and 1-MT enhanced the antitumor activity of the vaccine, as evidenced by delayed tumor development and induction of enhanced splenic cytotoxic T lymphocyte (CTL) responses. Most recently, it was shown in a B16 melanoma model that the combination of 1-MT with an anti-tumor vaccine resulted in the conversion of T_{regs} to a T-helper Th17-like phenotype with concomitant $CD8^+$ T cell activation and enhanced anti-tumor efficacy [98]. Also, in a *ret* transgenic mouse tumor model, 1-MT enhanced the activity of a RET peptide-based vaccine to control spontaneous tumor development [99]. Collectively, these results suggest that IDO inhibition can enhance the efficacy of both chemotherapeutic and immunotherapeutic approaches.

IDO may also play a part in tumor resistance to cytokine-based treatments. In a recent study utilizing immunocompetent and nude mice bearing the RMA lymphoma, B16F melanoma, or WEHI-164 fibrosarcoma, frequent administration of an IFNγ-NGR (a tumor neovasculature homing peptide) fusion protein resulted in reduced efficacy and tumor resistance [100]. Notably, IDO activity was increased in lymphoma homogenates after multiple treatments with IFNγ-NGR, but not after a single treatment. Co-administration of 1-MT increased tumor responses to multiple treatments with IFNγ-NGR in all tumor models. No synergism between IFNγ-NGR and 1-MT was observed *in vitro* in tumor cell proliferation assays or in tumor-bearing nude mice, implying that the potentiating effect was mediated by host T cells. The authors suggested that the IDO-mediated tumor resistance could be caused by excessive stimulation of tryptophan catabolism.

Instead of relying on IDO inhibitors such as 1-MT, several studies have utilized IDO-specific small interfering RNA (siRNA) to show the benefits of IDO inhibition in relevant models. Specifically, Zheng *et al.* [101] showed that IDO siRNA treatment of B16 tumor cells *in vitro* inhibited tumor cell growth and enhanced tumor-specific killing. More recently, it was shown that skin delivery of IDO siRNA inhibited tumor growth and prolonged survival in both the MBT-2 murine bladder and CT-26 colon tumor models [102]. Concurrently, IDO expression was down-regulated in $CD11c^+$ lymphocytes, and the number of infiltrating T cells and neutrophils increased at tumor sites. T cells may be mainly responsible for the tumor rejection because the effect was abolished by $CD8^+$ T cell depletion. In addition, in a *neu*-overexpressing MBT-2 tumor model, IDO siRNA enhanced the efficacy of a HER-2/Neu DNA vaccine. The data suggest that antitumor immunity can be effectively elicited by IDO-specific siRNAs as well as small molecule inhibitors, and the results further confirm that IDO inhibition can potentiate cancer vaccines.

DEVELOPMENT OF IDO INHIBITORS

Given the substantial evidence supporting the role of IDO in regulating tumor immune tolerance and other relevant medical conditions, there is a growing interest in developing pharmaceutically suitable IDO inhibitors for therapeutic utility. Several IDO inhibitors or compound scaffolds have been previously reported in the literature, as listed in Table **2**. Some are structurally related tryptophan analogs, such as 1-MT and methythiohydantoin-tryptophan (MTH-trp). However, most of them possess fairly weak enzymatic and cellular activities, as well as properties unfavorable for pharmaceutical development. Recently, additional medicinal chemistry efforts have been undertaken to discover more suitable inhibitors and significant progress has been made [103, 104]. Among all IDO inhibitors reported to date, 1-MT is the most well-studied. In this section, we review 1-MT and other reported IDO inhibitors from a development perspective.

Table 2: Reported IDO Inhibitors*

Agent	Developer	Comments	Refs.
Clinical			
D-1-MT	NewLink Genetics	Phase I trials in patients with various tumors	[105, 107, 108]
IDO inhibitor	Incyte	IND approved for oncology indications	[103, 104]
Preclinical			
MTH-Trp			[30, 96]
Phenylimidazole-based			[109]
Naphthoquinone-based			[110]
Brassinin			[112, 113]
Exiguamine A			[114-116]
Diindolmethane			FN #5
NSC401366			[117]

* Data as of August 2009. FN: Footnote.

1-MT has been used in most preclinical studies and exists as two stereoisomers, D and L. These isomers exhibit differential activities in assays performed with different cell types [105]. The L isomer has been reported to be more potent against the purified enzyme and in HeLa cell-based assays. The D isomer, on the other hand, was more effective in reversing the suppression of T cell proliferation by IDO$^+$ DCs, using both human monocyte-derived DCs and murine DCs isolated directly from TDLNs. Further, the D isomer was more efficacious *in vivo* as an anticancer agent either alone or in combination with cytotoxic agents. It was originally believed that the D isomer specifically targets the IDO pathway based on the fact that the antitumor effect of D-1-MT is completely lost in *INDO* knockout mice. However, the D isomer has recently been shown to be largely inactive against the IDO enzyme and in several experimental systems that measure tryptophan to kynurenine conversion [19, 20, 22]. Moreover, 1-MT has been shown to exhibit activity in dendritic cells independent of IDO inhibition [106]. Clearly, there are conflicting data regarding the precise roles of the individual 1-MT isomers in the regulation of the IDO pathway that need to be resolved. Nevertheless, an effort to develop D-1-MT in the clinic has been undertaken. Preclinical evaluation of the pharmacokinetics (PK) and toxicology of D-1-MT in rats and dogs suggests that the compound has low protein binding, high exposure, a long half-life, and low clearance in both species. In addition, oral administration of the compound at close to saturating doses in both species for 28 consecutive days was well tolerated with no mortality, adverse events, histopathological lesions or significant changes in hematology, clinical chemistries, and body weight [107]. These data suggest that D-1-MT has an overall safe profile in preclinical species. D-1-MT is currently being investigated in clinical trials aimed at assessing the utility of IDO inhibition to block host-mediated immunosuppression and enhance antitumor immunity [105]. Given the conflicting data regarding the activity of D-1-MT against IDO and a lack of solid evidence of IDO2 biological function, it remains a question whether this compound will adequately test the hypothesis of IDO inhibition in cancer patients.

Four phase I trials are currently ongoing in the United States (US) to evaluate D-1-MT in advanced cancer patients with various solid tumors [108]. Interestingly, an abstract from the 2006 American Society of Clinical Oncology (ASCO) annual meeting described a small study on the effects of an autologous thermostable hemoderivative vaccine (ATHV) with and without 1-MT in metastatic prostate cancer patients (n=30) (Lasalvia-Prisco EM *et al.*[3]). The patients were randomized into three groups subjected to different treatments: I, only sympthomatic; II, ATHV and III, ATHV + simultaneous subcutaneous administration of 1-MT, and trp to kyn conversion was monitored to assess IDO inhibition. The study found that tumor growth was significantly slower in Group II and III than in Group I ($p<0.01$ and $p<0.005$). Tumor growth was also significantly slower in Group III than in Group II ($p<0.02$). IDO inhibition was confirmed only in Group III. No severe toxicities were reported. Although the authors did not disclose which isomer was used, if L-1-MT was used this preliminary result would support that breaking immune tolerance *via* IDO inhibition may enhance the tumor growth inhibition exerted by a cancer vaccine. In addition, an ongoing phase I trial conducted in the US has recently reported early evidence of antitumor activity of D-1-MT as a single agent in patients with solid tumors at a well tolerated dose (Soliman HH *et al.*[4]). However, one has to be cautious in interpreting these findings because they were reports from scientific conferences and have not been subjected to vigorous scientific scrutiny.

Recently, Incyte Corporation disclosed their identification of a novel, potent IDO inhibitor that has completed preclinical pharmacological, PK and safety assessments, and has been cleared by the US Food and Drug Administration (FDA) for human testing [103]. A compound from the same series was shown to be a competitive inhibitor with low nM cellular potency (IC_{50} = 19 nM) and demonstrated potent *in vivo* antitumor activity in the GM-CSF-expressing B16 mouse melanoma tumor model [104]. Overall, this novel series of compounds are significantly more potent than all other IDO inhibitors previously reported and exhibit impressive activities in various relevant *in vitro* and *in vivo* systems. In addition, these compounds possess excellent PK properties and safety profile. Given the controversy surrounding 1-MT, a true IDO inhibitor with favorable

[3] Lasalvia-Prisco, E. M.; Garcia-Giralt, E.; Cucchi, S.; Larranaga, J.; Wagner, D. Prostate cancer: Autologous immunotherapy optimized by indoleamine-2,3-dioxygenase (IDO)-inhibitor as immune-tolerance breaker. *Journal of Clinical Oncology, 2006 ASCO Annual Meeting Proceedings*. **2006**, 24 (18S), 12509.

[4] Soliman, H. H.; Antonia, S.; Sullivan, D.; Vanahanian, N.; Link, C.; Lee, H. Overcoming tumor antigen anergy in human malignancies using the novel indoleamine 2,3-dioxygenase (IDO) enzyme inhibitor, 1-methyl-D-tryptophan (1MT). *Journal of Clinical Oncology, 2009 ASCO Annual Meeting Proceedings*. **2009**, 27 (15S), 3004.

pharmacological properties would be of great value to better understand the role of IDO and to further explore the therapeutic potential of IDO inhibition in the clinic.

In addition to the compounds described above, there are a number of preclinical IDO inhibitors that have been reported. MTH-Trp, a *de novo* IDO enzyme inhibitor, is more active than 1-MT. An *in vitro* recombinant human IDO enzyme assay showed that MTH-trp was a competitive inhibitor with K_i = 11.6 μM while 1-MT was about 3-fold less potent (K_i = 34.3 μM). Additionally, MTH-trp was shown to be approximately 20-fold more potent than 1-MT in a cell-based assay. The thiohydantoin side chain is probably a mimetic of the amino acid backbone in tryptophan. Preliminary data indicated that MTH-trp was more soluble in aqueous solution than 1-MT but was also more rapidly cleared from serum. MTH-trp is orally active and like 1-MT, MTH-trp also slowed tumor growth and potentiated cytotoxic agent such as paclitaxel in the MMTV-*Neu* tumor model [30, 96].

Recently, 4-phenylimidazole (4-PI) derivatives were described as IDO inhibitors. Based on the reported crystal structure of IDO and computational modeling, several 4-PI analogues interacting with IDO at different sites such as the active site entrance, the interior of the active site or the heme iron binding site were tested. The three most potent inhibitors from this series had single digit μM enzyme potency [109]. The same group also reported a different class of naphthoquinone-based IDO inhibitors [110]. Mendione, an example of the class, exhibited similar antitumor activity to previously characterized IDO inhibitors in mouse tumor models. Efforts were taken to increase the potency of this series of compounds and a pyranonaphthoquinone-based analogue was identified as the most potent compound with a K_i= 61-70 nM against the IDO enzyme. However, its cellular potency was around 7 μM. Nevertheless, synthetic accessibility of these compounds will facilitate preclinical SAR analysis as well as further optimization of their pharmacological properties.

Several natural products have also been identified as IDO inhibitors. Brassinin is a phytoalexin, a natural product from cruciferous plants. Brassinin has chemopreventive activity in preclinical models but the underlying mechanisms are largely unknown [111]. The original natural product brassinin was found to be a moderately active competitive IDO inhibitor (*K*i = 97.7 μM). A search of its structural analogues led to further understanding of the structure-activity relationship (SAR) and the identification of compounds (*e.g.*, *K*i = 11.6 μM) that are more potent than 1-MT [112]. Another recent study showed that brassinin and a synthetic derivative 5-bromo-brassinin (5-Br-brassinin) are bioavailable IDO inhibitors [113]. Both compounds, when combined with chemotherapy, caused regression of mammary gland tumors in MMTV-*Neu* mice. In addition, growth of highly aggressive melanoma isograft tumors was suppressed by 5-Br-brassinin treatment alone. This effect was not observed in athymic mice, indicating the participation of host T cell immunity, or in IDO knockout mice, supporting that IDO inhibition is essential to the antitumor mechanism of 5-Br-brassinin. Thus, the natural product brassinin represents a new class of compounds with IDO inhibitory activity.

Exiguamine A is another natural product that inhibits IDO enzyme (*K*i = 41 nM). However, its cellular activity has not been reported. Nevertheless, this compound might represent an appealing lead structure for the further development of synthetic IDO inhibitors. Indeed, progress has been made in synthesizing its analogues *via* a simpler synthetic route while retaining compound activity against IDO [114-116]. The nutritional supplement, indole-3-carbinol and its metabolite, 3,3'-diindolylmethane (DIM), are indole-containing compounds with structural similarity to tryptophan. A report showed that DIM competitively inhibited tryptophan metabolism in SKBR-3 breast cancer cells treated with human IFN-γ. The potency was estimated to be around 25 μM. DIM did not inhibit tryptophan metabolism in human liver cytosolic preparations, indicating that it does not inhibit TDO. Thus, DIM is an IDO-specific inhibitor with moderate activity (Cao D *et al.*[5]). Finally, a targeted-based screen has also identified NSC 401366 (imidodicarbonimidic diamide, N-methyl-N'-9-phenanthrenyl-, monohydrochloride) as a relatively potent (K_i = 1.5 μM) and competitive nonindolic IDO inhibitor [117].

CONCLUSION AND PATH FORWARD

Although cancer is a disease initiated with normal cells that acquire a series of (epi)genetic and biochemical changes, there is a growing consensus that various

[5]Cao, D.; Ward, B.; Desta, Z.; Roberts, T.; Badve, S.; Bigsby, R.; Wilkes, D.; Skaar, T. C. Diindolylmethane inhibits indoleamine 2,3-dioxygenase activity in breast cancer cells. *The 96th AACR Annual Meeting*. **2005**, Abstract # 2461.

components of the tumor microenvironment, including the immune system, also play a critical role in promoting tumor development and progression. The fact that currently approved cancer drugs, including cytotoxic agents and target-based therapies, eventually are associated with the development of resistance in most if not all patients underscores the urgent need to develop more effective treatments that could better control the disease and also overcome resistance. Due to the extreme plasticity of tumor cells, a treatment based on targeting a particular tumor-promoting gene/protein or even several tumor-promoting genes/proteins simultaneously within tumor cells will inevitably lead to tumor cells adapting an alternative route(s) for growth and/or survival, and ultimately developing resistance. Further, tumor cells that have emerged under treatment pressure are usually more aggressive and more difficult to treat. Therefore, instead of targeting tumor cells directly, one prevailing concept in modern cancer drug development is to target the microenvironment components critical for supporting tumor cell growth and survival. The belief is that unlike tumor cells, resistance to such therapies will be less likely to emerge because cells from the tumor environment are considered "normal" and thus are less prone to genetic changes. Among the many attempts within this strategy, anti-angiogenesis drugs, which block the formation of new blood vessels at the tumor site, have shown considerable success in the clinic and are a powerful testament to this concept. A therapeutic strategy that tackles the immune system would fall into the same category.

The overwhelming evidence supporting a critical role of the immune system in tumor regulation has led to tremendous efforts aimed at harnessing its power to combat cancer. The success or failure of the immune system to reject a tumor depends on the delicate balance of forces between tumor immunity and immune tolerance. Frequently, the negative regulation of tumor immunity has been considered the culprit that allows tumor cells to escape host immune surveillance during tumor development as well as for the unsuccessful development of many immunotherapies aimed at activating the immune system. As described in this review, IDO can suppress the local immune response by reducing tryptophan that is essential for, and by producing tryptophan metabolites that are toxic to, tumor-reactive lymphocytes. This hypothesis is supported by numerous observations from preclinical tumor models and patients' samples of various tumor types.

Based on this biology, inhibition of IDO activity or expression has exhibited antitumor activity in a variety of relevant tumor models. Importantly, combinations of IDO inhibition with various cytotoxic agents or immune based therapies have further demonstrated superior antitumor activity compared to the individual agents alone. Noticeably, it has been well documented that some cytotoxic agents can modulate immune responses *via* a variety of mechanisms and thus there is a real potential to develop effective treatments combining chemo- and immunotherapies in the clinic [118, 119]. These findings, together with data showing that increased IDO expression is an independent prognostic variable for reduced overall survival in cancer patients, suggest that IDO is one of the key regulators of tumor immune tolerance and that IDO inhibition may represent an effective strategy to treat cancer, either alone or in combination with chemotherapeutics or other immune based therapies.

From a drug development perspective, IDO is an attractive target. *INDO*$^{-/-}$ knockout mice are viable and apparently healthy [120], implying that IDO inhibition may not cause severe mechanism-based toxicities in the clinic. In addition, IDO chemistry is well defined and its crystal structure has been solved which will help to better understand the SAR during lead optimization. The only other closely related protein IDO2 is structurally different. Moreover, IDO inhibitors reported in the literature could serve as leads for further development. Lastly, the clinical pharmacodynamic (PD) effect of an IDO inhibitor can be determined by monitoring levels of kyn and trp, as well as kyn/trp ratio in patients' blood as reported in previous studies [63, 65, 79, 82].

Given that few immune based anti-cancer therapies have been approved by regulatory authorities, the overarching issue in developing an effective treatment would ultimately rely on testing the right drugs or drug combinations in the right patient population. It is clear that successful control of most if not all cancers will require the application of multiple agents that effectively target different pro-cancer mechanisms. One might imagine that one rational combination could involve the destruction of tumor cells by a chemotherapeutic agent and/or a target-based therapy, followed by an active immunotherapy that specifically boosts the anti-tumor immune response and/or an agent like an IDO inhibitor that would remove the immune suppression in the tumor and its microenvironment.

Clinical trials will also need to address the question of who will benefit the most from such a treatment regimen by determining whether IDO inhibition significantly improves the overall efficacy of the treatment, and whether IDO expression or activation indeed plays a role in the tumor development in the studied patient populations. Based on all the emerging findings regarding IDO involvement in human cancers, an IDO inhibitor has the potential to provide an additional important complement to the current stable of oncology agents.

ACKNOWLEDGEMENTS

None declared.

CONFLICT OF INTEREST

The authors confirm that this chapter contents have no conflict of interest.

DISCLOSURE

The chapter submitted for the eBook Series entitled **"Advances in Cancer Drug Targets, Volume 2"** is an update of our article in **Current Cancer Drug Targets, Volume 9, Issue 8, 2009, pp. 938-952,** with additional text and references.

REFERENCES

[1] Peters JC. Tryptophan nutrition and metabolism: an overview. Adv Exp Med Biol 1991; 294: 345-58.

[2] Ruddick JP, Evans AK, Nutt DJ, Lightman SL, Rook GA, Lowry CA. Tryptophan metabolism in the central nervous system: medical implications. Expert Rev Mol Med 2006; 8: 1-27.

[3] Takikawa O. Biochemical and medical aspects of the indoleamine 2,3-dioxygenase-initiated L-tryptophan metabolism. Biochem Biophys Res Commun 2005; 338: 12-9.

[4] Higuchi K, Hayaishi O. Enzymic formation of D-kynurenine from D-tryptophan. Arch Biochem Biophys 1967; 120: 397-03.

[5] Taylor MW, Feng GS. Relationship between interferon-gamma, indoleamine 2,3-dioxygenase, and tryptophan catabolism. FASEB J 1991; 5: 2516-22.

[6] Mellor AL, Munn DH. IDO expression by dendritic cells: tolerance and tryptophan catabolism. Nat Rev Immunol 2004; 4: 762-74.

[7] Hayaishi O. Indoleamine 2,3-dioxygenase--with special reference to the mechanism of interferon action. Biken J 1985; 28: 39-49.

[8] Däubener W, MacKenzie CR. IFN-gamma activated indoleamine 2,3-dioxygenase activity in human cells is an antiparasitic and an antibacterial effector mechanism. Adv Exp Med Biol 1999; 467: 517-24.

[9] Munn DH, Zhou M, Attwood JT, *et al.* Prevention of allogeneic fetal rejection by tryptophan catabolism. Science 1998; 281: 1191-3.

[10] Kadoya A, Tone S, Maeda H, Minatogawa Y, Kido R. Gene structure of human indoleamine 2,3-dioxygenase. Biochem Biophys Res Commun 1992; 189: 530-6.

[11] Najfeld V, Menninger J, Muhleman D, Comings DE, Gupta SL. Localization of indoleamine 2,3-dioxygenase gene (INDO) to chromosome 8p12-->p11 by fluorescent in situ hybridization. Cytogenet Cell Genet 1993; 64: 231-2.

[12] Sugimoto H, Oda S, Otsuki T, Hino T, Yoshida T, Shiro Y. Crystal structure of human indoleamine 2,3-dioxygenase: catalytic mechanism of O2 incorporation by a heme-containing dioxygenase. Proc Natl Acad Sci USA 2006; 103: 2611-6.

[13] Macchiarulo A, Nuti R, Bellocchi D, Camaioni E, Pellicciari R. Molecular docking and spatial coarse graining simulations as tools to investigate substrate recognition, enhancer binding and conformational transitions in indoleamine-2,3-dioxygenase (IDO). Biochim Biophys Acta 2007; 1774: 1058-68.

[14] Thomas SR, Stocker R. Redox reactions related to indoleamine 2,3-dioxygenase and tryptophan metabolism along the kynurenine pathway. Redox Rep 1999; 4: 199-220.

[15] Sono M, Roach MP, Coulter ED, Dawson JH. Heme-Containing Oxygenases. Chem Rev 1996; 96: 2841-88.

[16] Shimizu T, Nomiyama S, Hirata F, Hayaishi O. Indoleamine 2,3-dioxygenase. Purification and some properties. J Biol Chem 1978; 253: 4700-06.

[17] Ball HJ, Sanchez-Perez A, Weiser S, *et al.* Characterization of an indoleamine 2,3-dioxygenase-like protein found in humans and mice. Gene 2007; 396: 203-13.

[18] Ball HJ, Yuasa HJ, Austin CJ, Weiser S, Hunt NH. Indoleamine 2,3-dioxygenase-2; a new enzyme in the kynurenine pathway. Int J Biochem Cell Biol 2009; 41: 467-71.

[19] Metz R, Duhadaway JB, Kamasani U, Laury-Kleintop L, Muller AJ, Prendergast GC. Novel tryptophan catabolic enzyme IDO2 is the preferred biochemical target of the antitumor indoleamine 2,3-dioxygenase inhibitory compound D-1-methyl-tryptophan. Cancer Res 2007; 67: 7082-87.

[20] Lob S, Konigsrainer A, Schafer R, Rammensee HG, Opelz G, Terness P. Levo- but not dextro-1-methyl tryptophan abrogates the IDO activity of human dendritic cells. Blood 2008 ; 111 : 2152-4.

[21] Qian F, Villella J, Wallace PK, *et al.* Efficacy of levo-1-methyl tryptophan and dextro-1-methyl tryptophan in reversing indoleamine-2,3-dioxygenase-mediated arrest of T-cell proliferation in human epithelial ovarian cancer. Cancer Res 2009; 69: 5498-04.

[22] Lob S, Konigsrainer A, Zieker D, *et al.* IDO1 and IDO2 are expressed in human tumors: levo- but not dextro-1-methyl tryptophan inhibits tryptophan catabolism. Cancer Immunol Immunother 2009; 58: 153-7.

[23] Belladonna ML, Orabona C, Grohmann U, Puccetti P. TGF-beta and kynurenines as the key to infectious tolerance. Trends Mol Med 2009; 15: 41-9.

[24] Baban B, Hansen AM, Chandler PR, *et al.* A minor population of splenic dendritic cells expressing CD19 mediates IDO-dependent T cell suppression *via* type I IFN signaling following B7 ligation. Int Immunol 2005; 17: 909-19.

[25] Belladonna ML, Volpi C, Bianchi R, *et al.* Cutting edge: Autocrine TGF-beta sustains default tolerogenesis by IDO-competent dendritic cells. J Immunol 2008; 181: 5194-8.

[26] Braun D, Longman RS, Albert ML. A two-step induction of indoleamine 2,3 dioxygenase (IDO) activity during dendritic-cell maturation. Blood 2005; 106: 2375-81.

[27] Musso T, Gusella GL, Brooks A, Longo DL, Varesio L. Interleukin-4 inhibits indoleamine 2,3-dioxygenase expression in human monocytes. Blood 1994; 83: 1408-11.

[28] MacKenzie CR, González RG, Kniep E, Roch S, Däubener W. Cytokine mediated regulation of interferon-gamma-induced IDO activation. Adv Exp Med Biol 1999; 467: 533-9.

[29] Chiarugi A, Rovida E, Dello Sbarba P, Moroni F. Tryptophan availability selectively limits NO-synthase induction in macrophages. J Leukoc Biol 2003; 73: 172-7.

[30] Okamoto T, Toné S, Kanouchi H, Miyawaki C, Ono S, Minatogawa Y. Transcriptional regulation of indoleamine 2,3-dioxygenase (IDO) by tryptophan and its analogue : Down-regulation of the indoleamine 2,3-dioxygenase (IDO) transcription by tryptophan and its analogue. Cytotechnology 2007; 54: 107-13.

[31] Grohmann U, Orabona C, Fallarino F, *et al.* CTLA-4-Ig regulates tryptophan catabolism *in vivo*. Nat Immunol 2002; 3: 1097-101.

[32] Tas SW, Vervoordeldonk MJ, Hajji N, *et al.* Noncanonical NF-kappaB signaling in dendritic cells is required for indoleamine 2,3-dioxygenase (IDO) induction and immune regulation. Blood 2007; 110: 1540-9.

[33] Kim YH, Choi BK, Kang WJ, *et al.* IFN-{gamma}-indoleamine-2,3 dioxygenase acts as a major suppressive factor in 4-1BB-mediated immune suppression *in vivo*. J Leukoc Biol 2009; 85: 817-25.

[34] Fallarino F, Grohmann U, Hwang KW, *et al.* Modulation of tryptophan catabolism by regulatory T cells. Nat Immunol 2003; 4: 1206-12.

[35] Orabona C, Grohmann U, Belladonna ML, *et al.* CD28 induces immunostimulatory signals in dendritic cells *via* CD80 and CD86. Nat Immunol 2004; 5: 1134-42.

[36] Fallarino F, Vacca C, Orabona C, *et al.* Functional expression of indoleamine 2,3-dioxygenase by murine CD8 alpha(+) dendritic cells. Int Immunol 2002; 14: 65-8.

[37] Thomas SR, Salahifar H, Mashima R, Hunt NH, Richardson DR, Stocker R. Antioxidants inhibit indoleamine 2,3-dioxygenase in IFN-gamma-activated human macrophages: posttranslational regulation by pyrrolidine dithiocarbamate. J Immunol 2001; 166: 6332-40.

[38] Orabona C, Puccetti P, Vacca C Bicciato, S, *et al.* Toward the identification of a tolerogenic signature in IDO-competent dendritic cells. Blood 2006; 107: 2846-54.

[39] Orabona C, Pallotta MT, Volpi C, *et al.* SOCS3 drives proteasomal degradation of indoleamine 2,3-dioxygenase (IDO) and antagonizes IDO-dependent tolerogenesis. Proc Natl Acad Sci USA 2008; 105: 20828-33.

[40] Munn DH, Shafizadeh E, Attwood JT, Bondarev I, Pashine A, Mellor AL. Inhibition of T cell proliferation by macrophage tryptophan catabolism. J Exp Med 1999; 189: 1363-72.

[41] Grohmann U, Bianchi R, Belladonna ML, *et al.* IFN-gamma inhibits presentation of a tumor/self peptide by CD8 alpha- dendritic cells *via* potentiation of the CD8 alpha+ subset. J Immunol 2000; 165: 1357-63.

[42] Grohmann U, Bianchi R, Orabona C, *et al.* Functional plasticity of dendritic cell subsets as mediated by CD40 *versus* B7 activation. J Immunol 2003; 171: 2581-7.

[43] Fallarino F, Bianchi R, Orabona C, *et al.* CTLA-4-Ig activates forkhead transcription factors and protects dendritic cells from oxidative stress in nonobese diabetic mice. J Exp Med 2004; 200: 1051-62.

[44] Mellor AL, Baban B, Chandler P, *et al.* Cutting edge: induced indoleamine 2,3 dioxygenase expression in dendritic cell subsets suppresses T cell clonal expansion. J Immunol 2003; 171: 1652-5.

[45] Logan GJ, Smyth CM, Earl JW, *et al.* HeLa cells cocultured with peripheral blood lymphocytes acquire an immuno-inhibitory phenotype through up-regulation of indoleamine 2,3-dioxygenase activity. Immunology 2002; 105: 478-87.

[46] Orabona C, Belladonna ML, Vacca C, *et al.* Cutting edge: silencing suppressor of cytokine signaling 3 expression in dendritic cells turns CD28-Ig from immune adjuvant to suppressant. J Immunol 2005; 174: 6582-6.

[47] Hwu P, Du MX, Lapointe R, Do M, Taylor MW, Young HA. Indoleamine 2,3-dioxygenase production by human dendritic cells results in the inhibition of T cell proliferation. J Immunol 2000; 164: 3596-9.

[48] Mellor AL, Keskin DB, Johnson T, Chandler P, Munn DH. Cells expressing indoleamine 2,3-dioxygenase inhibit T cell responses. J Immunol 2002; 168: 3771-6.

[49] Frumento G, Rotondo R, Tonetti M, Damonte G, Benatti U, Ferrara GB. Tryptophan-derived catabolites are responsible for inhibition of T and natural killer cell proliferation induced by indoleamine 2,3-dioxygenase J Exp Med 2002; 196: 459-68.

[50] Fallarino F, Grohmann U, Vacca C, *et al.* T cell apoptosis by tryptophan catabolism. Cell Death Differ 2002; 9: 1069-77.

[51] Munn DH, Sharma MD, Baban B, *et al.* GCN2 kinase in T cells mediates proliferative arrest and anergy induction in response to indoleamine 2,3-dioxygenase. Immunity 2005; 22: 633-42.

[52] Fallarino F, Grohmann U, You S, *et al.* The combined effects of tryptophan starvation and tryptophan catabolites down-regulate T cell receptor zeta-chain and induce a regulatory phenotype in naive T cells. J Immunol 2006; 176: 6752-61.

[53] Curti A, Pandolfi S, Valzasina B, *et al.* Modulation of tryptophan catabolism by human leukemic cells results in the conversion of CD25- into CD25+ T regulatory cells. Blood 2007; 109: 2871-7.

[54] Hill M, Tanguy-Royer S, Royer P, *et al.* IDO expands human CD4+CD25high regulatory T cells by promoting maturation of LPS-treated dendritic cells. Eur J Immunol 2007; 37: 3054-62.

[55] Sharma MD, Baban B, Chandler P, *et al.* Plasmacytoid dendritic cells from mouse tumor-draining lymph nodes directly activate mature Tregs *via* indoleamine 2,3-dioxygenase. J Clin Invest 2007; 117: 2570-82.

[56] Myint AM, Schwarz MJ, Steinbusch HW, Leonard BE. Neuropsychiatric disorders related to interferon and interleukins treatment. Metab Brain Dis 2009; 24: 55-68.

[57] Brandacher G, Hoeller E, Fuchs D, Weiss HG. Chronic immune activation underlies morbid obesity: is IDO a key player? Curr Drug Metab 2007; 8: 289-95.

[58] Curti A, Trabanelli S, Salvestrini V, Baccarani M, Lemoli RM. The role of indoleamine 2,3-dioxygenase in the induction of immune tolerance: focus on hematology. Blood 2009; 113: 2394-401.

[59] Quan J, Tan PH, MacDonald A, *et al*. Manipulation of indoleamine 2,3-dioxygenase (IDO) for clinical transplantation: promises and challenges. Expert Opin Biol Ther 2008; 8: 1705-19.

[60] Pertovaara M, Raitala A, Juonala M, *et al*. Indoleamine 2,3-dioxygenase enzyme activity correlates with risk factors for atherosclerosis: the Cardiovascular Risk in Young Finns Study. Clin Exp Immunol 2007; 148: 106-11.

[61] Schroecksnadel K, Frick B, Winkler C, Fuchs D. Crucial role of interferon-gamma and stimulated macrophages in cardiovascular disease. Curr Vasc Pharmcol 2006; 4: 205-13.

[62] Uyttenhove C, Pilotte L, Theate I, *et al*. Evidence for a tumoral immune resistance mechanism based on tryptophan degradation by indoleamine 2,3-dioxygenase. Nat Med 2003; 9: 1269-74.

[63] Feder-Mengus C, Wyler S, Hudolin T, *et al*. High expression of indoleamine 2,3-dioxygenase gene in prostate cancer. Eur J Cancer 2008; 44: 2266-75.

[64] Sadun RE, Sachsman SM, Chen X, *et al*. Immune signatures of murine and human cancers reveal unique mechanisms of tumor escape and new targets for cancer immunotherapy. Clin Cancer Res 2007; 13: 4016-25.

[65] Schroecksnadel K, Winkler C, Fuith LC, Fuchs D. Tryptophan degradation in patients with gynecological cancer correlates with immune activation. Cancer Lett 2005; 223: 323-9.

[66] Nakamura T, Shima T, Saeki A, *et al*. Expression of indoleamine 2, 3-dioxygenase and the recruitment of Foxp3-expressing regulatory T cells in the development and progression of uterine cervical cancer. Cancer Sci 2007; 98: 874-81.

[67] Astigiano S, Morandi B, Costa R, *et al*. Eosinophil granulocytes account for indoleamine 2,3-dioxygenase-mediated immune escape in human non-small cell lung cancer. Neoplasia 2005; 7: 390-6.

[68] Ino K, Yamamoto E, Shibata K, *et al*. Inverse correlation between tumoral indoleamine 2,3-dioxygenase expression and tumor-infiltrating lymphocytes in endometrial cancer: its association with disease progression and survival. Clin Cancer Res 2008; 14: 2310-7.

[69] Ino K, Yoshida N, Kajiyama H, *et al*. Indoleamine 2,3-dioxygenase is a novel prognostic indicator for endometrial cancer. Br J Cancer 2006; 95: 1555-61.

[70] Brandacher G, Perathoner A, Ladurner R, *et al*. Prognostic value of indoleamine 2,3-dioxygenase expression in colorectal cancer: Effect of tumor infiltrating T cells. Clin Cancer Res 2006; 12: 1144-51.

[71] Huang A, Fuchs D, Widner B, Glover C, Henderson DC, Allen-Mersh TG. Serum trytophan decrease correlates with immune activation and impaired quality of life in colorectal cancer. Br J Cancer 2002; 86: 1691-6.

[72] Witkiewicz A, Williams TK, Cozzitorto J, *et al*. Expression of indoleamine 2,3-dioxygenase in metastatic pancreatic ductal adenocarcinoma recruits regulatory T cells to avoid immune detection. J Am Coll Surg 2008; 206: 849-54.

[73] Takao M, Okamoto A, Nikaido T, *et al*. Increased synthesis of indoleamine-2,3-dioxygenase protein is positively associated with impaired survival in patients with serous-type, but not with other types of ovarian cancer. Oncol Rep 2007; 17: 1333-9.

[74] Okamoto A, Nikaido T, Ochiai K, *et al*. Indoleamine 2,3-dioxygenase serves as a marker of poor prognosis in gene expression profiles of serous ovarian cancer cells. Clin. Cancer Res 2005 ; 11 : 6030-9.

[75] Polak ME, Borthwick NJ, Gabriel FG, *et al*. Mechanisms of local immunosuppression in cutaneous melanoma. Br J Cancer 2007; 96: 1879-87.

[76] Munn DH, Sharma MD, Hou D, *et al.* Expression of indoleamine 2,3-dioxygenase by plasmacytoid dendritic cells in tumor-draining lymph nodes. J Clin Invest 2004; 114: 280-90.

[77] Lee JR, Dalton RR, Messina JL, *et al.* Pattern of recruitment of immunoregulatory antigen-presenting cells in malignant melanoma. Lab Invest 2003; 83: 1457-66.

[78] Wobser M, Voigt H, Houben R, *et al.* Dendritic cell based antitumor vaccination: impact of functional indoleamine 2,3-dioxygenase expression. Cancer Immunol Immunother 2007; 56: 1017-24.

[79] Weinlich G, Murr C, Richardsen L, Winkler C, Fuchs D. Decreased serum tryptophan concentration predicts poor prognosis in malignant melanoma patients. Dermatology 2007; 214: 8-14.

[80] Sun JX, Zhang WG, Chen YX, *et al.* Indoleamine 2, 3-dioxygenase expression in cells of human acute monocyte leukemia (M(5)) and acute lymphocyte leukemia and therapeutic effect of its inhibitor 1-methyl tryptophan. Zhongguo Shi Yan Xue Ye Za Zhi 2007; 15: 478-82.

[81] Curti A, Aluigi M, Pandolfi S, *et al.* Acute myeloid leukemia cells constitutively express the immunoregulatory enzyme indoleamine 2,3-dioxygenase. Leukemia 2007; 21: 353-5.

[82] Corm S, Berthon C, Imbenotte M, *et al.* Indoleamine 2,3-dioxygenase activity of acute myeloid leukemia cells can be measured from patients' sera by HPLC and is inducible by IFN-gamma. Leuk Res 2009; 33: 490-4.

[83] Hoshi M, Ito H, Fujigaki H, *et al.* Indoleamine 2,3-dioxygenase is highly expressed in human adult T-cell leukemia/lymphoma and chemotherapy changes tryptophan catabolism in serum and reduced activity. Leuk Res 2009; 33: 39-45.

[84] Karanikas V, Zamanakou M, Kerenidi T, *et al.* Indoleamine 2,3-dioxygenase (IDO) expression in lung cancer. Cancer Biol Ther 2007; 6: 1258-62.

[85] Pan K, Wang H, Chen MS, *et al.* Expression and prognosis role of indoleamine 2,3-dioxygenase in hepatocellular carcinoma. J Cancer Res Clin Oncol 2008; 134: 1247-53.

[86] Ishio T, Goto S, Tahara K, Tone S, Kawano K, Kitano S. Immunoactivative role of indoleamine 2,3-dioxygenase in human hepatocellular carcinoma. J Gastroenterol Hepatol 2004; 19: 319-26.

[87] Riesenberg R, Weiler C, Spring O, *et al.* Expression of indoleamine 2,3-dioxygenase in tumor endothelial cells correlates with long-term survival of patients with renal cell carcinoma. Clin Cancer Res 2007; 13: 6993-7002.

[88] Musajo L, Benassi CA, Parpajola A. Excretion and isolation of kynurenine and 3-hydroxykynurenine from human pathological urine. Clin Chim Acta 1956; 1: 229-35.

[89] Spacek M. Kynurenine in disease, with particular reference to cancer. Can Med Assoc J 1955; 73: 198-201.

[90] Leklem JE, Brown RR. Abnormal tryptophan metabolism in a family with a history of bladder cancer. J Natl Cancer Inst 1976; 56: 1101-4.

[91] Wolf H, Brown RR. Tryptophan metabolism in bladder cancer patients from Copenhagen. Scand J Urol Nephrol 1979; 13: 143-8.

[92] Carlin JM, Ozaki Y, Byrne GI, Brown RR, Borden EC. Interferons and indoleamine 2,3-dioxygenase: role in antimicrobial and antitumor effects. Experientia 1989; 45: 535-41.

[93] Friberg M, Jennings R, Alsarraj M, *et al.* Indoleamine 2,3-dioxygenase contributes to tumor cell evasion of T cell-mediated rejection. Int J Cancer 2002; 101: 151-5.

[94] Yoshida N, Ino K, Ishida Y, *et al.* Overexpression of indoleamine 2,3-dioxygenase in human endometrial carcinoma cells induces rapid tumor growth in a mouse xenograft model. Clin Cancer Res 2008; 14: 7251-9.

[95] Miyazaki T, Moritake K, Yamada K, *et al.* Indoleamine 2,3-dioxygenase as a new target for malignant glioma therapy. J Neurosurg 2009; 111: 230-7.

[96] Muller AJ, DuHadaway JB, Donover PS, Sutanto-Ward E, Prendergast GC. Inhibition of indoleamine 2,3-dioxygenase, an immunoregulatory target of the cancer suppression gene Bin1, potentiates cancer chemotherapy. Nat Med 2005; 11: 312-9.

[97] Ou X, Cai S, Liu P, *et al.* Enhancement of dendritic cell-tumor fusion vaccine potency by indoleamine-pyrrole 2,3-dioxygenase inhibitor, 1-MT. J Cancer Res Clin Oncol 2008; 134: 525-33.

[98] Sharma MD, Hou DY, Liu Y, *et al.* Indoleamine 2,3-dioxygenase controls conversion of Foxp3+ Tregs to TH17-like cells in tumor-draining lymph nodes. Blood 2009; 113: 6102-11.

[99] Zeng J, Cai S, Yi Y, *et al.* Prevention of spontaneous tumor development in a ret transgenic mouse model by ret peptide vaccination with indoleamine 2,3-dioxygenase inhibitor 1-methyl tryptophan. Cancer Res 2009; 69: 3963-70.

[100] Gasparri AM, Jachetti E, Colombo B, *et al.* Critical role of indoleamine 2,3-dioxygenase in tumor resistance to repeated treatments with targeted IFNgamma. Mol Cancer Ther 2008; 7: 3859-66.

[101] Zheng X, Koropatnick J, Li M, *et al.* Reinstalling antitumor immunity by inhibiting tumor-derived immunosuppressive molecule IDO through RNA interference. J Immunol 2006; 177: 5639-46.

[102] Yen MC, Lin CC, Chen YL, *et al.* A novel cancer therapy by skin delivery of indoleamine 2,3-dioxygenase siRNA. Clin Cancer Res 2009; 15: 641-9.

[103] Incyte Corporation [Homepage on the internet]. Delaware: Incyte Corporation. Available from: http://www.incyte.com/

[104] Yue EW, Bouty B, Wayland B, *et al.* Discovery of potent competitive inhibitors of indoleamine 2,3- dioxygenase with *in vivo* pharmacodynamic activity and efficacy in a mouse melanoma model. J Med Chem 2009; 52: 7364-7.

[105] Hou DY, Muller AJ, Sharma MD, *et al.* Inhibition of indoleamine 2,3-dioxygenase in dendritic cells by stereoisomers of 1-methyl-tryptophan correlates with antitumor responses. Cancer Res 2007; 67: 792-801.

[106] Agaugué S, Perrin-Cocon L, Coutant F, André P, Lotteau V. 1-Methyl-tryptophan can interfere with TLR signaling in dendritic cells independently of IDO activity. J Immunol 2006; 177: 2061-71.

[107] Jia L, Schweikart K, Tomaszewski J, *et al.* Toxicology and pharmacokinetics of 1-methyl-d-tryptophan: absence of toxicity due to saturating absorption. Food Chem Toxicol 2008; 46: 203-11.

[108] ClinicalTrials.gov. Available from: http://clinicaltrials.gov/ct2/results?term=1-methyl-D-tryptophan

[109] Kumar S, Jaller D, Patel B, *et al.* Structure based development of phenylimidazole-derived inhibitors of indoleamine 2,3-dioxygenase. J Med Chem 2008; 51: 4968-77.

[110] Kumar S Malachowski WP, DuHadaway JB, *et al.* Indoleamine 2,3-dioxygenase is the anticancer target for a novel series of potent naphthoquinone-based inhibitors. J Med Chem 2008; 51: 1706-18.

[111] Mehta RG, Pezzuto JM. Discovery of cancer preventive agents from natural products: from plants to prevention. Curr Oncol Rep 2002; 4: 478-86.

[112] Gaspari P, Banerjee T, Malachowski WP, *et al.* Structure-activity study of brassinin derivatives as indoleamine 2,3-dioxygenase inhibitors. J Med Chem 2006; 49: 684-92.

[113] Banerjee T, Duhadaway JB, Gaspari P, *et al.* A key *in vivo* antitumor mechanism of action of natural product-based brassinins is inhibition of indoleamine 2,3-dioxygenase. Oncogene 2008; 27: 2851-7.

[114] Carr G, Chung MK, Mauk AG, Andersen RJ. Synthesis of indoleamine 2,3-dioxygenase inhibitory analogues of the sponge alkaloid exiguamine A. J Med Chem 2008; 51: 2634-7.

[115] Volgraf M, Lumb JP, Brastianos HC, *et al.* Biomimetic synthesis of the IDO inhibitors exiguamine A and B. Nat Chem Biol 2008; 4: 535-7.

[116] Brastianos HC, Vottero E, Patrick BO, *et al.* Exiguamine A, an indoleamine-2,3-dioxygenase (IDO) inhibitor isolated from the marine sponge Neopetrosia exigua. J Am Chem Soc 2006; 128: 16046-7.

[117] Vottero E, Balgi A, Woods K, *et al.* Inhibitors of human indoleamine 2,3-dioxygenase identified with a target-based screen in yeast. Biotechnol J 2006; 1: 282-8.

[118] Haynes NM, van der Most RG, Lake RA, Smyth MJ. Immunogenic anti-cancer chemotherapy as an emerging concept. Curr Opin Immunol 2008; 20: 545-57.

[119] Zitvogel L, Apetoh L, Ghiringhelli F, Kroemer G. Immunological aspects of cancer chemotherapy. Nat Rev Immunol 2008; 8: 59-73

[120] Baban B, Chandler P, McCool D, Marshall B, Munn DH, Mellor AL. Indoleamine 2,3-dioxygenase expression is restricted to fetal trophoblast giant cells during murine gestation and is maternal genome specific. J Reprod Immunol 2004; 61: 67-77.

CHAPTER 9

p53 Plays a Key Role in Exporting Bid from the Nucleus to Induce Cell Death in Response to Etoposide Treatment

George G. Chen[*,1], Gang Song[1,2], Baoguang Hu[1,3], Liping Liu[1,4] and Paul B.S. Lai[1]

[1]Department of Surgery, Faculty of Medicine, The Chinese University of Hong, Kong, Hong Kong, China; [2]Cancer Research Center, Medical College of Xiamen University, Xiamen, People's Republic of China; [3]Department of Gastrointestinal Surgery, the Affiliated Hospital of Binzhou Medical University, Binzhou, Shandong, China; [4]Department of Hepatobiliary and Pancreas Department of Hepatobiliary Surgery, the Second Clinical Medical College of Jinan University (Shenzhen People's Hospital), Shenzhen, Guangdong Province, China

Abstract: Appropriate subcellular localization of proteins is crucial for regulating their functions. Both p53 and the BH3-only Bid play roles in the development and the treatment of hepatocellular carcinoma. Bid genomic loci contain p53-binding DNA response elements and Bid can mediate p53-dependent transactivation. However, how these molecules function in the liver cells is not completely known. In this study, liver cells were stimulated by etoposide to damage DNA, and the location and the interaction of Bid and p53 were examined by Western blot, immonocchemical staining, immunoprecipitation and siRNA methods. Our data showed that etoposide-induced DNA damage significantly induced p53 and Bid nuclear export. When cells were stimulated by etoposide, p53 could, through the interaction with Bid, cause translocation of Bid from the nucleus to the cytoplasm and on to its ultimate location in the mitochondria. Moreover, p53 physically associated with Bid, and both p53 and Bid cooperatively promoted cell death induced by etoposide. Knockdown of Bid expression notably attenuated cell death induced by etoposide and also released p53 from the mitochondria. In conclusion, these findings reveal a novel mechanism how p53 facilitates Bid nuclear export and how both of them interact in the nucleus and the mitochondria to induce apoptosis in response to etoposide-induced DNA damage.

Keywords: Bid, cell death, etoposide, hepatocellular carcinoma, mitochondria, nucleus, p53.

***Corresponding Author George G. Chen:** Department of Surgery, Prince of Wales Hospital, Shatin, Hong Kong; Tel: 852 26323934; Fax: 852 26450605; E-mail: gchen@cuhk.edu.hk

INTRODUCTION

Bid, a Bcl-2 family protein, is a BH3 domain-only agonist [1,2]. Specific proximal death signals, such as Fas and TNF-α, are connected with the BH3–only pro-apoptotic members to interact with the multidomain molecules of Bak and Bax, which in turn serve as a pathway towards the amplification loop of the intrinsic mitochondrial-mediated apoptotic pathway. In response to death signals by receptor-mediated activation of Fas-signaling, caspase 8 is activated from the cleavage of procaspase 8, which eventually cleaves Bid into a p15 form of tBid. tBid is modified by myristoylation and translocated into mitochondria where it activates oligomerization of Bak or Bax and induces cytochrome *c* release. Cytochrome *c* then activates the apoptotic cascade of caspases 9 and 3 leading to cell death [3,4]. On the other hand, evidence has shown that the cleavage of Bid may not be an absolute requirement for Bid to be pro-apoptotic [5-7]. Studies on mutant Bid that lacks the caspase 8 cleavage site have found that it can still kill cells [6], and Bid has been shown to translocate to the mitochondria without cleavage [7]. Recent studies have also demonstrated that the physiological role of Bid in development and cellular homeostasis may be cell-type specific. Bid-deficient mice are devoid of Fas-stimulated apoptosis. Bid$^{-/-}$ mice showed normal growth at the embryonic and infant stages, but developed myeloproliferative disorder, which resembles the lethal chronic myleomonocytic leukaemia. This implies that Bid plays a role in regulating myeloid homeostasis and suppressing leukaemogenesis [8]. However, Bid$^{-/-}$ mice did not experience accelerated development of liver cancer following treatment with diethylnitrosamine in a mouse HCC model. Instead the delayed development of tumors was manifested, with the decreased level of cell death in the affected livers [9].

Full-length Bid is also involved in DNA damage response. Upon DNA damage by stimuli such as etoposide or irradiation, DNA-damage kinase ATM is activated by phosphorylation in the nucleus, which in turn phosphorylates Bid at serine 61 (in mouse Bid) and serine 78 (in mouse and human Bid). Phosphorylated Bid participates in cell cycle arrest in S phase and DNA repair [10,11]. The majority of currently identified substrates of ATM are nuclear proteins and a portion of Bid localizes to the nucleus [10-12]. Therefore it is most likely that Bid is phosphorylated in the nucleus. Oberkovita G, *et al.* [13] reported that etoposide and ionizing radiation induced the exit of Bid from nucleus and raised a novel possibility that Bid may be activated in the nucleus and that its activity in the DNA damage pathway requires nuclear export. The amino acid sequence of Bid does not have any obvious nuclear localization signals (NLS), but carries nuclear export signals (NES). However, mutating Bid NES does not affect the nuclear exit of Bid [13], suggesting that Bid NES does not seem to function as an NES. Therefore, Bid is transported into the nucleus and its export is probably mediated by other NES-carrying proteins.

The tumor suppressor p53 is a crucial mediator of cell cycle arrest and apoptosis in response to DNA damage or other cellular stresses. p53 transactivates various target genes, including p21 [14], Bax [15], Bad [16], Bid [17], Puma [18], and many others [19,20]. In unstressed cells, murinc double minute-2 (MDM2) binds to the transactivation domain of p53 and inhibits its transcriptional activity, shuttles p53 out of the nucleus, and targets p53 for ubiquitin-mediated proteolysis [21]. p53 can also function in the transcription-independent pathway to induce apoptosis. Although a detailed mechanism of the transcription-independent function of p53 has not yet been determined, recent studies have revealed that upon an apoptotic stimulus, p53 translocates into mitochondria to interact directly with Bcl-2 or Bcl-x_L to displace and activate proapoptotic Bax or Bak signaling [22,23]. Appropriate subcellular localization is crucial for regulating p53 function. p53 nuclear export is mediated by a highly conserved leucine-rich NES located in its tetramerization domain. Mutation of NES residues prevents p53 export and hampers tetramer formation [24]. Sax JK, *et al.* have showed that both the human and the mouse Bid genomic loci contain p53-binding DNA response elements that bind p53 and mediate p53-dependent transactivation [17]. In this study, we further studied the relationship between p53 and Bid following etoposide-induced DNA damage. We found that p53 shuttled between the nucleus and the cytoplasm and that etoposide could significantly induce its nuclear export. We also showed that when stimulated by etoposide, p53 could, through the interaction with Bid, cause translocation of Bid from the nucleus to the cytoplasm and on to its ultimate location in the mitochondria. Knockdown of Bid expression notably attenuated cell death induced by etoposide and also released p53 from the mitochondria. These findings reveal a novel mechanism how p53 facilitates Bid nuclear export and how both of them interact in the mitochondria to induce apoptosis in response to etoposide-induced DNA damage.

MATERIALS AND METHODS

Cell Culture and DNA Constructs

Chang liver cell line and hepatocellular carcinoma (HCC) cell lines PLC/PRF/5 and Hep3B were obtained from the American Type Culture Collection (Rockville, MD), and cultured as previously described [25,26]. Human Bid and wild-type p53 genes were cloned from a cDNA expression library of the human hepatoblastoma cell line HepG2, and the construction of Bid/pcDNA3.1 (+) and p53/pcDNA3.1 (+) expression plasmids was carried out as our previous publication [25]. For the construct of the FLAG-Bid expression vector, the Bid gene was amplified by the sense primer containing the Hind III restriction site and the FLAG sequence, and the anti-sense primer with the XbaI restriction site. The sequence of these two primers was as follows: Sense primer: ACGTAAGCTTATGGATTACAAGGAT GACGACGATAAGATGTGCAGCGGTGCTGGGGTC. Anti-sense primer: AC GTTCTAGATCAGTCCATCCCATTGGC. The amplified PCR product was cloned into pcDNA3.1 (+). Positive clones were confirmed by DNA sequencing. For the construct of the GFP-Bid expression vector, the Bid gene was amplified using the sense primer containing the KpnI restriction site (ACGTGGTACC ATGTGCAGCGGTGCTGGGGTC), and the anti-sense primer with the ApaI restriction site (ACGGGGCCCTCAGTCCATCCCATTTCTGGC). The amplified PCR product was cloned into pEGFP-C1 and positive clones were confirmed by DNA sequencing. For the construct of the GFP-p53 expression vcctor, the p53 insert was excised from p53/pcDNA3.1 (+) by KpnI and ApaI. The excised insert was cloned into pEGFP-C1 excised by KpnI and ApaI. Clones were confirmed by DNA sequencing. NLS-Bid-GFP was a gift from Dr. Atan Gross [13].

Cell Viability Assays

Bid/PLC/PRF/5 cells, vector/PLC/PRF/5 cells or Chang liver cells were transfected with corresponding constructs and the cells were incubated with 150 μM etoposide (Calbiochem, San Diego, CA). After exposure to etoposide, the cells were observed under a phase-contrast microscope and the cell numbers were determined after trypan blue staining of viable cells in parallel plates. The experiment was repeated at least three times for each test. Triplicate assays were performed for each group of cells and data are expressed as mean ± SD.

Generation of Bid/PLC/PRF/5 Stable Clones and Transient Transfection

The Bid/pcDNA3.1 plasmid or empty vector was introduced into the PLC/PRF/5 HCC cells, and the stable cell clones were obtained by the addition of 500 μg/ml of G418 into the culture. Bid-expressing clones and control clones were chosen for the subsequent experiments. Transient transfection was performed by using lipofectamine™ 2000 (Invitrogen, Carlsbad, CA).

RNA Interference

Chang liver cells were cultured to subconfluence and transiently transfected with small interfering RNA (siRNA) against Bid (Invitrogen) by using Lipofectamine™ 2000 (Invitrogen). At 24 h posttransfection, the culture medium was replaced with fresh one, followed by addition of 150 μM etoposide. After 36 h of incubation, both floating and adherent cells were used for the subsequent experiments.

Immunofluorescence Double Staining

Immunofluorescence double staining was performed as our previous description [27]. Briefly, cells were grown on 25 mm diameter glass coverslips placed in six-well plates. After treatment by experimental conditions, cells were fixed and permeabilized. The fixed and permeabilized cells were first incubated for 1 h at room temperature with the first primary antibody. The cells were then washed with PBS and subsequently incubated with both FITC-conjugated goat anti-mouse and TRITC-conjugated goat anti-rabbit secondary antibodies. The cells were washed by PBS and labeled with 600 nM DAPI in PBS for 5 min. After washing with PBS, the cells were mounted in ProLong Antifade solution onto glass slides. For fluorescence microscopy, stained cells were examined with a Zeiss Spot camera and Spot Camera Imaging System (Carl Zeiss, Jena, Germany). Negative controls were prepared by replacing the primary antibody with PBS.

Cytosolic, Nuclear, and Mitochondrial Protein Isolation

The cytosolic, nuclear, and mitochondrial protein fractions were isolated according to the previously reported procedure and tubulin, lamin B and Cox 4/Hsp60 proteins were respectively measured to indicate the purity of cellular fractions [28,30]. Briefly, after cells were treated as indicated, the cells were immediately washed with ice-cold PBS, and scraped with a rubber policeman in ice-cold homogenization buffer. The cells were then enriched and resuspended in ice-cold extract buffer A containing Protease Inhibitor Cocktail. The re-suspended cells were homogenized and the homogenates were centrifuged to obtain the mitochondria pellets. Pellet was resuspended in buffer A. The supernatants were further centrifuged at 100,000 *g* for 1 h at 4°C to collect the supernatants (the cytosolic fraction). For the isolation of the nuclear protein, 500 μl ice-cold extract buffer B was added to the pellet obtained after centrifugation. The pellet and the buffer B were mixed and centrifuged at 10,000 *g* for 30 sec at 4°C. The supernatant was discarded and the pellet was resuspended in 50 ml ice-cold extract buffer C. The pellet was homogenized with 10 strokes of Teflon homogenizer and then centrifuged at 10,000 *g* for 20 min at 4°C to collect the supernatant (the nuclear fraction).

Western Blot Analysis

Western blot was performed as previous publications [25,26]. The anti-Flag M2 monoclonal antibody was obtained from Sigma (Sigma, St. Louis, MO). All other antibodies were provided by Santa Cruz (Santa Cruz, CA). Nuclear protein Lamin B, cytosolic protein tubulin and mitochondrial protein Cox 4 were detected by their respective antibodies and used as protein loading controls in relevant tests.

Immunoprecipitation

All immunoprecipitation procedures were carried out at 4°C. Cell lysates were isolated and incubated with the appropriate antibody for 1 h, and subsequently incubated with protein A-Sepharose beads (Santa Cruz) or anti-Flag M2 beads (Sigma) for 1 h. The protein–antibody complexes that were recovered on beads were subjected to Western blot analysis after separation by SDS–PAGE.

RESULTS

Etoposide-Induced DNA Damage Results in p53 and Bid Nuclear Export

Appropriate subcellular localization of p53 and Bid is crucial for regulating their functions. To explore the functional relationship between p53 and Bid in response to etoposide-induced DNA damage, the colocalization of endogenous p53 and Bid was analyzed by immunofluorescence double staining following treatment with etoposide. We first evaluated the subcellular localization of p53 and Bid in Chang liver cells either with or without etoposide treatment. In untreated cells, we found that p53 and a portion of the Bid protein were localized in the nucleus (Fig. **1A**, top panels). However, after treatment with 150 μM of etoposide, most of p53 and Bid proteins were colocalized in the cytoplasm, and little was observed in the nucleus (Fig. **1A**, bottom panels). This difference in the subcellular localization of p53 and Bid in the cells that are treated with or without etoposide, indicates that the colocation of p53 and Bid in cells may be important for the execution of proapoptotic functions. To further assess the subcellular localization of Bid in Chang liver cells, we performed Western blotting analysis of the subcellular fractionations (Fig. **1B**). After the exposure of Chang liver cells to 150 μM of etoposide for 2 h, both the endogenous levels of p53 and Bid translocated from the nucleus to the cytoplasm. This is in agreement with the localization of Bid that was observed from the immunofluorescence staining.

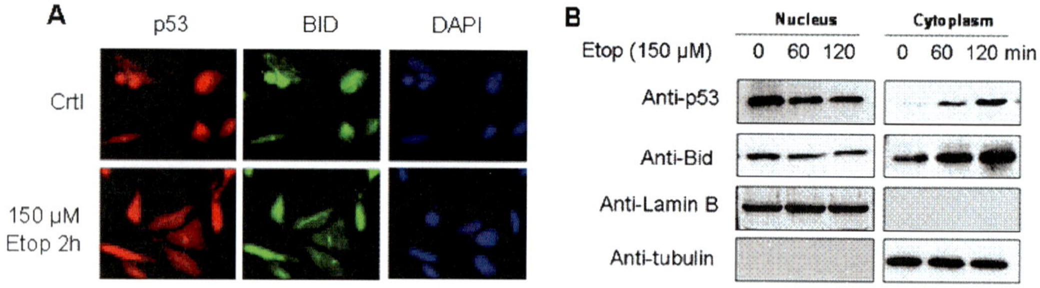

Fig. (1): Colocalization of endogenous p53 and Bid in response to etoposide-induced DNA damage. **A**. Chang liver cells were treated with 150 μM etoposide for 0, 60 and 120 min and then immunostained with anti-p53 and anti-Bid antibodies followed by the corresponding TRITC-, and FITC-conjugated secondary antibodies to show the presence of p53 and Bid proteins simultaneously. DAPI was used for the counter-staining of the nucleus. The fluorescent images were visualized with a fluorescence microscope (×200). **B**. Distribution of p53 and Bid in Chang liver cells. Nuclear and cytosolic fractions were prepared as described in Materials and Methods, and the expression of p53 and Bid in response to etoposide at different time points was determined by Western blotting. Nuclear protein Lamin B and cytosolic protein tubulin were detected as protein loading controls.

To further demonstrate whether DNA damage induced a change in the cellular location of p53 and Bid, we generated constructs that link the green fluorescent protein (GFP) to the N-terminus of p53 and Bid to test their subcellular localizations in Chang liver cells either with or without etoposide treatment. In untreated cells, most of the GFP-p53 fluorescence appeared in the nucleus (Fig. **2A**, top left panel). 60 minutes after etoposide treatment, there was an increase in the cytosolic fluorescence of GFP-p53, and at 120 min after treatment there was a further increase in this fluorescence (Fig. **2A**, top right panels and Fig. **2B**). Similar results were obtained with cells transfected with GFP-Bid (Fig. **2A**, middle panels and Fig. **2C**). The finding confirmed the immunofluorescence staining result shown in Fig. (**1**).

Bid does not carry a classical NLS. We also found that NLS-Bid-GFP drove Bid-GFP to the nucleus, and that DNA damage did not result in the nuclear export of NLS-Bid-GFP (Fig. **2A**, bottom panels), confirming the ability of NLS to retain the Bid in the nucleus [13]. Previous studies showed that mutating NES motif of Bid did not affect its nuclear export [13], indicating that the NES of Bid does not seem to function as an NES, and Bid nuclear export is probably mediated by other NES-carrying proteins in a passive way. Our results suggest that p53 may be a candidate protein to fulfill this function.

Bid Physically Interacts with p53

It is known that both the human and the mouse Bid genomic loci contain p53-binding DNA response elements that bind p53 and mediate p53-dependent transactivation of a reporter gene [17]. However, whether p53 physically interacts with Bid has not yet been reported. We therefore performed coimmunoprecipitation experiments (Fig. **3**). The specific association of endogenous Bid with endogenous p53 was detected in the Chang liver ($p53^{+/+}$) cells either with or without etoposide (Fig. **3A**). Etoposide up-regulated p53 expression in Chang liver cells, but not in p53 deficient Hep3B ($p53^{-/-}$) cells (Fig. **3A**). To further understand whether p53 directly binds to Bid, Hep3B ($p53^{-/-}$) and Chang liver ($p53^{+/+}$) cells were cotransfected with GFP-p53 and with either Flag-Bid or the control plasmid, the cell lysates were isolated from these transfected cells followed by immunoprecipitation with anti-Flag antibody. Similar to endogenous Bid and p53, the exogenous Flag-Bid and exogenous GFP-p53 showed a specific binding interaction (Fig. **3B**). Collectively, these data support the conclusion that Bid physically associates with p53.

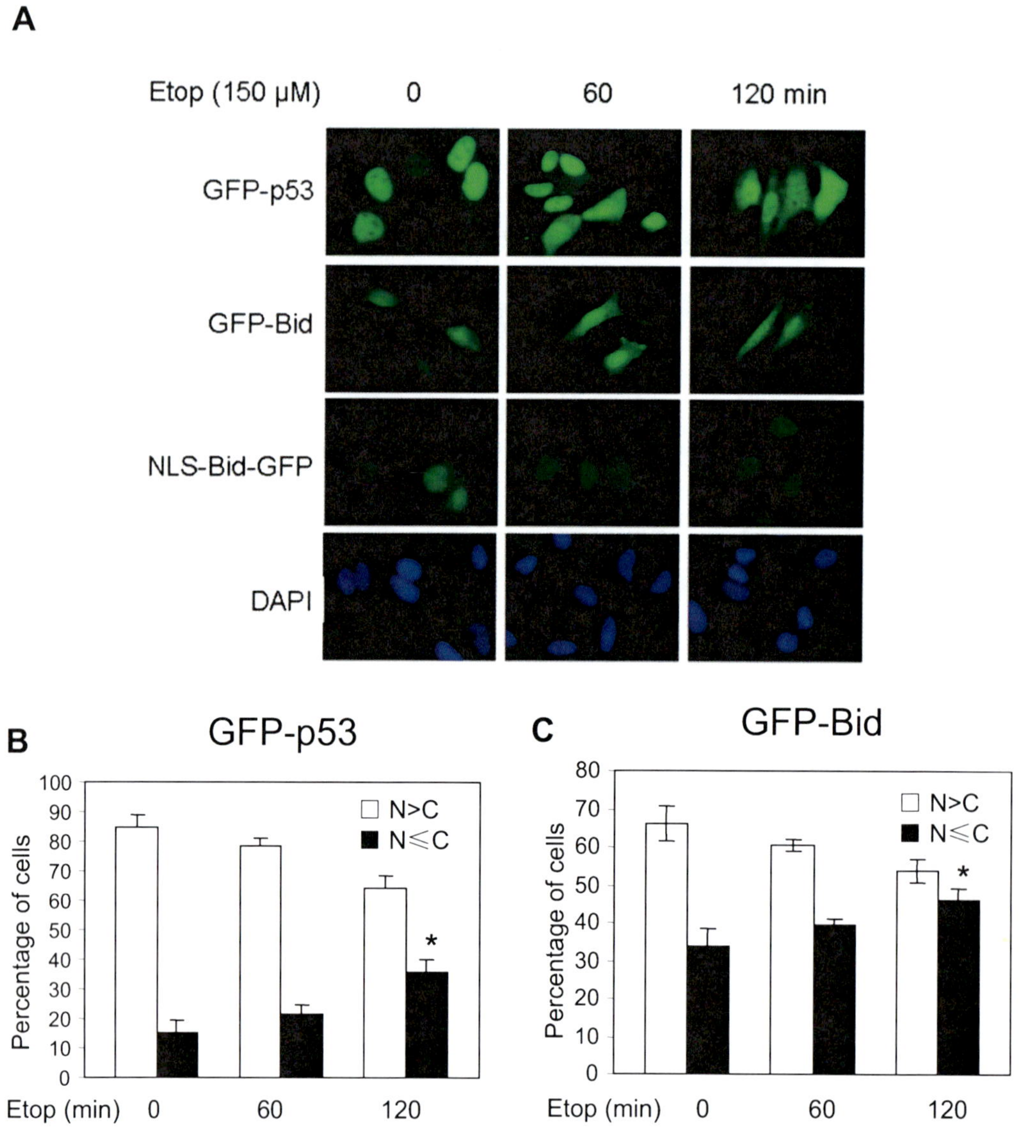

Fig. (2): Etoposide-induced DNA damage results in p53 and Bid nuclear export. **A**. DNA damage results in the nuclear exit of GFP-p53 and GFP–BID. Chang liver cells were grown on coverslips and transfected with a GFP-p53 or a GFP–BID construct. At 24 h or 16 h post–transfection, the cells were treated with or without 150 μM etoposide. At the indicated time points after etoposide treatment, the cells were fixed and pictures were taken using a fluorescence microscope (×200). The bottom panels showed fusing Bid to a NLS significantly drove Bid into the nucleus when the cells were treated by etoposide. **B** and **C**. The histograms represent the percentage of cells that show a prevalence of GFP-p53 and GFP–BID in the nucleus (N>C) or the distribution of GFP-p53 and GFP–BID in the nucleus equal or less than in cytoplasm (N≤C). The data are expressed as the means ± SD of three independent experiments in which 60 cells were analyzed each time.

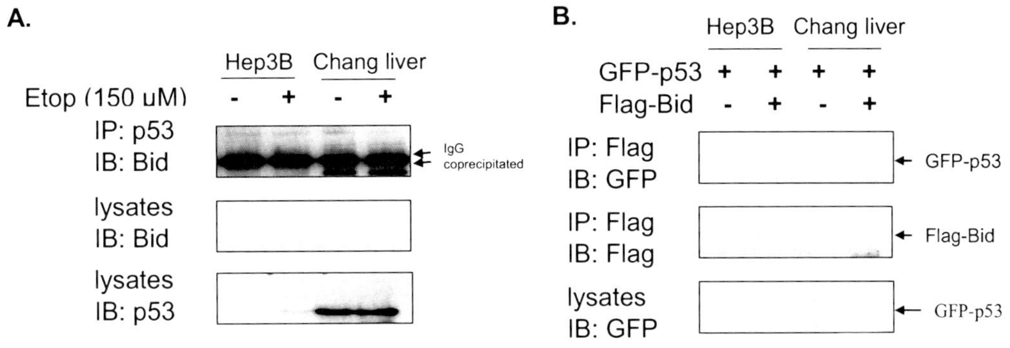

Fig. (3): Bid physically interacts with p53. **A**. Whole-cell extracts from Hep3B ($p53^{-/-}$) and Chang liver ($p53^{+/+}$) cells, pretreated with etoposide (150 μM) or without, were immunoprecipitated (IP) with anti-p53 antibody, followed by immunoblotting with anti-Bid antibody. The coprecipitated Bid was indicated (top panel). The bottom panel (control) shows p53 undetectable in Hep3B ($p53^{-/-}$) cells but detectable in Chang liver ($p53^{+/+}$) cells. **B**. Hep3B ($p53^{-/-}$) and Chang liver ($p53^{+/+}$) cells were cotransfected with GFP-p53 and with either Flag-Bid or control plasmid, followed by immunoprecipitation with anti-Flag antibody. Immunoblotting was performed to detect Flag-Bid-associated p53.

p53 was Associated with Bid in Mitochondria to Induce Cell Death Following Etoposide Treatment

Mitochondria, the target of numerous pro-apoptotic signal molecules, play a major role in apoptosis triggered by many stimuli. To examine whether p53 and Bid was associated with each other at the mitochondria in response to etoposide-induced DNA damage, plasmids GFP-p53, GFP-Bid, GFP-Bid plus p53, and NLS-Bid-GFP plus p53 were transfected into PLC/PRF/5 (p53 mutant and no transcriptional activity) separately, and their fluorescence distribution patterns were compared. A portion of p53 and Bid were found diffused across the cytoplasm following etoposide-induced DNA damage (Fig. **4A**, left two panels). Moreover, coexpression of GFP-Bid and p53 gave rise to an image characteristic of mitochondrial punctiform particles formed at an early apoptotic stage (Fig. **4A**, the fourth and fifth panels). However, coexpression of NLS-Bid-GFP and p53, the NLS-Bid-GFP was localized in the nucleus (Fig. **4A**, the third panel). These results implied that the nucleus-localized p53 associated with at least a portion of Bid if not all, and directed it to the mitochondria from the nucleus in response to etoposide-induced DNA damage. Etoposide did not significantly influence Bid in p53-negative Hep 3B cells. In order to evaluate the effect of the p53-associated Bid on etoposide-induced cell death, we generated a single stable clone Bid/PLC/PRF/5 and the cells were transfected with p53. Without etoposide treatment, there was no significant difference of cell death between the Bid/PLC/PRF/5 group and empty vector control in the presence or absence of p53. However, when the cells were treated with etoposide we found that in the presence of p53 the Bid/PLC/PRF/5 group showed higher level of cell death compared to the empty vector group (Fig. **4B**). Taken together, these results demonstrate that etoposide induces much more apoptotic cells in the presence of both p53 and Bid than in the absence of either p53 or Bid, indicating that both p53 and Bid are required for etoposide to induce cell death in liver cancer cells tested.

The mitochondrion is an important organelle for apoptosis initiation. To validate whether p53 is able to direct Bid to mitochondria, Bid/PLC/PRF/5 (p53 mutant) were transfected with p53 followed by etoposide treatment. Mitochondrial fraction was prepared for western blotting analyses. As shown in Fig. (**4C**), the presence of p53 caused more Bid accumulated in the mitochondrial fraction, implying that p53 was able to direct Bid to mitochondria. To further investigate in detail the possibility that p53 interacts with Bid in the mitochondria, a coimmunoprecipitation experiment was performed. As shown in Fig. (**4D**), the association of p53 and Bid was detected in the mitochondria as well as in the total cell lysate after etoposide treatment. Therefore, the physical association between p53 and Bid, which is initially formed in the nucleus (Fig. **4A**), is also presented in the cytoplasm and in the mitochondria (Fig. **4**), indicating that p53 is associated with Bid and located to the mitochondria *via* the physical interaction.

Block of Bid Reduces Mitochondrial Fraction of p53 and Attenuates Cell Death

In order to further investigate the relationship between Bid and p53 and their roles in apoptosis, we inhibited Bid expression in Chang liver ($p53^{+/+}$) cells by RNA interference. At 24 h after Bid siRNA transfection, the cells were treated with or without etoposide (150 μM) for 36 h. To detect cell death the cells were observed under a phase-contrast microscope and the number of the cells was determined

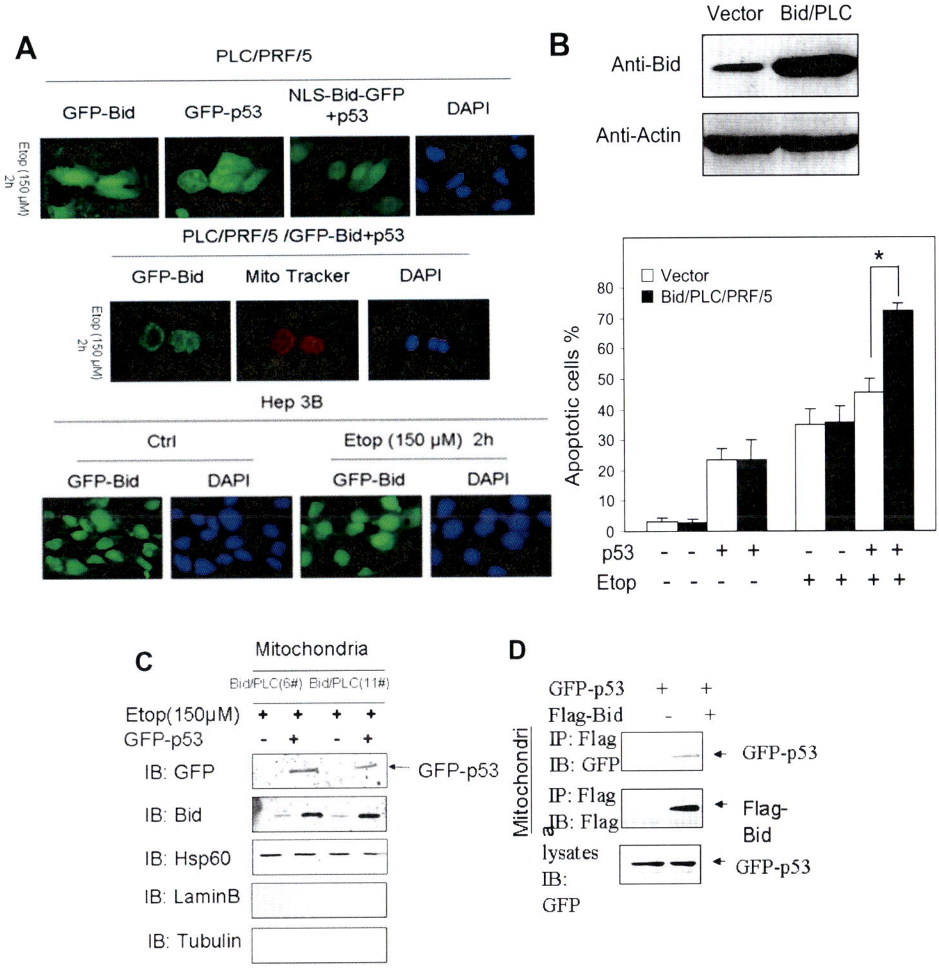

Fig. (4): p53 and Bid interact in the mitochondria to induce cell death in response to etoposide-induced DNA damage. **A**. PLC/PRF/5 cells were transfected with GFP-Bid, GFP-p53, GFP-Bid plus p53, or NLS-Bid-GFP plus p53, and 24 h later, cells were fixed and visualized by fluorescence microscopy (×200). Hep 3B cells (p53 negative) were set up as the control. Hep 3B cells were transfected with GFP-Bid and treated with or without etoposide. **B**. PLC/PRF/5 cells stably expressing Bid (Bid/PLC), or carrying an empty vector were transfected with p53 or without. 24 h later, cells were treated with 150 μM etoposide for another 36 h, and the cell numbers were counted after trypan blue staining of viable cells. The data are expressed as the means ± SD of three independent experiments. **C**. Bid/PLC /PRF/5 cells were transfected with p53, followed by etoposide treatment. Mitochondrial fractions were prepared as described in Materials and Methods, and the expression of GFP-p53 and Bid was determined by Western blotting. Mitochondrial protein Cox4 was detected as protein loading controls (please refer to Fig. **5B**). **D**. PLC/PRF/5 cells were transfected with GFP-p53 and with either Flag-Bid or vector plasmid, and mitochondrial fractions followed by immunoprecipitation with anti-Flag antibody. Immunoblotting was performed to detect Flag-Bid-associated GFP-p53.

after trypan blue staining of viable cells in parallel plates. Chang liver ($p53^{+/+}$) cells with Bid depletion were found to be more resistant to etoposide-induced cell death than control cells (Fig. **5A**). These results further demonstrated that both p53 and Bid were needed for the maximal effect of etoposide on cell death. To study whether p53 subcellular localization is affected by Bid, nuclear, cytosolic, and mitochondrial fractions were prepared from Bid siRNA-treated Chang liver($p53^{+/+}$) cells for Western blot analysis. Bid siRNA suppressed more than

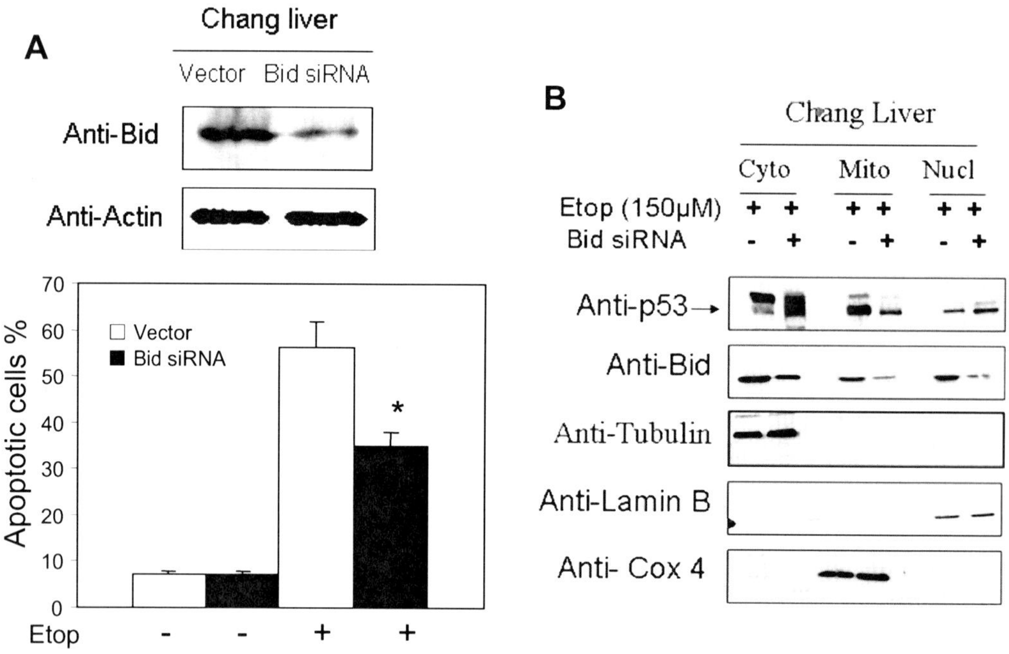

Fig. (5): Block of Bid decreases the mitochondrial fraction of p53 and attenuates cell death. **A**. Cells with depleted Bid are more resistant to etoposide-induced apoptosis. Chang Liver cells were transfected with Bid siRNA. At 48 h posttransfection, cell lysates were subjected to immunoblot analysis for assessing how efficiently the Bid siRNA inhibited the expression of Bid. Chang liver cells were transfected with either mock or Bid-specific siRNA. 24 h after the transfection, etoposide (150 μM) was added and the cells were incubated for another 36 h. At the end of the incubation, the number of the cells was counted after trypan blue staining of viable cells. The data are expressed as the means ± SD of three independent experiments. **B**. Block of Bid expression reduces the mitochondrial localization of p53. Chang Liver cells were transfected with either Bid siRNA or control siRNA. At 24 h after transfection, the cells were treated with etoposide (150 μM) for another 36 h, followed by cell fractionation and immunoblotting analysis. Nuclear protein Lamin B, cytosolic protein tubulin and mitochondrial protein Cox 4 were detected as protein loading controls.

60% of Bid (Fig. **5B**). The level of the mitochondrial p53 was significantly reduced in Bid siRNA-treated cells compared to control siRNA-treated cells, However, the level of the nuclear p53 was increased. The increased nuclear p53 was probably due to more Bid-free cytosolic p53 available for entering the nucleus when Bid was blocked by its siRNA.

DISCUSSION

The BH3-only pro-apoptotic members, full-length Bid and its truncated form (tBid), link the extrinsic death receptor pathway and intrinsic mitochondrial apoptotic pathway [2]. Recently, the non-apoptotic role of Bid in the DNA damage response has been described, and this role does not require its BH3 domain [10,11]. However, another study reports that Bid is not always implicated in DNA damage and replicative stress-induced apoptosis or cell cycle arrest [29]. Our recent study showed that Bid exhibits S phase checkpoint activation and plays a pro-apoptotic role in response to different degrees of etoposide-induced DNA damage in HCC cells [30]. Previous studies have demonstrated that a portion of Bid localizes in the nucleus where Bid is phosphorylated by ATM or ATR [10,11,13]. Our present study confirms the nuclear localization of Bid, and further demonstrates that the subcellular location of Bid defines the role of Bid in the processing of DNA damage by showing that the nucleocytoplasmic shuttling of Bid is important for its functions in response to DNA damage. Recent studies have shown that Bid NES does not seem to function to export Bid from the nucleus [13], suggesting that there are other NES-carrying proteins to help Bid to enter or exit the nucleus. As a well-characterized transcription factor, p53 functions indisputably in the nucleus. More importantly, p53 carries typical NES, and recent studies have shown that p53 plays a distinct cytoplasmic role in the regulation of the mitochondrial pathway [23,31]. p53 is known to function at the upstream of Bid as its transcriptional activator [17]. In the present study, we demonstrated that p53 was involved in Bid nuclear export following etoposide-induced DNA damage and that p53 could, through interaction with Bid, cause translocation of Bid from the nucleus to the mitochondria to induce cell death. Therefore, we believe that p53 can function as a Bid carrier to export Bid from the nucleus.

Nuclear export has been recognized as an important cellular process that regulates many proteins [32]. This process may be achieved by a group of proteins acting as carriers for cargo delivery between the nucleus and the cytoplasm, and coordinating the activation and inactivation of regulatory factors involved in cell cycle and apoptosis. The proteins that undergo nucleocytoplasmic shuttling change their subcellular compartments in response to diverse signals. It has been demonstrated that p53 was able to translocate from the nucleus into the cytoplasm and even onto the mitochondria during DNA damage-induced and p53-dependent apoptosis [22,23,31]. Our present study indicates that p53 shuttling may play a carrier role in the regulation of Bid function. DNA damage results in the physical association of p53 with Bid in the nucleus and the export of p53 and Bid in combination form the nucleus. In PLC/PRF/5 (p53 mutant) cells transfected GFP-Bid alone, most cells displayed a nuclear distribution of Bid after etoposide treatment, whereas cotransfection of GFP-Bid and p53 significantly induced Bid translocation into the cytoplasm, supporting that p53 can facilitate the Bid export from the nucleus. Moreover, if Bid is trapped in the nucleus by NLS [13], p53 was not able to induce Bid nuclear export even in the presence of etoposide (Fig. **4A**). Our result reveals that p53 has a novel function by serving as a carrier for nucleocytoplasmic translocation of Bid. This new concept is also supported by the fact that Bid genomic loci contain p53-binding DNA response elements [17]. In addition, our experiment suggests that this novel function of the nucleocytoplasmic transport may remain inactive without a proper stimulus since the cells without etoposide treatment neither the physical association between p53 and Bid nor the export of Bid from the nucleus will occur. Therefore, in order to export Bid from the nucleus both p53 and a proper stimulus such as etoposide are required.

Although p53 is mainly functional in the nucleus to regulate other molecules, it can present in the mitochondria to assist or influence other molecules such as Bid [23,30,31].

Our result has shown that the repression of Bid reduces the level of p53 in the mitochondria but increase p53 in the cytoplasm and the nucleus (Fig. **5B**). This interesting observation may fit into the model of p53 nucleocytoplasmic shuttling of Bid and may serve as a piece of evidence to support the close relationship between Bid and p53 in the mitochondria. Classically or traditionally DNA-damage agents will induce p53 expression and the translocation of p53 from cytoplasm to nucleus will regulate its target gene expression and cause cell growth arrest and apoptosis. However, increasing evidence has indicated that genotoxic stress or DNA-damage agents can also trigger a rapid translocation of p53 to the mitochondria, contributing to apoptosis in a transcription-independent manner [33-37]. Our finding that etoposide causes the translocation of p53 and Bid to the mitochondria is another piece of evidence to support that p53 can mediate apoptosis in a transcription-independent manner.

Previous data suggest that several members of Bcl-2 family may contribute to p53-induced apoptosis, yet no molecular mechanism has been clearly proposed for the observations [37, 38]. Recently, we and other groups have observed that the full length Bid can localize to the mitochondria and induce apoptosis in response to the apoptotic stimuli [5,30]. More importantly, in the present study, we have found that p53 can directly associate with Bid and that both of them can co-operatively promote apoptosis induced by DNA damage agent etoposide. These data strongly suggest that the interaction between p53 and Bid is one of the important mechanisms responsible for DNA damage-induced apoptosis. However, it is noted that such an interaction is not a sole mechanism that responsible for Etop-mediated apoptosis since etoposide can still induce a significant number of apoptotic cells in the absence of p53. It is known that etoposide can induce apoptosis *via* the activation of Bax [39,40]. Nevertheless, our result is consistent with a recent report showing that full-length Bid translocation is sufficient for the activation of mitochondrial cell death pathway [5]. Moreover, inhibition of Bid expression in Chang liver ($p53^{+/+}$) cells by RNA interference results in the reduction of mitochondrial p53 level and an increase in cell resistance to etoposide. Sax *et al.* have reported that upon treatment with chemotherapeutic agents adriamycin and the nucleotide analogue 5-fluorouracil, $Bid^{-/-}$ mouse embryonic fibroblast cells (MEFs) show much less apoptosis than wild-type MEFs and that both chemotherapeutic agents can stabilize endogenous p53 [17]. Our present finding is generally in line with their result and we have further demonstrated that the physical association and the functional collaboration between p53 and Bid are involved in the mitochondrion-mediated cell death of liver cells induced by etoposide.

CONCLUDING REMARKS

We have revealed a novel p53 nucleocytoplasmic shuttling function, which plays an important role in assisting Bid translocation from the nucleus to the cytoplasm/ mitochondria through the interaction with Bid following the stimulation of etoposide. Such an interaction occurs at physical level in the nucleus and the mitochondria to facilitate the intrinsic mitochondrion-mediated apoptotic pathway. Since p53 is frequently mutated in HCC, future studies should examine whether mutant p53 can still be able to associate with Bid to relocate it to the mitochondria.

ACKNOWLEDGEMENTS

None declared.

CONFLICT OF INTEREST

The authors confirm that this chapter contents have no conflict of interest.

DISCLOSURE

The chapter submitted for the eBook Series entitled **"Advances in Cancer Drug Targets, Volume 2"** is an update of our article in **Current Cancer Drug Targets, Volume 9, Issue 7, 2009, pp. 871-880,** with additional text and references.

REFERENCES

[1] Wang K, Yin XM, Chao DT, Milliman CL, Korsmeyer SJ. BID: a novel BH3 domain-only death agonist. Genes Dev 1996, 10, 2859-69.

[2] Yin XM. Bid, a BH3-only multi-functional molecule, is at the cross road of life and death. Gene 2006, 369, 7-19.

[3] Li H, Zhu H, Xu CJ, Yuan J. Cleavage of BID by caspase 8 mediates the mitochondrial damage in the Fas pathway of apoptosis. Cell 1998, 94, 491-501.

[4] Luo X, Budihardjo I, Zou H, Slaughter C, Wang X. Bid, a Bcl2 interacting protein, mediates cytochrome c release from mitochondria in response to activation of cell surface death receptors. Cell 1998, 94, 481-90.

[5] Konig HG, Rehm M, Gudorf D, Krajewski S, Gross A, Ward MW, Prehn JH. Full length Bid is sufficient to induce apoptosis of cultured rat hippocampal neurons. BMC Cell Biol 2007, 8, 7-14.

[6] Sarig R, Zaltsman Y, Marcellus RC, Flavell R, Mak TW, Gross A. BID-D59A is a potent inducer of apoptosis in primary embryonic fibroblasts. J Biol Chem 2003, 278, 10707-15.

[7] Valentijn AJ, Gilmore AP. Translocation of full-length Bid to mitochondria during anoikis. J Biol Chem.2004, 279, 32848-57.

[8] Zinkel SS, Ong CC, Ferguson DO, Iwasaki H, Akashi K, Bronson RT, Kutok JL, Alt FW, Korsmeyer SJ. Proapoptotic BID is required for myeloid homeostasis and tumor suppression. Genes Dev 2003, 17, 229-39.

[9] Bai L, Ni HM, Chen X, Difrancesca D, Yin XM. Deletion of bid impedes cell proliferation and hepatic carcinogenesis. Am J Pathol 2005, 166, 1523-32.

[10] Zinkel SS, Hurov KE, Ong C, Abtahi FM, Gross A, Korsmeyer SJ. A role for proapoptotic BID in the DNA-damage response. Cell 2005, 122, 579-91.

[11] Kamer I, Sarig R, Zaltsman Y, Niv H, Oberkovitz G, Regev L, Haimovich G, Lerenthal Y, Marcellus RC, Gross AProapoptotic BID is an ATM effector in the DNA-damage response. Cell 2005, 122, 593-603.

[12] Lavin MF, Kozlov S. ATM activation and DNA damage response. Cell Cycle 2007, 6, 931-42.

[13] Oberkovitz G, Regev L, Gross A. Nucleocytoplasmic shuttling of BID is involved in regulating its activities in the DNA-damage response. Cell Death Differ 2007, 14, 1628-34.

[14] el-Deiry WS, Tokino T, Velculescu VE, Levy DB, Parsons R, Trent JM, Lin D, Mercer WE, Kinzler KW, Vogelstein BWAF1, a potential mediator of p53 tumor suppression. Cell 1993, 75, 817-25.

[15] Miyashita T, Reed JC. The tumor suppressor p53 is a direct transcriptional activator of the human bax gene. Cell 1995, 80, 293-9.

[16] Jiang P, Du W, Heese K, Wu M. The Bad guy cooperates with good cop p53: Bad is transcriptionally up-regulated by p53 and forms a Bad/p53 complex at the mitochondria to induce apoptosis. Mol Cell Biol. 2006, 26, 9071-82.

[17] Sax JK, Fei P, Murphy ME, Bernhard E, Korsmeyer SJ, El-Deiry WS. BID regulation by p53 contributes to chemosensitivity. Nat Cell Biol 2002, 4, 842-9.

[18] Nakano K, Vousden K. H. PUMA, a novel proapoptotic gene, is induced by p53. Mol Cell 2001, 7, 683-94.

[19] Okamura S, Arakawa H, Tanaka T, Nakanishi H, Ng CC, Taya Y, Monden M, Nakamura Y. p53DINP1, a p53-inducible gene, regulates p53-dependent apoptosis. Mol Cell 2001, 8, 85-94.

[20] Schuler M, Green DR. Transcription, apoptosis and p53: catch-22. Trends Genet 2005, 21, 182-7.

[21] Prives C. Signaling to p53: breaking the MDM2-p53 circuit. Cell 1998, 95, 5-8.

[22] Chipuk JE, Kuwana T, Bouchier-Hayes L, Droin NM, Newmeyer DD, Schuler M, Green DR. Direct activation of Bax by p53 mediates mitochondrial membrane permeabilization and apoptosis. Science 2004, 303, 1010-4.

[23] Mihara M, Erster S, Zaika A, Petrenko O, ChittendenT, Pancoska P, Moll UM. p53 has a direct apoptogenic role at the mitochondria. Mol Cell 2003, 11, 577-90.

[24] Stommel JM, Marchenko ND, Jimenez GS, Moll UM, Hope TJ, Wahl GM. A leucine-rich nuclear export signal in the p53 tetramerization domain: regulation of subcellular localization and p53 activity by NES masking. EMBO J 1999, 18, 1660-72.

[25] Miao J, Chen GG, Chun SY, Chak EC, Lai PB. Bid sensitizes apoptosis induced by chemotherapeutic drugs in hepatocellular carcinoma. Int J Oncol 2004, 25, 651-9.
[26] Miao J, Chen GG, Chun SY, Yun JP, Chak EC, Ho RL, Lai PB. Adenovirus-mediated tBid overexpression results in therapeutic effects on p53-resistant hepatocellular carcinoma. Int J Cancer 2006, 119, 1985-93.
[27] Li M, Lee TW, Yim AP, Mok TS, Chen GG. Apoptosis induced by troglitazone is both peroxisome proliferator-activated receptor-gamma- and ERK-dependent in human non-small lung cancer cells. J Cell Physiol 2006, 209, 428-38.
[28] Liu Z, Ng E.K, Liang NC, Deng YF, Leung BC, Chen GG. Cell death induced by Pteris semipinnata L. is associated with p53 and oxidant stress in gastric cancer cells. FEBS Lett 2005, 579, 1477-87.
[29] Kaufmann T, Tai L, Ekert PG, Huang DC, Norris F, Lindemann RK, Johnstone RW, Dixit VM, Strasser A. The BH3-only protein bid is dispensable for DNA damage- and replicative stress-induced apoptosis or cell-cycle arrest. Cell 2007, 129, 423-33.
[30] Song G, Chen GG, Chau KJ, Miao J, Lai BS. Bid exhibits S phase checkpoint activation and plays a pro-apoptotic role in response to etoposide-induced DNA damage in human hepatoma cells. Apoptosis 2008, 13, 693-701.
[31] Baptiste N, Prives C. p53 in the cytoplasm: a question of overkill? Cell 2004, 116, 487-9.
[32] Komeili A, O'Shea EK. Nuclear transport and transcription. Curr Opin Cell Biol 2000, 12, 355-60.
[33] Erster S, Mihara M, Kim RH, Petrenko O, Moll UM. *In vivo* mitochondrial p53 translocation triggers a rapid first wave of cell death in response to DNA damage that can precede p53 target gene activation. Mol Cell Biol 2004, 24, 6728-41.
[34] Endo H, Kamada H, Nito C, Nishi T, Chan PH. Mitochondrial translocation of p53 mediates release of cytochrome c and hippocampal CA1 neuronal death after transient global cerebral ischemia in rats. J Neurosci 2006, 26, 7974-83.
[35] Wolff S, Erster S, Palacios G, Moll UM. p53's mitochondrial translocation and MOMP action is independent of Puma and Bax and severely disrupts mitochondrial membrane integrity. Cell Res 2008, 18, 733-44.
[36] Guan L, Huang F, Li Z, Han B, Jiang Q, Ren Y, Yang Y, Xu C. P53 transcription-independent activity mediates selenite-induced acute promyelocytic leukemia NB4 cell apoptosis. BMB Reports 2008, 41, 745-50.
[37] Bonini P, Cicconi S, Cardinale A, Vitale C, Serafino AL, Ciotti MT, Marlier LN. Oxidative stress induces p53-mediated apoptosis in glia: p53 transcription-independent way to die. J Neurosci Res 2004, 75, 83-95.
[38] Biswas G, Guha M, Avadnoni NG. Mitochondria-to nucleus stress signaling in mammalian cells: nature of nuclear gene targets, transcription regulation, and induced resistance to apoptosis. Gene 2005, 354, 132-9.
[39] Albihn A, Lovén J, Ohlsson J, Osorio LM, Henriksson M. c-Myc-dependent etoposide-induced apoptosis involves activation of Bax and caspases, and PKCdelta signaling. J Cell Biochem 2006, 98, 1597-614.
[40] Choi JS, Shin S, Jin, YH, Yim H, Koo KT, Chun KH, Oh YT, Lee WH, Lee SK. Cyclin-dependent protein kinase 2 activity is required for mitochondrial translocation of Bax and disruption of mitochondrial transmembrane potential during etoposide-induced apoptosis. Apoptosis 2007, 12, 1229-41.

Advances in Cancer Drug Targets, Vol. 2, 2014, 347-357

CHAPTER 10

Fibrates Action in Daunorubicin Chemical Reaction

Ganesaratnam K. Balendiran*

Department of Chemistry, Youngstown State University, One University Plaza, Youngstown, OH 44555, USA

Abstract: Anthracyclines are an important reagent in many chemotherapy regimes for treating a wide range of tumors. One of the primary mechanisms by which anthracycline acts involves DNA damage caused by inhibition of topoisomerase II. Enzymatic detoxification of anthracycline is a critical factor in determining anthracycline resistance. The natural product, daunorubicin, a toxic analogue of anthracycline, is reduced to the less toxic daunorubicinol by the catalytic action of AKR1B10, which is overexpressed in most cases of smoking associated squamous cell carcinoma (SCC) and adenocarcinoma. In addition, AKR1B10 was discovered as an enzyme overexpressed in human liver, cervical, and endometrial cancer cases in samples from uterine cancer patients. The expression of AKR1B10 was also found to be associated with tumor recurrence after surgery and with keratinization of squamous cell carcinoma in cervical cancer. It is estimated to have the potential as a tumor intervention target for colorectal cancer cells (HCT-8) and as a diagnostic marker for non-small-cell lung cancer. This chapter presents the chemical mechanism of action of daunorubicin and a method to improve the effectiveness of daunorubicin by modulating the catalytic activity of AKR1B10.

Keywords: AKR, AKR1B10, cancer, daunorubicin, fibrate.

INTRODUCTION

The mechanism of chemical action of a molecular target is important for the efficacy of a drug. It is equally important for obtaining clinical approval for its use. Aldose reductase [1] and aldose reductase like protein, AKR1B10 [2, 3], are molecular targets for antilipidemic drug action. Fibrates have demonstrated clinical use in reducing lipid level. Expression of these proteins reduces the drug resistance due to their catalytic ability for daunorubicin [4]. This article focuses

***Corresponding Author Ganesaratnam K. Balendiran:** Department of Chemistry, Youngstown State University, One University Plaza, Youngstown, OH 44555, USA; Tel: 13309417103; Fax: 13309411579; E-mails: pl_note@yahoo.com; gkbalendiran@ysu.edu

on an approach to increase the chemotherapeutic benefits of daunorubicin with the combined application of fibrates.

ANTHRACYCLINES AND THEIR THERAPEUTIC APPLICATION

Natural products like daunorubicin are traditionally produced from the microorganisms *Streptomyces peucetius* and *Streptomyces coeruleorubidus* by a fermentation process [5, 6]. Daunorubicin is an antitumor antibiotic with proven clinical use as a powerful agent in leukemias, lymphomas, sarcomas, and solid breast, ovary, and lung tumors [7]. This is a compound with a glycoside bond linking a tetracyclic aglycone possessing a substituted anthraquinone chromophore and an aminosugar [5]. Anthracyclines are routinely employed in combination with other groups of medications. Each drug exhibits a different mechanism of action, thus maximizing tumor cell killing while minimizing resistance at the same time.

MECHANISM OF ANTHRACYCLINE ACTION

The mechanism of action and the cytotoxicity caused by daunorubicin analogues are not completely understood. However, multiple mechanisms are beginning to be recognized for anthracyclines derivatives. Some of them are: (1) induction of topoisomerase II mediated DNA strand breaks, (2) generation of reactive oxygen species (ROS) mediated lipid peroxidation, and (3) topoisomerase II independent doxazolidine mediated apoptosis.

The nucleic acid topology is modified through various nuclear processes such as replication, transcription, chromatin remodeling, chromosome condensation and decondensation, and recombination and repair by DNA topoisomerases [8-10]. Though DNA topoisomerases can introduce breaks into DNA segments, topoisomerase II transports a double helix through a double-stranded cut of another duplex. Topoisomerase activity can be harmful to cells due to the action of small compounds [9, 11-13], known as topoisomerase poisons which transform topoisomerase II into a lethal DNA-damaging agent by stabilizing an enzyme-DNA complex [9, 11, 14].

UPREGULATION OF AKR1B10 IN TUMOR

Biomarker, AKR1B10, an Aldo-Keto Reductase (AKR) protein family member, is overexpressed in most instances of squamous cell carcinoma (SCC) and adenocarcinoma. Both SCC and adenocarcinoma are associated with the metabolism of tobacco carcinogens [15]. The AKR1B10, which belongs to the aldose reductase (AR) subfamily (AKR1B), was discovered as an enzyme upregulated in human liver cancers [16-19] and detected in 20.0% of cervical cancer cases and 15.8% of endometrial cancer cases in samples from uterine cancer patients [20]. In addition, statistical analysis indicated that AKR1B10 expression was associated with tumor recurrence after surgery and keratinization of squamous cell carcinoma in cervical cancer [20]. AKR1B10 is upregulated during tumorigenic transformation of human mammary epithelial cells [21]. Also, bioinformatics analysis of the public gene expression data and validation of clinical specimens reveal AKR1B10 as a potential diagnostic marker for non-small-cell lung cancer [22]. Moreover, studies on the effect of small interfering RNA (siRNA)-mediated downregulation of AKR1B10 on proliferation of colorectal cancer cells (HCT-8) estimated its potential as a tumor intervention target [23]. Moreover, AKR1B10 is a novel regulator of the biosynthesis of fatty acid, an essential component of the cell membrane in breast cancer cells [21].

AKR1B10 ACTIVITY

Daunorubicin, utilized in the treatment of lung cancer, is reduced by AKR1B10 in the presence of NADPH with the catalytic efficiencies of $k_{cat}/K_m = 1.3\ mM^{-1}\ min^{-1}$. This AKR1B10 catalyzed reduction of the carbonyl group in daunorubicin results in the formation of the corresponding alcohol at atom position 13 (Fig. **1**). The alcohol that is formed, daunorubicinol, is inactive towards interacting with topoisomerase II. The reduction of anthracycline activity leads to drug resistance. This is largely because the alcohol metabolites of anthracyclines have been shown to exhibit significantly reduced anticancer properties [24, 25]. Furthermore, the toxic effects on the heart associated with anthracycline-based cancer treatment are largely attributable to the anthracycline alcohol metabolite(s) that form and accumulate in cardiac cells. These metabolites are known to disrupt several key processes in heart muscle and thus impair heart function [26].

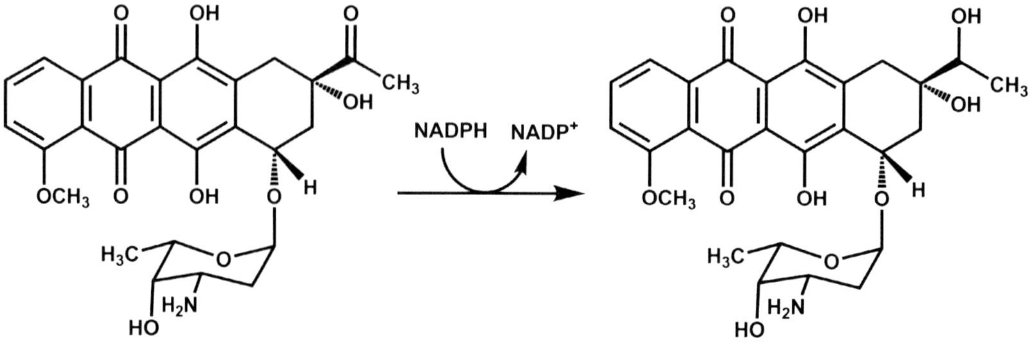

Fig. (1): AKR1B10 catalyzed reduction of daunorubicin. Ketone moiety not in the tetracyclic ring is converted to alcohol in the presence of NADPH.

SIDE EFFECTS OF ANTHRACYCLINES

Serious side effects of anthracyclines include acute cardiac injury and chronic congestive heart failure [27]. Acute toxicity is known to develop immediately after anthracycline treatment begins and consists of brief and usually manageable arrhythmias and hypotension [28]. Other cardiac effects are irreversible and limit the dosage of anthracycline, restricting lifetime cumulative dose [29]. Also, decreases in the left ventricular ejection fraction (LVEF) seen in studies involving treatment of childhood cancer have been correlated with high dosage of anthracycline. Furthermore, a clinical study indicated that an estimated cumulative 26% of patients would experience anthracycline-related Congestive Heart Failure at a cumulative dose of 550 mg/m^2 [30]. Anthracyclines induce acute cardiac lesions through effects on the sarcoplasmic reticulum (SR) in adults. Anthracyclines exhibit effects similar to those of caffeine, an agent known to render the SR nonfunctional by the depletion of the releasable SR calcium pool [31]. The most severe damage is cardiomyopathy, which has permanent effects and is related to high peak plasma anthracycline [32]. Cardiomyopathy develops from defense against free radical damage to the myocytes and repeated damage to the mitochondria [33, 34].

ACTIVE SITE AND SUBSTRATE SPECIFICITY OF AKR1B10

Aromatic interactions play a role in the binding of the tetracyclic moiety of daunorubicin in the ARK1B10 active site (Fig. **2**). The cavity made by residues

Gly19, Thr20, Trp21, Lys22, Asp44, Tyr49, Lys78, Trp80, His111, Trp112, Gln114, Phe116, Phe123, Lys125, Gly129, Ser160, Asn161, Gln184, Tyr210, Ser211, Pro212, Leu213, Ser215, Pro216, Asp217, Pro219, Leu229, Trp220, Ala246, Ile261, Pro262, Lys263, Ser264, Thr266, Arg269, Glu272, Cys299, Val301, Gln303 and Ser304 creates space for the binding of cofactor and substrate in AKR1B10. The substrate binding pocket is encompassed by the nicotinamide ring of $NADP^+$ and residues Trp21, Val48, Tyr49, Lys78, Trp80, Pro81, Thr82, His111, Trp112, Gln114, Phe116, Phe123, Lys125, Ala131, Asn161, Tyr210, Cys299, Val301, Gln303 and Ser304. In addition to the polar and van der Waals interactions, aromatic interactions play a critical role in the binding of daunorubicin to AKR1B10.

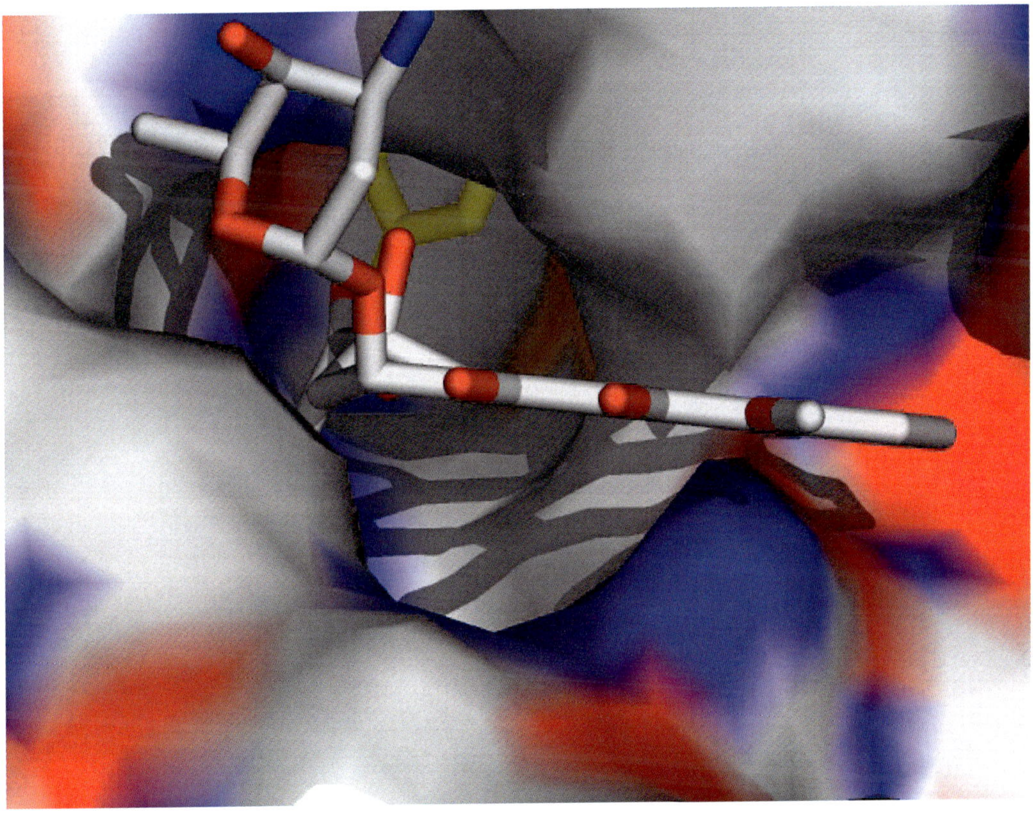

Fig. (2): Binding of daunorubicin in the active site cavity of AKR1B10. Active site of AKR1B10 is shown in the surface representation and color corded in white, red and blue to reflect the neutral, negative and positive residues. Nicotinamide ring of the cofactor in yellow and the daunorubicin in white are presented with N and O atoms in blue and red respectively.

CATALYTIC MECHANISM OF AKR1B10

The catalytic mechanism of AKR1B10 is anticipated to involve a stereo specific transfer of the pro-R hydride from C4 position of the nicotinamide. The regiospecific transfer of the hydride to the re-face of the substrate carbonyl carbon atom of the carbonyl double bond leads to the formation of alcoholate anion. This hydride transfer is followed by protonation of the substrate carbonyl oxygen anion by an enzyme functional group. Based on the site-directed mutagenesis, kinetic, structural, quantum mechanical, and molecular mechanics studies performed on aldose reductase it is proposed that the proton is donated from Tyr48. The Tyr48-mediated proton donation is facilitated by an extended network of hydrogen bonding interactions involving residues Asp43 and Lys77 in aldose reductase. If a similar mechanism is in operation in AKR1B10, the corresponding residues are Asp43, Tyr49 and Lys79. Also, in AKR1B10, the N_Z atom of Lys78 is at 2.7Å and 3.1Å from the O_{D2} atom of Asp44 and OH group of Tyr49, respectively. Therefore, it is conceivable that the proton transfer to the substrates takes place through Tyr49 in AKR1B10.

IMPROVING THE EFFECTIVENESS OF ANTHRACYCLINES BY VIRTUE OF INHIBITORS

Fibrates, ciprofibrate, fenofibrate, fenofibric acid, and Wy 14,643 inhibit the reduction of daunorubicin by 35-40% that is catalyzed by AKR1B10 (Fig. **3** and Table **1**) [1, 2]. Although fenofibrate and Wy 14,643 have a comparable inhibition potential, ciprofibrate and fenofibric acid show lower potential. Importantly, the prodrug, fenofibrate, is 25-fold more effective than its hydrolyzed fibrate derivative, fenofibric acid, in inhibiting the AKR1B10 catalyzed reduction of daunorubicin. Both fenofibrate and fenofibric acid demonstrate the same level of inhibition in the ARK1B10 catalyzed reduction of daunorubicin using 20 and 500 μM concentrations of fenofibrate and fenofibric acid, respectively. This indicates that the prodrug, fenofibrate, which is the isopropyl ester of fenofibric acid, has a higher potency than the hydrolyzed acid form. This structurally divergent class of compounds including ciprofibrate, fenofibric acid and fenofibrate are antilipidemic drugs which have shown beneficial clinical use for the treatment of hyperglycemia [35, 36, 40]. Fibrates show several attractive pharmacological properties [37-39]. Consequently, the undesired activity of ARK1B10 in the chemical action of anthracycline could be modulated by the exploitation of ciprofibrate, fenofibrate, fenofibric acid, gemfibrozil, and Wy 14,643.

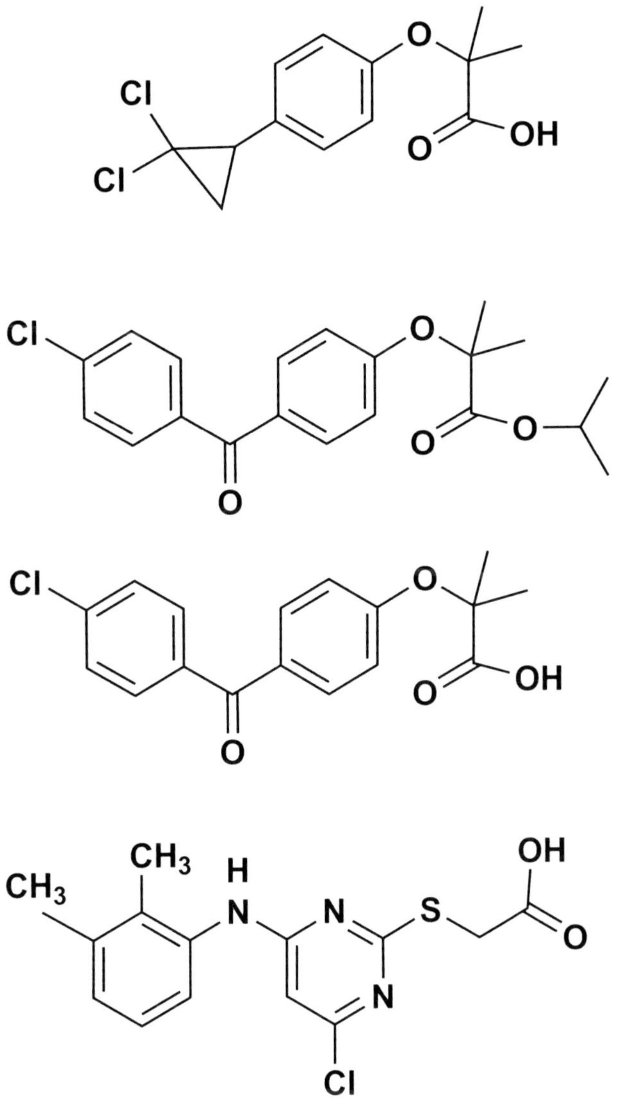

Fig. (3): Chemical structures of the inhibitors capable of modulating AKR1B10 catalyzed inactivation of daunorubicin reaction. Ciprofibrate is 2-[p-(2,2-dichlorocyclopropyl)-phenoxy]-2-methylpropanoic acid, Fenofibrate is isopropyl ester of 2-[4-(4-chlorobenzoyl)-phenoxy]-2-methylpropanoic acid, Fenofibric acid is 2-[4-(4-chlorobenzoyl)-phenoxy]-2-methylpropanoic acid and Wy 14,643 is 4-Chloro-6-(2,3-xylidino)-2-pyrimidinylthioacetic acid.

Table 1: **Percentage Inhibition of Fibrates in the AKR1B10 Catalyzed Reduction of Daunorubicin**

Inhibitors	Concentration (μM)	Inhibition (%)
Ciprofibrate	250	33
	500	39
Fenofibrate	20	35
Fenofibric Acid	250	25
	500	35
Wy 14,643	250	37
	500	50

CONCLUSIONS AND FUTURE PROSPECTIVE

Fibrates are a class of synthetic compounds with varied chemical structures and known pharmacological properties. They could be used alone or in Statin-fibrate combination therapy to reduce incidences of cardiovascular disease in patients with Type 2 diabetes, decrease serum triglycerides, lower insulin resistance and fasting blood glucose levels in non-obese Japanese Type 2 diabetic patients, decrease concentrations of circulating, small, low density lipoproteins (LDL), increase high density lipoproteins (HDL), and improve glucose tolerance, resulting in favorable effects on blood coagulation and global fibrinolytic function as well as to reduce the lipid content of intermediate density lipoprotein in Type 1 diabetes. Because of the fact that the metabolite, fenofibric acid, is less potent than the pro-drug fenofibrate in modulating the AKR1B10 catalyzed reduction of anthracyclines because it is necessary to design and generate a derivative that is less hydrolysable and more stable in the biophase.

ACKNOWLEDGEMENTS

This work was supported by funding DK085496 from the National Institute of Diabetes and Digestive and Kidney Diseases, the American Diabetes Association, and Dean's Reassign time.

CONFLICT OF INTEREST

The author confirms that this chapter contents have no conflict of interest.

DISCLOSURE

The chapter submitted for the eBook Series entitled **"Advances in Cancer Drug Targets, Volume 2"** is an update of our article in **Current Cancer Drug Targets, Volume 9, Issue 3, 2009, pp. 366-369,** with additional text and references.

REFERENCES

[1] Balendiran GK, Verma M, Perry E. Chemistory of Fibrates. Current Chemical Biology 2007; 1(3): 311-316.

[2] Balendiran GK, Martin HJ, El-Hawari Y, Maser E. Cancer biomarker AKR1B10 and carbonyl metabolism. Chem Biol Interact 2009; 178(1-3): 134-7.

[3] Verma M, Martin H-J, Haq W, O'Connor TR, Maser E, Balendiran GK. Inhibiting wild-type and C299S mutant AKR1B10; a homologue of aldose reductase upregulated in cancers. European Journal of Pharmacology 2008; 584: 213-221.

[4] Martin HJ, Breyer-Pfaff U, Wsol V, Venz S, Block S, Maser E. Purification and characterization of akr1b10 from human liver: role in carbonyl reduction of xenobiotics. Drug Metab Dispos 2006; 34(3): 464-70.

[5] Arcamone F, Franceschi G, Orezzi P, Cassinelli G, Barbieri W, Mondelli R. Daunomycin. I. The structure of daunomycione. Journal of the American Chemical Society 1964; 86: 5334-5.

[6] Arcamone F, Franceschi G, Penco S, Selva A. Adridmycin (14-hydroxydaunomycin), a novel antitumor antibiotic. Tetrahedron Letters 1969; 13: 1007-10.

[7] Dimarco A, Gaetani M, Orezzi P, Scarpinato BM, Silvestrini R, Soldati M, *et al.* 'Daunomycin', A New Antibiotic Of The Rhodomycin Group. Nature 1964; 201: 706-7.

[8] Wang JC. Cellular roles of DNA topoisomerases: a molecular perspective. Nat Rev Mol Cell Biol 2002; 3(6): 430-40.

[9] Pommier Y, Pourquier P, Fan Y, Strumberg D. Mechanism of action of eukaryotic DNA topoisomerase I and drugs targeted to the enzyme. Biochim Biophys Acta 1998; 1400(1-3): 83-105.

[10] Nitiss JL. Roles of DNA topoisomerases in chromosomal replication and segregation. Adv Pharmacol 1994; 29A: 103-34.

[11] Liu LF. DNA topoisomerase poisons as antitumor drugs. Annu Rev Biochem 1989; 58: 351-75.

[12] Froelich-Ammon SJ, Osheroff N. Topoisomerase poisons: harnessing the dark side of enzyme mechanism. J Biol Chem 1995; 270(37): 21429-32.

[13] Capranico G, Binaschi M, Borgnetto ME, Zunino F, Palumbo M. A protein-mediated mechanism for the DNA sequence-specific action of topoisomerase II poisons. Trends Pharmacol Sci 1997; 18(9): 323-9.

[14] Wang JC. DNA topoisomerases. Annu Rev Biochem 1996; 65: 635-92.

[15] Fukumoto S, Yamauchi N, Moriguchi H, Hippo Y, Watanabe A, Shibahara J, *et al.* Overexpression of the aldo-keto reductase family protein AKR1B10 is highly correlated with smokers' non-small cell lung carcinomas. Clin Cancer Res 2005; 11(5): 1776-85.

[16] Jez JM, Flynn TG, Penning TM. A new nomenclature for the aldo-keto reductase superfamily. Biochem Pharmacol 1997; 54(6): 639-47.
[17] Cao D, Fan ST, Chung SS. Identification and characterization of a novel human aldose reductase-like gene. J Biol Chem 1998; 273(19): 11429-35.
[18] Hyndman DJ, Flynn TG. Sequence and expression levels in human tissues of a new member of the aldo-keto reductase family. Biochim Biophys Acta 1998; 1399(2-3): 198-202.
[19] Scuric Z, Stain SC, Anderson WF, Hwang JJ. New member of aldose reductase family proteins overexpressed in human hepatocellular carcinoma. Hepatology 1998; 27(4): 943-50.
[20] Yoshitake H, Takahashi M, Ishikawa H, Nojima M, Iwanari H, Watanabe A, *et al.* Aldo-keto reductase family 1, member B10 in uterine carcinomas: a potential risk factor of recurrence after surgical therapy in cervical cancer. Int J Gynecol Cancer 2007; 17(6): 1300-1306.
[21] Ma J, Yan R, Zu X, Cheng JM, Rao K, Liao DF, *et al.* Aldo-keto reductase family 1 B10 affects fatty acid synthesis by regulating the stability of acetyl-coa carboxylase-alpha in breast cancer cells. J Biol Chem 2008; 283(6): 3418-23.
[22] Kim B, Lee HJ, Choi HY, Shin Y, Nam S, Seo G, *et al.* Clinical validity of the lung cancer biomarkers identified by bioinformatics analysis of public expression data. Cancer Res 2007; 67(15): 7431-8.
[23] Yan R, Zu X, Ma J, Liu Z, Adeyanju M, Cao D. Aldo-keto reductase family 1 B10 gene silencing results in growth inhibition of colorectal cancer cells: Implication for cancer intervention. Int J Cancer 2007; 121(10): 2301-2306.
[24] Tanaka M, Bateman R, Rauh D, Vaisberg E, Ramachandani S, Zhang C, *et al.* An unbiased cell morphology-based screen for new, biologically active small molecules. PLoS Biol 2005; 3(5): e128.
[25] Ax W, Soldan M, Koch L, Maser E. Development of daunorubicin resistance in tumour cells by induction of carbonyl reduction. Biochem Pharmacol 2000; 59(3): 293-300.
[26] Minotti G, Menna P, Salvatorelli E, Cairo G, Gianni L. Anthracyclines: molecular advances and pharmacologic developments in antitumor activity and cardiotoxicity. Pharmacol Rev 2004; 56(2): 185-229.
[27] Olson LE, Bedja D, Alvey SJ, Cardounel AJ, Gabrielson KL, Reeves RH. Protection from doxorubicin-induced cardiac toxicity in mice with a null allele of carbonyl reductase 1. Cancer Res 2003; 63(20): 6602-6.
[28] Mordente A, Minotti G, Martorana GE, Silvestrini A, Giardina B, Meucci E. Anthracycline secondary alcohol metabolite formation in human or rabbit heart: biochemical aspects and pharmacologic implications. Biochem Pharmacol 2003; 66(6): 989-98.
[29] Safra T. Cardiac safety of liposomal anthracyclines. Oncologist 2003; 8 Suppl 2: 17-24.
[30] Swain SM, Whaley FS, Ewer MS. Congestive heart failure in patients treated with doxorubicin: a retrospective analysis of three trials. Cancer 2003; 97(11): 2869-79.
[31] Burke BE, Mushlin PS, Cusack BJ, Olson SJ, Gambliel HA, Olson RD. Decreased sensitivity of neonatal rabbit sarcoplasmic reticulum to anthracycline cardiotoxicity. Cardiovasc Toxicol 2002; 2(1): 41-51.
[32] Maluf FC, Spriggs D. Anthracyclines in the treatment of gynecologic malignancies. Gynecol Oncol 2002; 85(1): 18-31.

[33] Hortobagyi GN. Anthracyclines in the treatment of cancer. An overview. Drugs 1997; 54 Suppl 4: 1-7.

[34] Legha SS, Benjamin RS, Mackay B, Ewer M, Wallace S, Valdivieso M, *et al.* Reduction of doxorubicin cardiotoxicity by prolonged continuous intravenous infusion. Ann Intern Med 1982; 96(2): 133-9.

[35] Miller DB, Spence JD. Clinical pharmacokinetics of fibric acid derivatives (fibrates). Clin Pharmacokinet 1998; 34(2): 155-62.

[36] Forcheron F, Cachefo A, Thevenon S, Pinteur C, Beylot M. Mechanisms of the triglyceride- and cholesterol-lowering effect of fenofibrate in hyperlipidemic type 2 diabetic patients. Diabetes 2002; 51(12): 3486-91.

[37] Jones IR, Swai A, Taylor R, Miller M, Laker MF, Alberti KG. Lowering of plasma glucose concentrations with bezafibrate in patients with moderately controlled NIDDM. Diabetes Care 1990; 13(8): 855-63.

[38] Fruchart JC, Brewer HB, Jr., Leitersdorf E. Consensus for the use of fibrates in the treatment of dyslipoproteinemia and coronary heart disease. Fibrate Consensus Group. Am J Cardiol 1998; 81(7): 912-7.

[39] Rubins HB, Robins SJ, Collins D, Fye CL, Anderson JW, Elam MB, *et al.* Gemfibrozil for the secondary prevention of coronary heart disease in men with low levels of high-density lipoprotein cholesterol. Veterans Affairs High-Density Lipoprotein Cholesterol Intervention Trial Study Group. N Engl J Med 1999; 341(6): 410-8.

[40] Balendiran GK. Fibrates in the chemical action of daunorubicin. Curr Cancer Drug Targets 2009; 9(3): 366-9.

INDEX

A

Atta-ur-Rahman (Ed)

B

C

D

E

F

H

I

K

L

M

N

O

P

Q

R

T

V

Z

Made in United States
North Haven, CT
04 November 2026

21719574R00215